AIDS IN ASIA

AIDS IN ASIA

A Continent in Peril

Susan S. Hunter

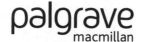

AIDS IN ASIA
Copyright © Susan S. Hunter, 2005.

First published 2005 by
PALGRAVE MACMILLAN™
175 Fifth Avenue, New York, N.Y. 10010 and
Houndmills, Basingstoke, Hampshire, England RG21 6XS.
Companies and representatives throughout the world.

PALGRAVE MACMILLAN is the global academic imprint of the Palgrave Macmillan division of St. Martin's Press, LLC and of Palgrave Macmillan Ltd. Macmillan® is a registered trademark in the United States, United Kingdom and other countries. Palgrave is a registered trademark in the European Union and other countries.

ISBN 1–4039–6774–1

Library of Congress Cataloging-in-Publication Data
Hunter, Susan S.
AIDS in Asia : a continent in peril / Susan Hunter.
     p.   cm.
   Includes bibliographical references and index.
   ISBN 1–4039–6774–1
   1. AIDS (Disease)—Asia.   I. Title.

RA643.86.A78H86   2004
362.196'9792'0095—dc22

                                                            2004053467

A catalogue record for this book is available from the British Library.

Design by Letra Libre, Inc.

First edition: January 2005
10   9   8   7   6   5   4   3   2   1

Printed in the United States of America.

To my beloved husband and best friend, Arlin Greene

CONTENTS

Preface   ix

Chapter 1 Asian Peril, Global Peril   1

Chapter 2 AIDS in Asia:
           The Looming Mushroom Clouds of Infection   21

Chapter 3 The Origin of Asia's States of AIDS:
           Empire and Overthrow   53

Chapter 4 Chaining the Elephant:
           The Impact of Colonialism   97

Chapter 5 Asia and the World Drug Industry   137

Chapter 6 Gender, Religion, and Economics in the East   179

Chapter 7 Fulfilling Heaven's Mandate:
           The Impact of AIDS on Children   217

Chapter 8 As Asia Goes, . . .   253

Notes   269
Index   285

PREFACE

IT IS ESPECIALLY FITTING THAT I AM WRITING THE PREFACE to *AIDS in Asia: A Continent in Peril* in a hotel in Port Moresby, Papua New Guinea, after concluding one of my last days of work on the design of a national assessment of families and children affected by HIV/AIDS. While PNG is a small country of little more than 5 million people, it has the sad distinction of being the fourth country in Asia considered by experts to have a generalized AIDS epidemic. This means that the epidemic has moved from core groups of infected persons—in PNG's case, poor women who are forced to turn to sex work in order to survive and feed their children—to the general population. As you read the ensuing chapters, the meaning of these words will become clearer and you will know that many other countries in Asia have also already exceeded this level although their official reporting systems do not reflect that fact. For now, suffice it to say that PNG is facing a fast growing epidemic that promises to have catastrophic effects on the social and economic fabric of a country already struggling with massive problems of development.

In July 2004, a leading Australian AIDS expert, Dr. David Cooper from Sydney's St. Vincent's Hospital and a co-chair of the scientific meetings at the International AIDS Conference in Bangkok, warned that Papua New Guinea faces the threat of an AIDS pandemic of Sub-Saharan Africa proportions unless enormous efforts are taken to stem the virus's spread. While Papuan society has severe problems stemming from the stress of extreme poverty—prominent among them widespread and spine tingling levels of violence against women and children that make it impossible for me to do much but work and return to my hotel room under close surveillance—the professionals I work with here are charming and capable people committed to resolve the problems stemming from their colonial legacy and move on to higher levels of achievement for themselves, their families, and their countries. AIDS will make that daunting task even more difficult, if not impossible, and set a country that had already acknowledged the impossibility of meeting global goals for children even further behind on the road to modernity. But PNG, as you will see from this book, will not be alone for long when the truth about epidemics in other Asian countries, including the region's largest, most populous, and most modernized, is known.

As I wrote the body of this book on AIDS in Asia, I had the same chilling and heart rending experience that I had had in writing my book about AIDS in Africa. I began like any author does, accumulating mounds of data about Asian history and social structure, and then set to the task of knitting it together and making sense of it relative to the HIV/AIDS pandemic. As I wove the material together and the lines of the book began to emerge, I was startled and distressed by what I saw in my work. Not only is the epidemic huge and growing unrestrained in most Asian countries, but when the underlying social, political and economic patterns that fuel its growth are brought together and analyzed, it is quite clear that there is little standing in the way of catastrophic impact. Doubt about the severity of the epidemic in Asia turned to certainty for me, and I hope that as you read this work, I succeed in convincing you that this conclusion is reasonable and that action is needed on your part and by the global community to face this future realistically, compassionately, and effectively.

I hope, too, that you are moved to understanding and compassion by the stories of HIV/AIDS affected young people that begin each chapter of this work. They are drawn from the experiences of actual children I have met in my work and I have included them to personalize the tragedy that is AIDS for young people, the fastest growing age group of infected individuals, who are helpless unless we take steps to protect them from the epidemic. I am told by readers of *Black Death* that the stories of AIDS-affected women that run through that work and tie it together were key in broadening their minds and opening their hearts to those who are personally affected by this tragedy. A colleague of mine in Malawi who recently read *Black Death* e-mailed me to say that the stories brought him to tears because they brought back many of his own experiences and memories of helping impoverished, AIDS-burdened communities torn apart by this disease.

Over the past five years, I have had the privilege of working with hundreds of incredibly courageous people who are fighting this epidemic in Asia. Some are internationally known; hundreds more contribute to their countries, regions, or villages. Big or little, I have seen them perform miracles. Thank God for that. AIDS demands every ounce of courage and creativity that humans have. To respond to the disease and its impact, individuals must literally rethink and restructure the societies in which they live and confront and change long-standing social institutions and relationships, often at great personal expense. The work is long, heart-breaking, unforgiving, and demands all the courage they have as human beings. Let us all stand up and give them a hand, a prayer, and some real assistance to rebuild their lives.

When my editor asked me to write a book about HIV/AIDS in Asia shortly after I'd finished my first book on HIV/AIDS in Africa, I was brought to a standstill. I had thought that *Black Death: AIDS in Africa* would be my one and only book about the global AIDS pandemic, but she argued that the upsurge of Asia's epidemics also deserved book length treatment. Exhausted by writing *Black Death*, I wondered how I could possibly go on to produce a second book in such a short period of time.

I soon realized that in *Black Death* I had barely skimmed the surface of many important issues affecting the global pandemic. I had presented very little information on an especially key topic determining epidemic growth: the vulnerability and lack of entitlement of women. I had also, ironically enough, talked very little about that aspect of the epidemic which is my principal professional specialty: the impact of HIV/AIDS on children and young people. I have been working in that area since 1989, when I became involved in the world's first special census of orphans of HIV/AIDS in Uganda. where I was working as a Rockefeller Foundation Social Science Research Fellow and lecturer at Makerere University in Kampala. That work led eventually to the first comprehensive international study of orphans and AIDS-affected children, *Children on the Brink*, in 1997, which has become a biennial publication supported by the global AIDS community. Since that time, I have worked twice at UNICEF headquarters developing global policy and with seventeen countries in Africa, the Caribbean, and Asia organizing national assessments of children affected by HIV/AIDS. Much of what I have learned is reflected in chapter 7 of this book.

AIDS in Asia is also fundamentally more political than *Black Death*, which focused on science and evolutionary biology. Because of this, I know I have stepped on many toes, and presented a very one-sided picture of societies in the Asian region. A book about AIDS will inevitably focus on much that is wrong and problematic. Please do not forget that there is much that is good, noble, and, indeed, awe-inspiring about Asia that has been neglected in this work. No civilization is perfect, and as we lean together to confront the problems that make the epidemic of HIV/AIDS possible, we will succeed in creating space for more of the good things to flourish.

My task is now finished. I have only one more thing to do, and that is to thank all the many people that have made this work possible. The first person to thank is my editor, Gabriella Pearce, who set me to this daunting task. Her vision about the impact and meaning of the global HIV/AIDS pandemic is extraordinary, and her grace under pressure has been a comfort to me. My sisters,

Joyce Devine and Margaret Bellucci, took time out of their busy lives to read an earlier version of this work and make insightful comments to help me restructure it. Thank you both! Many AIDS and Asia experts graciously gave of their time to read this book in its early stages, offer suggestions for improving it, and endorsed it. Thanks one and all. And to all the AIDS and community experts in each of the twenty-five countries where I have worked—recognized and not—I would like to express my thanks and admiration. Without you, the lives of millions of people would be much harder than they already are. And last but not least, I would like to thank my husband, Arlin Greene, who never failed to support me during the six-month, non-stop, round-the-clock period that I worked to meet the deadlines for this book.

ONE

ASIAN PERIL, GLOBAL PERIL

"I CAME TO BANGKOK WHEN I WAS ONLY FOURTEEN," he said softly. Rageena leaned forward to see his face more clearly. Black eyes gleamed from features as jagged as the mountains of her Nepali homeland, but he was so big and rugged-looking he could have passed for a Tibetan, she thought. Most Lao people were small, like Nepalis, not big like Phet. He'd been HIV-positive for eight years and still looked very healthy. She sighed. Maybe there was hope.

"I slipped across the Lao border into Thailand for the first time when I was twelve," Phet continued. "My friends and I took a boat across the Mekong. We were crossing illegally, but it didn't matter to us. We were only children and we were looking for adventure as much as we were looking for work." His hands were folded quietly in his lap, his arms lay still at his sides. He spoke easily, but Rageena knew what tension underlay his composure. Each person in the group was to tell the story of how they'd become infected with HIV. She'd known that when she agreed to come to the conference, but didn't look forward to it. Phet had volunteered to go first. He's like a Bodhisattva, she thought, a saint who has stayed here to help us with our troubles. She was drawn to his face, so calm and radiant and open.

"It was the dry season," Phet said. "That's a very slow season for rice farmers, and my friends and I were bored. We'd seen lots of Thai people in Savannkhet. It's a small city on the border near our village that attracts traders from Thailand and Vietnam." She nodded. Like Pakri, the lowland border town between Nepal and India where she came from.

"We'd seen the Thais on television, too, a few times in the city. They were so beautiful and so rich, like big actors from Hollywood. They had all the things we wanted in life. The women, the cars and motorcycles, and houses like we'd never seen before. So we went one night. Our parents had warned us not to do it. The recruiters had come through our small village many times, looking for cheap Lao labor for Thai factories. Many people in our village had gone before, and they warned us, but we were young and didn't believe their stories. We thought they were just telling us lies to scare us, so they could keep us at home to labor in the rice fields. 'How difficult can this be?' we thought.

"The first time we went it was okay. We did well. We worked for a pig farmer, and while it was hard work, he treated us well and promised us work for the next season. We even eluded the guards at the border on the way back by hiring a little boat to take us across, and came back to the village with some money for our parents. It was a rite of passage, and we thought we'd made it through.

"The next season, when it came time to travel again, we decided the pig farmer was too small for us and we'd go with the recruiters. They said factory work would be easier than the farmwork we'd done and would pay better. They scoffed at our pig farmer, and pretty soon they had us believing that we deserved better than what he was offering.

"They came to our village later that morning and four of us climbed in the truck. There were already five boys in the back under the tarpaulin. They were from Kengkok, the little village next door to us, and were all much younger, eleven or twelve at the most. They looked very frightened. As we drove off, I could see the face of my sweetheart. She was crying, and I shouted to her that I would return very soon." He paused.

"We stopped in another three villages and picked up at least twenty more people. When we came near the border, the truck pulled over to a farmer's field and he shoveled water buffalo manure on the tarpaulin. The labor recruiters laughed when the young boys cried out. 'Shut your bloody mouths,' they shouted. 'This manure will keep you quiet enough to get past the border, and it sure will keep the guards from looking too deep.'

"My friend gasped for breath while we waited in the line at the border. The recruiter pounded on the side of the truck. 'Keep him quiet,' he barked. I cradled his head and tried to create an airspace for him by curling around him. He quieted and was breathing better. I could hear the gang boss making his excuses and then his deals with the border guards. They knew what was under the manure, but only charged him the usual tax and put the rest in their pockets. They never checked on our papers or even pulled the tarpaulin back to see if we were alive.

"By the time we reached our destination—where we had come to in Thailand was unknown to me—I had fallen asleep. The guards woke us by banging on the side panels. They freed two boys from the back who shoveled us out. By then my friend was barely breathing, and he gagged on the huge drafts of night air we drew into our lungs. One of the boys from Kengkok wasn't moving, and I could see that his terrified friends were weeping. The guards slapped them and herded us all into a barracks of sorts. The guard ordered us to sleep and ignored our pleas for food and water. 'Tomorrow,' he said, 'you'll get your share tomorrow.' When I heard the large padlock slap shut, I was surer than ever I'd made a mistake. The pig farmer had never locked us in, and we ate with his family every night. We had decent places to sleep in the barn with the pigs.

"In the morning, when the boys asked for their friend, the boss told them that he had gone back to Thailand. In fact, they had buried him and poured quicklime on his body, but we didn't know that until later, when the Thai police raided the labor camp. There were lots of camps like this, not only on the border between Thailand and Laos, but on the Burmese border, too. The same week, five young women being smuggled from northern Burma to Bangkok suffocated under the load of flowers hiding them. The driver found a quiet spot on the road where he lifted the rear of his dump truck. The bodies slid out on the side of the road, covered by the mound of flowers. They weren't found until two days later, when the stench of human decay began to overshadow the flowers' riotous odors. One woman was still living, imprisoned under her friends' bodies.

"I found out later that there had been so many instances of abuse and corruption that the Thai government began an official investigation of their police. Near the farm where we worked, seven Burmese illegals were hacked to death, and their bodies disappeared, disintegrated with quicklime like the young boy's. Like us, they weren't being paid, and although they were scared of the bosses, their hunger finally drove them to protest. They asked for more food, but the owner just laughed. 'Go to the police,' he told them, knowing that without immigration papers, they would be deported and the authorities in Myanmar[1] would imprison them in forced labor worse than the Thai rice farm.

"It was the same problem for us. Immigration is illegal in Laos, so it was impossible for us to get papers. When the abuse started, we had nowhere to run. Even if we could have." He smiled to himself. "We were locked in at night and worked under armed guard during the day. We had no papers, so we couldn't have gone to the police even if we could have escaped. We dreamed about running back to Laos, but we didn't even know where we were. And we were hungry all the time.

"After we had been there three days, the guard locked us up with no food at dinnertime. When the smallest of my three friends, Khamhoung, complained, the guard laughed and said he had been chosen for dinner by the owner of the farm. He leered at us when he said it. 'Well,' I told Khamhoung. 'You go. It's better than not eating.' Four hours later, he was back. We gathered around to hear his story, but he refused to talk. He just laid on his bed. It was funny because he was someone who joked all the time, and kept us in good spirits even when things were at their worst. I noticed, though, when he rolled over on his side, that the back of his trousers were stained and a little bloody.

"I grabbed him by the shoulders and forced him to look at me. I shook him. 'What happened?' I shouted, terrified. 'The owner had a table full of food,' he said. 'I was very happy when I saw that because we haven't eaten much in three days. But he told me that I had to be his woman before he would let me eat. He told me he'd be gentle with me, that I would like it.' Khamhoung curled up, covering his face. 'I was so hungry,' he moaned."

Phet stopped, exhausted and disheartened by his story. Rageena feared what he would say next, but prayed he would go on, wanting to hear more. Somehow she was pleased to hear him say these terrible things. It was her story. A different country, perhaps, but her story nonetheless. She was astounded that a man from a country so many miles away had suffered from the same brutality she had fallen prey to as a young girl in Nepal. She had always assumed that men would be the aggressors and that women were born for suffering. That is what the ancient Hindu texts said, after all. Especially women who had lost their virginity or were not married. But as he struggled, she held her sleeve across her face to hide her tears.

"The next night it was me," Phet continued. "He took us each in turn. It was the only way we could get food. Gradually, we just did it without thinking about it. I know you think it's horrible," he said sadly. "It was horrible. But the worst for me was still to come."

By the age of fifty-four she'd come close to dying at least a dozen times, but her brushes with eternity were for no mean cause. "We are fighting," Emmeline Pankhurst declared in 1914, "for a time when every little girl born into the world will have an equal chance with her brothers, when we shall put an end to foul outrages upon our sex, when our streets shall be safe for the girlhood of our race, when every man shall look upon every woman as his own sister." [2]

Despite her striking physical beauty—Emmeline had raven black hair that set off expressive, deep violet eyes under delicately penciled brows, a magnificent carriage, and a melodious voice—her loving marriage, and the demands of raising five children, Pankhurst was no clinging vine. With more than enough lives for a cat, she defied the antiquarian British stance toward women so often that Parliament passed the infamous "Cat and Mouse" Act in 1913 (officially called the Prisoners Temporary Discharge for Ill-Health Bill) to lure her out of prison so she could regain her health and return to finish out her sentence. Violent protest was not an uncommon political weapon in European countries at the time, but it was especially shocking when wielded by a upper-middle-class woman with education and breeding. The Women's Social and Political Union (WSPU), which Emmeline led, was baited into violence by Herbert Gladstone, Britain's Home Secretary, who declared in 1908 that the WSPU had failed to convince him of the passion of their cause.

That year, thanks to the efforts of Pankhurst's WSPU and other women's suffrage groups around the country, a Women's Enfranchisement Bill had again come very close to passage by Parliament on February 28. Sleight of hand by the Parliament Speaker, who ruled that the bill could only be heard by the whole House, submerged it at the last minute for yet another year. Unsatisfied with that villainous triumph, Gladstone decided to have the last word. He enraged women suffrage partisans around Britain when he told them that argument alone would not be enough to convince the politicians. "There comes a time," he stated publicly, "when political dynamics are far more important than political argument." He admonished the women that men "know the necessity of demonstrating the greatness of their movement" and had brought about political change in the 1830s, 1860s, and 1890s by assembling in large numbers to demand their rights. "Of course," he said patronizingly, "it cannot be expected that women can assemble in such masses, but power belongs to the masses, and through this power a Government can be influenced into more effective action."

Discouraged but undiminished, the leadership of WSPU took Gladstone's words to heart. Besides starvation, Emmeline and her band of "unsexed viragoes" as they were called—ancient Anglo-Saxon for a she-wolf, Amazon, or manlike woman—routinely got themselves arrested by interrupting political gatherings to ask persistent, well-placed, and embarrassing questions about women's rights. They hurled insults and mockery at the lords of the land who were deaf to their demands, paraded on the street in their silk petticoats, and wielded other weapons of more violent protest including setting fires, smashing windows, and slashing pictures in the National Gallery. As many as 100,000 protestors joined their demonstrations and public meetings in London and other major English cities. "Shall us win?" they cried in Yorkshire.

"Shall us have the vote?" they asked in Leeds. "We shall!" was the rising rallying cry raised around the country.

Many early supporters of the WSPU doubted the need for militancy and
urged patience, but Emmeline felt she had been patient and ladylike for far too
long. Women had been pleading for Liberal Party support for their suffrage
campaign for more than thirty years with no results. The London *Daily Mirror*
asked, "By what means, but by screaming, knocking, and rioting, did men
themselves ever gain what they were pleased to call their rights?" Millicent
Fawcett, head of the National Union of Women's Suffrage Societies
(NUWSS), applauded the WSPU's militancy. "In my opinion," she said, "they
have done more during the last 12 months to bring [women's suffrage] within
the region of practical politics than we have been able to accomplish in the
same number of years."

<hr />

In the world today the story of AIDS, or acquired immunodeficiency disease syndrome, is overwhelmingly a story of power. It is the story of who has power and
who does not, the story of who lives and who dies, the story of who gets and who
does not, the story of who dines at the table of life and who starves. It is the story
of young people who are denied the right to education, food, and health. They
are denied the right to know how to protect themselves from this terrible disease,
like Phet and the other young people whose stories appear at the beginning of
each chapter of this book. Despite the work of Emmeline Pankhurst and thousands of other feminists who have sacrificed themselves for the cause of women's
rights for more than 100 years, AIDS is also the story of women who catch HIV,
the human immunodeficiency virus that causes AIDS, because they have no
power to resist. It is the story of men so marginal they are treated with perfidy
and maliciousness by fellow countrymen and their own governments, so marginal
their very lives are at stake from the moment of their births. It is the story of illicit
drugs, the story of sex for sale, and the story of armed rebellion. The story of
AIDS is not pretty, and it may be one we do not want to hear, but it has the power
to tell us the truth about the way the world works and our place in it.

Because this book focuses on AIDS in Asia, it includes many sad stories
of atrocities on the continent: the story of peasants selling blood in China so
that they can get something to eat; the story of children in Laos suffering
death and torture so they can earn a living; the story of orphans in Nepal
who are reviled by their family, friends, and neighbors; the story of Vietnamese children driven to the streets sniffing glue, shooting heroin, and sell-

ing their young bodies; the story of Indian children who go untreated for HIV because their government refuses free AIDS drugs offered by an Indian manufacturer that sells them abroad. At the same time, the story of AIDS on other continents has not come to an end. AIDS is also the story of young South African women getting infected at five times the rate of young South African men while economic and social chaos approaches on cat's paws; of Alabama prisoners denied treatment for HIV/AIDS and tuberculosis while their blood is being sold in Canada; of faithful women over fifty in developed countries whose husbands, armed with Viagra, are finding a new lease on life with other women.[3]

While we may not like it, it is important that we know the story of AIDS because the HIV/AIDS pandemic is rapidly getting worse all over the world. As you finish each sentence in this book, another person will have been infected with HIV. By 2001 HIV/AIDS had become the worst epidemic the world has ever known, and no area of the world is immune to it. By 2010 official projections say that more than 130 million people in the world will have been infected or have died from the disease. The problem is not just in Asia and Africa. From a handful of cases reported in the United States, Europe, and Africa in the early 1980s, AIDS has spread to millions of people in every country of the world. When HIV/AIDS first appeared, many parts of the world were "clean." By 1993 Poland, countries in Southeast Asia, and Greenland—formerly "clean"—reported infections, and by the turn of the twenty-first century there was not an infection-free state in the world. Measured by premature death, loss of human potential, disability, and use of scarce resources, HIV/AIDS is the biggest disease burden in the world. It creates losses for everyone, infected or not.

In late 2003 and early 2004 while this book was being written, the U.S. Centers for Disease Control (CDC) announced outbreaks of AIDS in two populations previously thought to be at extremely low risk: college students in the U.S. states of North Carolina and Florida, and U.S. women over fifty years of age.[4] In Los Angeles, California, the pornographic movie industry was shut down by an outbreak of HIV.[5] AIDS is the fifth leading cause of death among all Americans ages twenty-five to forty-four, the top cause of death of African American men in that age group, and according to CDC it is on the upswing again. The number of new HIV infections transmitted by people having unprotected sex in the United Kingdom—where a third of those currently infected are not aware that they have the disease—rose by 20 percent in 2003 alone, the largest increase ever recorded.[6] In 2003, 40,000 people were infected in Western Europe, also a historic rise, largely due to unsafe sex among young heterosexuals. In 2004 epidemiologists there had even more to worry about because the European Union opened its doors to Eastern European countries, where the epidemic is increasing at the fastest rate in the world.[7] In 2004 Edmonton, Canada, announced its largest syphilis outbreak since the 1980s and huge increases in gonorrhea and chlamydia because of casual sex without a condom. A new surge of HIV was on its way. [8]

The most important terrorist movement in the world today is not al Qaeda but a disease whose name we are just as tired of hearing about: HIV/AIDS. AIDS kills three times more people *each day* than died in the World Trade Center attack on September 11, 2001, and if we count those infected *each day*, it is five times more lethal. The disease is a pervasive security threat because it leads to growing poverty, food insecurity, economic and social collapse, deaths among the armed forces and police, increased criminal violence, and sudden power imbalances. The U.S. Central Intelligence Agency (CIA) called AIDS a security threat in 1999, and in January 2001, a U.S. National Intelligence Council report warned of massive loss of military capabilities and a 20 percent drop in sub-Saharan Africa's gross domestic product in less than ten years. African countries may not be able to uphold their peacekeeping commitments on the continent because of mounting deaths. In reverse, of course, war, chaos, and economic and social disruption create the perfect conditions for rapid HIV spread.

In sub-Saharan African countries where 20 to 40 percent of the population is infected and 60 percent of new infections occur in people under age twenty-four, AIDS not only kills the most productive people, but their deaths drain their families economically and psychologically. HIV/AIDS deaths and illnesses create huge demographic gaps and lost human potential. The epidemic creates vast political, economic, and social problems while it kills off the very people who can address them. Asia may soon suffer a food crisis similar to the one experienced in southern Africa over the past few years, where HIV/AIDS has reduced productivity while increasing the number of desperate individuals who are willing to violate social rules to get food and meet their other needs. Recent food emergencies in southern Africa have put 14.4 million people at risk of starvation, in part because 7 million agricultural workers had died of AIDS by 2002, most of them women.

HIV, the virus that causes AIDS after laying quiet within an individual for seven to ten years, currently infects 40 million people worldwide.[9] By the end of 2003, the disease had killed 31 million people and 3 million people now die from the disease each year. This is 8,200 per day. In total, more than 70 million people worldwide have been infected by HIV since the first cases were recorded in 1982 and at least 5 million additional people are being infected each year—some 15,000 per day. If these rates remain the same through the first decade of the twenty-first century, at least 52 million people will have died by 2010 and 78 million will be alive but infected with the virus, yielding a global total of infections and deaths that surpasses the world's two largest epidemics, the Black Death of the 1400s and the decimation of Native American populations in the 1500s.

But these rates will not remain the same. It is likely, given recent reports of infected blood transfusions in China and the looming HIV mushroom clouds in India, Russia, and other smaller but populous states in Asia, that global infection rates will soon soar even higher. In September 2002 the U.S. National Intelligence Council warned that the infected populations of five countries alone—Nigeria, Ethiopia, Russia, India, and China—would be 75 million by 2010. The global HIV reservoir is already huge and growing; by 2010, at the very minimum 130 million people will be what Gary Nable, director of the U.S. Vaccine Research Center, calls "incubators walking around with this virus, spreading it to other people." If AIDS takes off in Asia and the former states of the Soviet Union in the way experts believe it will, we can double or triple that estimate.

So far, the economic and political reverberations from AIDS have been relatively small. Although "Africa's AIDS catastrophe is a humanitarian disaster of world historic proportions," according to foreign policy expert Nicholas Eberstadt, it affects a continent that is marginal to global economic affairs, contributing less to the world economy on many measures than Switzerland. Eurasia, on the other hand, is home to three-fifths of the world's population and has a combined gross national product that exceeds either the United States or Europe. When it falls—or even if it merely stumbles—due to AIDS, the worldwide crisis will be greater than any experienced during Asia's 1997–1998 financial downturn. For not only will the death toll be staggering, but the economic costs around the world will be huge. The political reverberations could be downright dangerous. Half of the world's shipping passes through channels in Indonesia. Eurasia is home to four out of five of the world's standing armies of more than one million people, and it has four of the world's seven declared nuclear states.

Official statistics indicate that 11.3 million of the word's 41 million currently infected are in the region, but most experts feel the number is much, much higher. In November 2002 Eberstadt upped the ante on the HIV/AIDS epidemic in Asia, raising the world's eyebrows by declaring that infections and deaths in three of the region's most populous countries—China, India, and

Russia—will climb to well over 400 million by 2025.[10] His forecasts of altered Asian economic potential, shifting political might, and severe impacts on the global balance of power over the next two decades were all the more convincing because Eberstadt is not only a foreign policy pundit but a recognized authority in the field of demographics, or the science of predicting population change. His credentials include the chair of Harvard University's Center for Population and Development Studies and consultations with the U.S. Bureau of Census.

Although the world had already conditioned itself to AIDS deaths numbering in the tens of millions in Africa, predictions of several *hundred* million AIDS deaths in Asia, accompanied by shifts in political boundaries and economic chaos in the West's major trading partners, are less easy to shrug off. By 2010 the emerging Asian epidemics will vastly overshadow the epidemic's first run through Africa over the past three decades, exerting a much larger impact on the global economy because of the importance of these Asian tigers as trading and strategic partners to countries around the world. As frightening as Eberstadt's gloom-and-doom predictions for China, India, and Russia may be, they cannot be limited to only those states. HIV has taken a solid foothold in Asia's other very populous states. Indonesia, the fourth largest country in the world, with a population that is one-third the size of all sub-Saharan African countries put together and about 80 percent that of the United States, has a growing epidemic. The population of the five states of Southeast Asia—Cambodia, Laos, Myanmar, Thailand, and Vietnam—is almost as large. Even if Asia's three giants are removed, epidemic impact on the others could make deaths in sub-Saharan Africa look like very small potatoes indeed.

Severe epidemics in Asia are not only likely to occur; they are likely to occur much quicker than Eberstadt forecasts. In December 2003 UNAIDS, the United Nation's official epidemic coordinating agency, voiced its concern that much of HIV/AIDS in Asia is still hidden. The behavior that drives it—injecting drug use, commercial sex, and widespread same-sex behavior among men, both bisexual and homosexual—is illegal and remains clandestine. Many states currently reporting very low prevalence rates are using weak surveillance systems; epidemics could suddenly surge without any warning. Many experts, for example, feel that India is already at the rapid-growth stage of epidemic takeoff, a fact not acknowledged by that country's leaders. China officially reports less than one million infections, but conservative appraisals by well-documented sources indicate that the number is closer to 20 million. The horizon of Eberstadt's grim forecasts might be a lot closer than we think.

Since the fourteenth International AIDS Conference in Barcelona in mid-2002, epidemiological concern about the rapid explosion of AIDS in Asia has increased around the world. Eberstadt's more recent predictions have raised policymaker and public concern, fueling the launch of two global initiatives aimed at increasing HIV/AIDS prevention activities in Asia: the Asia Society's "AIDS in Asia" initiative funded by the Gates Foundation and the Global Business Council's campaign to raise AIDS awareness in the region spearheaded by former U.S. ambassador to the United Nations, Richard Holbrooke. Media and public interest is growing as well, including *Time Asia Magazine*'s 2002 cover stories "Stalking a Killer" and "Asia's Time Bomb." Human Rights Watch caused a major flurry in September 2003 with evidence that seven of China's provinces have high and growing infection rates due to a blood "donation" policy that not only spread the epidemic in China but is likely to have spread it to unsuspecting recipients of blood products exported by China around the world.

Central, East, South, and Southeast Asia have a combined population of 3.6 billion people. The continent has the highest number and proportion of persecuted women and children and the most people in poverty. Like Africa, AIDS epidemics in Asia have yet to hit their stride. The world was lulled into complacency by Thailand's early and effective control of HIV and by Cambodia's later successes, but these have contributed to a false sense of security. These two Asian states represent only 3 percent of the region's total population. They hardly constitute a basis for assuming that other states in the region have dealt with the disease. AIDS is not under control in the region's largest states; in fact, attempts at global management of the HIV/AIDS pandemic are backfiring because India and China refuse to acknowledge the extent of the disease within their borders or set up reliable means of monitoring and controlling it.

Few Asian governments have faced AIDS squarely. No Asian head of state spoke at the UN's special one-day session on AIDS in September 2003. Much of the data on AIDS in Asia is secret, incomplete, or has been manipulated, particularly in India and China. Epidemiologists hoped that outbreaks of sudden acute respiratory syndrome (SARS) over the past few years would motivate both to recognize the need to maintain their public health information systems and make their data public, but both have allowed their public health systems to go to shambles. Since clear data would expose substantial inequalities in underlying social and economic conditions, both countries have been slow to respond to international pressure to improve disease control.

Unless they act soon, the future is not bright. Although medical science responded rapidly in the early stages of the AIDS epidemic, progress in developing a cure or a vaccine has come to something of a standstill. In fact, halfway through the world's most promising vaccine trials, HIV mutated and recombined, forcing stunned scientists to modify the vaccine and hope for the best.[11] AIDS may take other internal and external forms or change the manner in which it is transmitted, behaving like the plague did in the 1300s and syphilis in the 1500s. Imagine, for a moment, if AIDS became a respiratory infection and could be transmitted by a sneeze, as the bubonic plague did when it became the Black Death in 1347. "No rule of nature contradicts such a possibility," says Joshua Lederberg, M.D., former president of New York City's Rockefeller University. "The proliferation of AIDS cases with secondary pneumonia multiplies the odds of such a mutant."[12] Although economists and politicians may be willing to risk that the infection will not move to "more valuable" populations, evolutionary biology suggests that delayed action against HIV/AIDS has produced an enormous reservoir of untamed microbes that are ready to burst forth at any minute and overrun the globe.

There are many small bright lights in the darkness that is AIDS, and one of the most important may be that it has turned into a rallying ground for the rights of the poor to their fair share of the world's resources. AIDS has made many more poor people aware that disease is not their innate fault but a predictable outcome in a world unwilling to allocate them sufficient resources to live decent lives. The wild and uncontrolled spread of the disease has shown us that "HIV and AIDS are part and parcel of a much broader social and economic configuration in which the processes of globalization, unequal capitalist development, and the politics of health are intertwined" in ways that will lead to death, disease, and starvation for billions of people in our world, says Brazilian AIDS expert Richard Parker.[13]

Thanks to the sense of urgency created by AIDS and the growing capabilities of molecular biology and genetics, we have learned more about the spread of diseases and the relationship between microbes and humans over the past twenty years than we had learned from the late 1800s until the 1980s. The HIV/AIDS epidemic has finally broken the illusion of medicine's control over epidemics and infections, cultivated in public-policy thinking since the 1950s. AIDS has shown us clearly that our economic and social decisions structure the spread of disease. AIDS has changed our perilously ignorant disrespect for the power of microbes and has shaken our conviction that we could wipe them from the face of the earth. We are forced to adopt a more reasonable and humble model of coexistence, acknowledging that ultimately we must learn how to live with our microbes. Many of them have positive benefits for us, but they will take advantage of every human fault and failing, every loss of humanitarian will, every denial of basic human rights, and every ounce of inequality that our thoughtlessness affords them.

The sense of urgency created by the rapid spread of HIV/AIDS across Asia and its continued escalation in other parts of the developing world is well deserved. According to Dr. David Morens of the University of Hawaii and National Institutes of Health, the news is not good. When seen from the point of view of evolution, "humans are standing at the edge of disaster. There are already 6 billion people on our planet, and the global population continues to grow at a great rate. Our societies haven't imploded yet only because most of the world lives at a level of privation Westerners would not accept, beyond the reach of the very resources Westerners cannot live without."[14] As one small example, the Netherlands sustains itself by drawing off the resources of an area fifteen times its actual size. British disease ecologist Tony McMichael says this "subsidy" is realized from the resource flows that rich countries established during colonial rule from the 1500s through the 1960s. Our longer life expectancies are another measure of the wealth we have acquired from less powerful populations by "borrowing," as McMichael phrases it, "against the environmental capital of future generations."[15]

The poor countries of the world suffer, among other things, higher rates of illness and shorter life expectancies as a result of this borrowing, and McMichael thinks that "in an increasingly unequal world (where the several hundred richest individuals today have a combined income equal to the world's poorest 3 billion people) one must conclude that the global economy is, in some ways, acting to the detriment of the health of large parts of the human population."[16] The global HIV/AIDS pandemic has come at a time when new findings in human biological and social evolution are converging, causing us to question and expand traditional views of disease and its agents, forcing us to restate our understanding of the relationship between human and natural agency in shaping epidemics. We are forced to reconsider our notion of ethics and of what we might owe to the poor of the world whose backbreaking labor finances our wealth and whose demise plays itself out before our very eyes.

The question of what to do about HIV/AIDS in Asia will not be resolved by science alone. We already know at least nine ways to prevent further spread of the disease and how to respond to its victims. Although a vaccine could avert total global disaster, it is far in the future and a little beside the point. We can stop this disease with prevention and treatment but hesitate because of the cost. What faces us now are questions of morality. We must address severe inequities in the distribution of global income, protect human rights, and provide access to care. A successful human response to the HIV/AIDS epidemic must, in the end, be composed of equal parts of science and economics and humanitarian concern for our future. AIDS may be the most serious challenge we have ever had to face, stretching our capacity to feel as well as think, our ability to balance scientific genius and economic considerations with our fundamental humanity in the face of human suffering and loss. The response must be measured in small steps and little ways, in acts of kindness and salvation by ordinary people, as much as it in giant steps of Nobel Prize-winning ingenuity.

History tells us that epidemics last a long, long time. HIV/AIDS will be around for at least the next two or three hundred years, a fact that management policies must keep in mind. The trajectory of HIV/AIDS growth that started in the late 1980s will continue until the middle of the twenty-first century, with peaks and valley occurring at different times on different continents. Then, after a long plateau, there will be a long drop, and AIDS will stabilize worldwide at a lower level and be with us permanently as an endemic, chronic disease. What will the epidemic look like as it gets worse? What will it feel like? What impact will it have? Imagine yourself in the middle of the Black Death, which killed one-quarter to one-third of the world's population during the fourteenth and fifteenth centuries. It completely changed social, economic, and political systems, religions, art, architecture, and the nature of interpersonal relations. HIV/AIDS will have the same effect over the next twenty to thirty years. Recent reports from Africa say that the much-anticipated worst day has already arrived on that continent. It is now Asia's turn.

Infection levels in Asia will soar over the next two decades, and the number of deaths will increase drastically until at least 2050 unless major changes are made in the way states are dealing with the epidemic. Tuberculosis and other related diseases will increase as well; in fact, world experts have long feared that the regular outbreaks of antibiotic-resistant strains of TB in Russia's prisons and in East and Central Asia and parts of China will spread to other areas of the world, making the disease virtually uncontrollable.[17] Karen Stanecki, chief of the Health Studies Branch of the U.S. Bureau of Census, says that the AIDS pandemic is dramatically changing the demographic makeup of African countries and will have similar effects in heavily hit Asian countries. By 2010 five countries will have negative population growth and eleven will have life expectancies lower than forty years, a statistic not seen since the end of the 1800s. Three countries that had life expectancies above 70 years of age before AIDS will have life expectances around 30 by 2010.[18] The same result is more than possible across the Asian continent.

There are many reasons why the largest epidemic human beings have ever known is not being controlled in Asia. Two are key. First, projections like Eberstadt's are roundly ignored, and second, many of the people most affected by the epidemic are viewed as marginal to their own societies and the global economy. Chapter 2 explores the interconnectedness of these two issues and other important dynamics in the spread of HIV/AIDS in Asia, including the continent's major "infection pumps": wildly inferior blood donation systems, roaming populations of migratory workers, booming drug and sex industries, and epidemiologically dangerous prison systems.

Many of the conditions that create and sustain AIDS in Asia are the fall-out of a collision between deeply authoritarian, tradition-bound societies and trends in the contemporary world. As the world's largest landmass, Asia has a diverse and complex history. Chapter 3 teases out some basic themes that help us better understand where Asia stands as it faces its biggest challenge yet, the HIV/AIDS epidemic. Asian societies were shaped by a series of nomadic incursions and peasant rebellions that continue today in other guises. Much of Asia is now in the grasp of destabilizing power plays between Islamic fundamentalists and governments that participate in the illicit drug and weapons industry to feed their armies while ignoring their commitments to meet the needs of their poor.

From the mid 1800s until 1950, much of Asia was held in suspended animation by European colonial exploitation, unfinished experiments in socialism, and World War II. European colonialists in Asia were the last in a series of brigands and pirates that took advantage of persistent instabilities in Asia's agrarian societies. They may not have been the most bloodthirsty or scurrilous, but they stole the region's vast wealth and sadly delayed democratic development and modernization in the region for 200 years. Chapter 4 explores colonialism and its contemporary sequels as the new nations of Asia attempt to find their footing in the world economic and political system, and chapter 5 takes a look at the role of international drug marketing in the development of Asian society since the 1600s.

With the threat of an irreversible disease disaster looming on the horizon, women are still denied equal rights, steadfastly held back by humanity's other half. Men control women not only politically, but in every other conceivable way: dress; access to information; economics; access to food and livelihood, affecting their energy for resistance; the level, type, and start date of their sexual careers; their privacy, residence, and mobility. Men also control women's access to spirituality and their very beliefs about their own natures, the source from which change in women's status is derived. In chapter 6 we take a closer look at why gender inequalities are still being perpetuated in Asia despite repeated proof of their lethal outcomes and economically damaging results. Religion will also be examined because it plays a major role in creating and reinforcing gender bias and myths about leadership and entitlement in the region. In this chapter, we also discuss another major engine in Asian economies, the illicit sex trade, booming in all countries. The danger of male sexuality that has no regard for female consequences is evident in the widespread exploitation of women and children.

In 1998 UNAIDS first reported that more women than men were becoming infected in sub-Saharan Africa, a pattern that is moving through Asia and other parts of the world at varying but rapid rates. Gender disparities in HIV transmission are solidly linked to intergenerational imbalances of power. Young people between fifteen and twenty-five are leading the world's age groups in new infection rates, another signal that the global epidemic has gone completely out of control. Chapter 7 explores how children and young people are exposed to HIV infection and what happens to them when they are orphaned and left vulnerable by their parents' deaths. It also discusses the larger issues of age-related exploitation and the role of children in the global economy.

AIDS in Asia takes the opportunity to explore in depth many themes that were only touched on in my earlier book, *Black Death: AIDS in Africa*,[19] which focused more on the science of the epidemic than on political issues. *AIDS in Asia* explores the most important political issue related to stopping the spread of HIV/AIDS: the realization of global human rights. The pandemic is shaping a new chapter in the global struggle for equity—between sexes, classes, and generations. The relationship between human rights violations and the spread of AIDS around the world is discussed in chapter 8. It also explores the implications of Asia's ripe and burgeoning epidemics and the inadequacy of the response. Each chapter uses a group of Asian nations to illustrate the main themes of the chapter; most Asian nations are covered over the course of the book.

Like *Black Death*, *AIDS in Asia* calls on the assistance of some memorable characters who are separated by many miles and many years of history. The stories of Phet, Rageena, and other Asian children of the epidemic, and Emmeline Pankhurst, the invincible Victorian feminist heroine, come at the beginning of each chapter. *Black Death* readers will be happy to know that several characters from that book also appear here. Darwin has some explaining to do about why he stole the theory of evolution from Alfred Russel Wallace, who discovered it in the jungles of Asia's Spice Islands. Molly has traveled from Uganda to lead a discussion group among young Asians living with HIV/AIDS at an international AIDS conference in Bangkok and give them a hand with developing community responses. Wherever I have traveled in Asia over the past four years, people want to know what Africans are doing to cope with the tragic impact of AIDS south of the Sahara. Those of you who know Molly will understand how she could not resist the opportunity to share her experiences in person and help these young Asians deal with their burden of infection and the despair that threatens their lives.

The Asian and African characters are composites of the many people who have told me their stories on my travels through these two continents, where I have worked on AIDS planning and policymaking for the past sixteen years. Emmeline Pankhurst, however, was a very real woman, an irrepressibly brave Victorian heroine with a mission that took all of her life, wisdom, and energy to fulfill. Known as Suffragettes, she and her contemporaries—and her daughters—took on the remarkably unpopular mission of making women's rights a reality in Britain at the turn of the twentieth century. Although I am sure she was pleased when equal rights were granted to the "other half" of the British population in 1918, I am equally sure she would be dismayed to know that almost 100 years later only a small fraction of her sisters on this planet share equal rights with men and have achieved anything even remotely parallel to what she achieved in Britain. This lingering inequality condemns millions of women to certain death through infection by their partners—people they trust and believe are mutually faithful—with the most terrible disease humans have ever known, HIV/AIDS.

HIV/AIDS affects every single person on the planet. First, and most immediately, there is an enormous and looming threat of infection, particularly for our young people. Not surprisingly—because the United States is one of the most sexually saturated and active cultures in the world—Americans are not excepted from the threat of HIV. AIDS is also an enormous challenge to human development all around the world. AIDS affects our supplier countries and trade partners in Europe, Asia, Latin America, the Caribbean, and Africa, which means it will dent worldwide standards of living. AIDS is contributing to the destruction of the environment and of the institutions that have supported ordinary social life for centuries of human existence. AIDS weakens armies and leaves borders exposed. And yet, by UNAIDS's own account, "the current pace and scope of the world's response to HIV/AIDS falls far short of what is required."

AIDS is increasing our foreign aid responsibility, but it must increase if we are to keep this disease at bay. The developed world can afford it. Right now, for example, the United States spends less than half of one percent of its gross domestic product on all foreign aid, the lowest of any developed country, and most of it goes to military aid and support for Israel, Egypt, Colombia, and Jordan. Public opinion polls across the developed world show that the average person is frightened and aware of the threats posed by HIV/AIDS and wants to increase support for developing countries struggling with the disease. But we have as yet to convince our elected leaders of our concern. AIDS is creating a permanent reservoir of shame among us because of our inaction. We are living through the worst holocaust the world has ever seen and not using our resources to stop it. The silence grows, and it is very dangerous to us all. Let us listen once again to the voices of Asians who are brave enough to speak out. But before we return to the group, let me tell you a little story from Nepal.

———————•◦•———————

"Alaska!" she shouted triumphantly, skipping up the brick cobbled lane. "A-L-A-S-K-A. Alaska has 571,951 square miles and is the biggest state in the United States. The capital is Anchorage, and the second largest city is Juniper. Do you want me to spell that, also?"

I hid my smile. "Uh, no. That's okay. But where'd you learn all this?" I asked. "Me?" she asked, pointing to her chest and raising her eyebrows mischievously, glancing behind her to see if I was talking to someone else. "Yes, you, you little scamp." She stiffened and planted her hands on her hips. "I am fourteen," Sumi said, looking like a tiny thundercloud. "I am not a little girl." Short and thin, I'd assumed she was only eight or ten, but like most poor Nepalis, her stature showed the effects of poor diet. "Well, that's clear to me," I said with a laugh, "because you know more about the United States that I do."

She brightened. "That may be true, but we can talk about that another day. Today you have come to my city, the most ancient and wonderful city in Nepal. And I know its history better than any guide. Shall I tell you more?" I nodded.

"Bhaktapur—that is B-H-A-K-T-A-P-U-R," she stated in a deep voice, throwing her head back and sweeping her arm in front of her theatrically—"is one of the oldest cities in the world. It is the seat of ancient kings, the ancestors of my race. It is a UNESCO World Heritage site and was formerly the capital of the Kathmandu Valley of Nepal." She ran ahead and pointed down a side street at the top floor of one of the medieval timber-and-brick houses. Her silver earrings caught the sunlight. "That is my house," she said proudly. "I will take you there one day, but today my brother must have quiet for his studies."

"What grade are you in? You know so much, your teacher must be very good."

The thundercloud returned. "My family sent me to school for five years, but then my father lost his job in India." She brightened. "I learn from books that tourists give me. Do you have a book for me?" Accepting the promise of an English-Nepali dictionary, she led me to the top of the street. "Look back," she ordered. The sweep of scenery was breathtaking, ancient tiered pagodas lying in the bowl of the high, snowcapped Himalayas. "Bhaktapur was founded by King Ananda Malla in the ninth century in the shape of Vishnu's conch shell," she continued. "It flourished on the ancient trade route to Tibet and is maintained today by our craftsmen, who continue to restore the ancient houses and temples. Now follow me, and I will show you the temples."

As Sumi turned, a boy emerged out of nowhere and grabbed her by the arm so hard she winced. His fingernails dug into her flesh, but she did not protest. "Why are you bothering this lady with your lies?" he demanded. She dropped her eyes from my face and, rubbing her arm, stepped away and melted into the crowd.

He smiled brightly at me. "You can call me Raj," he allowed. "Unlike my sister,"—he nodded at her disappearing back—"I have much deep knowledge of this site and am a very able guide. I am going to school while she stays home to help my mother. Come with me and I will take you to the shops where there are many fine things that tourists enjoy buying."

I held back from his grasp. "Just tell me one thing before we begin, Raj." He looked back. "How do you spell Alaska?"

TWO

AIDS IN ASIA

The Looming Mushroom Clouds of Infection

PHET LOOKED SO WEARY AND SAD MOLLY thought he would cry. If he did, she was going to bawl right along with him. He was only twenty-four, for heaven's sake, and he'd seen more of the bad side of life than most people see in a lifetime. Wasn't it true of all these children, she thought with a shake of her head, glancing around the circle.

Phet was still staring at his hands. "Hang on," Molly told the group, smiling. "Let's give Phet a rest. I feel a little guilty because I haven't told you anything about Africa yet. The conference organizers brought me here to do that, but you people talk so much I haven't had a chance." They laughed. "If you don't mind, Phet, I can do that now and you can catch your breath." He raised his eyes to her face and nodded his head.

"In Uganda, where I come from," she began, "men beat women if their dinner is not on the table on time. When there is dinner, that is." She smiled, acknowledging the group's laughter. "There's lots of starvation there, too. One of the main problems with administering AIDS drugs is that the patients don't have enough to eat and they can't take their pills on an empty stomach. Is that true here?" The group members murmured their agreement. "My friend Pauline's husband beat her all the time when he found out she was HIV positive. He blamed her when it was him that played around. Before AIDS came along, African men were expected to display their virility. Women, on the other hand, were expected to close their knees and pray. Pauline didn't start to have other partners until her husband left and there was no other way to support herself. She didn't know how the disease was transmitted then. No one did."

An older woman with streaks of gray in her hair shifted the folds of her sari. "In India the same is true. Women are ignorant and at the mercy of their husbands, fathers, and brothers. It is probably true in most countries in Asia, except for Japan and Singapore, countries where women work outside the home and have more respect."

"Not in Japan," said a young woman in the back. "Women have been housewives for too long. I think it happens, even in the U.S. In fact, I heard that old women there are getting it because the old men are taking Viagra and getting—what is it that the Americans say—a 'new lease on life.'" They all laughed. "We need a new women's revolution around the world!" She shook her head. "Sorry, guys, but it's true."

"I think it is true, too," said the Cambodian, "even though I'm a man." He grinned. "My organization has a program that trains sex workers in traditional weaving so they have some other source of income. I don't know of any women who haven't been very glad to get out of the sex trade. Most are very poor and are repeatedly beaten and misused."

Rageena narrowed her huge green eyes. "I had ten to twelve partners a day in Mumbai," Rageena said. "They kept me in a little cell, like a stall for an animal, and the men came one after another. They never washed, and they never said anything kind. If they had trouble with the sex, they beat me and said it was my fault. I spent nine years in that hell, then one day a cold caught me and I found myself with diarrhea and chest pains. When the doctor told the *didi*[1] I had the AIDS *rog*[2], she gave me 2,000 rupees and a train ticket home. I still did not know what was wrong with me. They sent me home with many bad diseases, but this one never got better. I finally had a blood exam. That is when I learned I had AIDS.[3]

"It wasn't until I came here that I began to understand just how unfair my position in Nepali society was. I thought my whole experience was my fault, that I had done something very bad in my past life or in this one. You know, we Nepalis believe that some diseases are from *kharab karma*, bad karma, like tuberculosis and leprosy. We also believe that disease results when you are off balance, become negligent, and don't take care of yourself. One form of negligence is when someone is *randi*, or sexually promiscuous. That is often said of females. Males are *rando*, but that is never used. Men are never sluts, only women, although in reality the opposite is true.

"So we were called *randi* and it was our fault, even though our fathers and brothers had sold us into prostitution. Many women were also tricked by promises of marriage. After too many days of backbreaking labor, they left their homes with a man who told them they were beautiful and promised them many wonderful things, like rides in fancy motorcars and visits to glittering towns. They were ensnared by evil men, who disappeared the minute they were out of sight of their parents. They had been sold by their own husbands. Sold. Right from their nuptial beds."

"Those beliefs and terms are the same in India," Gita said. "But the men always prefer you beautiful Nepali women, with your large eyes and fair skin," she teased.

"Oh, there were many Indian sisters in this life. There seems to be very little discrimination in the fate of the poor," Rageena shot back. "Or age discrimination, either. We all started very young in the trade."

"African girls do, too," Molly said. "We are 'equal opportunity bodies' all over the world. We think we have it bad in Africa because old men are raping children, hoping to cure themselves of AIDS. Wait until my friends hear how old men in Nepal think that the cure for AIDS is to have sex with 108 virgins because the wife of some one of these Hindu gods"—she could never remember their names; Christianity, she thought, was a lot more convenient in that respect—"hacked his penis into 108 pieces when he got angry because she wanted to take the top position for a change!"

For a fraction of a second all of their eyes grew wide and she could hear the sharp intake of collective breath. And then they started laughing hard. "You mean Parvati and Shiva," Rageena giggled.

"That's who I'm taking about!" Molly exclaimed. "Those are the ones I mean!" She grinned. "African men are very proud of their size, but I never heard of a man's penis getting so large it reached the clouds! I think the women would run for the hills." Even Phet was laughing at this point. "Let's take a break," Molly said. "Then I'll tell you about my friends and the community groups we started to help people living with AIDS in Uganda and take care of all the poor orphans."

———•◆•———

According to her birth certificate, Emmeline Goulden was not born on the auspicious day of July 14, 1858, as her legend holds, but on the day after. It was probably a small oversight because she was born near midnight, but Emmeline herself always maintained that the fourteenth of July was her true birth date. It was Bastille Day, the anniversary of the storming of the France's most celebrated prison and the beginning of the French Revolution in 1789, and a day that suited the fiery radical well. "I have always thought that the fact that I was born on that day had some kind of influence over my life," she wrote in 1908, on the eve of the revolution she was about to create in gender relations. She told readers of her broadside, *Votes for Women*, that "it was the women who gave the signal to spur on the crowd, and led to the final taking of that monument of tyranny, the Bastille, in Paris."

Emmeline was the oldest girl in a family of ten children born to Manchester cashier Robert Goulden and his wife, Sophie. Both were ardent socialists, ardent supporters of American abolitionists and antislavery campaigners in Britain, and advocates of equal rights for women. In the United States, suffragettes linked the emancipation of slaves and the campaign for women's rights in several ways. Enslavement of Africans in the American South had made the subordination of Southern white women possible, they argued, because the slaves' labor let the Southern tidewater plantation patriarchs treat their women as ornaments. On the other side of the coin, it was women, distressed as much by the sexual excesses of Southern white males as by their racism, who founded the American Anti-Slavery Society in the American North in 1833.

Protest was a Goulden family tradition. Robert and Sophie hosted American antislavery campaigner Henry Ward Beecher when he visited Manchester. Emmeline had been raised on bedtime reading that included his daughter Harriet Beecher Stowe's famous antislavery book, *Uncle Tom's Cabin*. When she was five, Emmeline helped her mother by collecting pennies at a large Manchester bazaar held to raise money for emancipated African slaves. "Young as I was," she recollected in her autobiography, "I knew perfectly well the meaning of the words slavery and emancipation." Activities like these, she said later, awakened "admiration for that spirit of fighting and heroic sacrifice by which alone the soul of civilisation is saved." Emmeline, who read by the age of three, said later that her favorite book was Thomas Carlyle's *History of the French Revolution*, which she read when she was nine years old.

Despite her parents' liberal views and Emmeline's evident gifts—her brothers called her "the dictionary"—Emmeline was sent to a boarding school that cultivated social skills to attract future suitors. But Manchester was at the center of the national campaign in Britain and the home of many important suffrage leaders, and in 1872, when she was fourteen, Emmeline attended her first suffrage meeting with her mother to hear Lydia Becker, Secretary of the Manchester National Society for Women's Suffrage. Already an avid reader of Becker's monthly *Women's Suffrage Journal*, she came away from the meeting "a conscious and confirmed" suffragist. At that point, her father relented and sent her to Paris with her sister Mary to attend the forward-thinking École Normale de Neuilly, one of the first schools in Europe to give young women the same education as young men. But when Mary's wealthy Parisian suitor asked for a dowry, Emmeline's outraged father called both the girls home to serve as his housekeepers while their mother went on holiday. They were urged to make the home attractive so their brothers would find suitable mates, but Emmeline refused to fetch her brother's slippers. "It used to puzzle me," she said, "why I was under such a particular obligation to make home attractive to my brothers. We were on excellent terms of friendship, but it was never suggested to them as a duty that they make home attractive to me."

Emmeline kept up with social issues and looked for a job. "I was always anxious to have outside work," said the budding feminist. "As a girl I felt strongly the necessity of women being trained to some profession or business which should enable them to be self-supporting." She was restless at the suppression of her independence, and attended many meetings and rallies. The main speaker at a pacifists' rally demanding British neutrality in the Turkish-Russian war, Richard Pankhurst, had remained a bachelor so he could devote himself to social causes but was swept off his feet by Emmeline's intelligence and activism and began to court her. Forty years her senior, the dashing idealist hated injustice of any kind and risked his law career by promoting the rights of the poor and equal rights for women. He opposed Britain's imperialistic foreign policy and advocated for the abolition of the House of Lords, disestablishment of the Church of England, home rule for Ireland, the nationalization of property, and free compulsory education. Counsel in an 1869 lawsuit claiming women's right to parliamentary vote on the basis of ancient precedents, the "Red Doctor" led the Manchester Women's Property Committee's campaign against the disenfranchisement of married women, who had no right to property or an independent legal identity.

Deflecting Emmeline's proposal that they skip the church ceremony and live together for a while "to try first how we should get on," Richard married her less than six months later with the pledge that "every struggling cause shall be ours." Less than three months later, in March 1880, she was named to the executive committee of the Manchester National Society for Women's Suffrage and took up her husband's radical causes in earnest. By September of that year Christabel Harriette Pankhurst, who became her mother's abiding companion and co-revolutionary after Richard's death, was born. Emmeline soon fell out with her father, whose business had suffered the brunt of rich Manchester's boycott against Richard's radical causes. She kept busy with her causes and her four children, who were told "If you do not grow up to help other people you will not have been worth the upbringing." She never saw her father again.

———•◆:•———

HIV/AIDS is fast becoming the worst human disaster the world has ever known. Even if a cure is found tomorrow, the toll of death and suffering by 2010 will far exceed any other recorded human catastrophe, any other previous epidemic, natural disaster, war, or incident of genocidal violence. On a timeline extending from A.D. 0 to 2010, three huge spikes of death loom. Two are just past the middle: the Black Death, which killed 93 million people worldwide by the early 1500s,[4] and the decimation of Native Americans by waves of multiple diseases brought by their European conquerors in the 1500s, which killed about 90 million people. At the other end of the timeline looms the impending disaster of AIDS, which will have killed or infected at least 130 million people by 2010. Everything in between is dwarfed by these gigantic disease disasters, including World War I, which killed 10 million people, the 1918–1919 influenza epidemic, which killed 20 million, and World War II, which killed 50 million people. Other events we commonly think of as catastrophic look relatively small next to these giants. The Vietnam War, for example, took 5 million lives on both sides; the U.S. Civil War, only 600,000. The huge death tolls in Russia under Stalin (20 million) and China under Mao (40 million) are dwarfed by AIDS. SARS, which has killed several hundred people, and other emerging diseases like Ebola do not even register on the time scale of major disasters.[5]

Based largely on official estimates for sub-Saharan Africa, the 2010 predictions do not factor in two important trends. For one thing, HIV has not stopped spreading in Africa, and AIDS deaths will not peak there for another decade. In some countries with very large populations (Angola, the Democratic Republic of the Congo, Liberia, Nigeria, and Ethiopia), HIV epidemics are just taking hold. For another thing, these projections do not include new estimates of epidemic impact in Asia, where the vast majority of human beings live. Epidemics on the Asian mainland—from Eastern Europe through Russia, Central Asia, east to the Pacific, and south to the Indian Ocean—and on the islands of the South China Sea and the Pacific Ocean have taken off more slowly than the African ones but are now rapidly accelerating.

As in Africa, the first Asian HIV cases appeared in the early to mid-1980s. The virus was initially detected in the early 1980s among men having sex with men in Australia, Japan, Malaysia, New Zealand, Singapore, and Hong Kong.

They were similar to contemporary outbreaks in the United States and Europe, from which the initial Asian cases are thought to have originated. By the mid-1980s, half or more of the sex workers in Mumbai (Bombay) and other parts of India and Thailand were also HIV-positive. High infection rates were also showing up among injecting drug users in the "Golden Triangle" (northern Thailand, Myanmar, Laos, northeast India, and parts of southern China), Nepal, and Vietnam. By the early 1990s, HIV had spread from these groups to heterosexual, non-drug using populations in Cambodia, parts of India, Myanmar, and Thailand. By late 1993 in Thailand, where more than one-fifth of all males patronized sex workers, 1.4 percent of pregnant women surveyed in public hospitals were HIV positive.[6]

While the groundwork for the spread of HIV in Asia had been laid by the mid- to late 1980s, the growth of AIDS there has been relatively slow compared to Africa. Between 1985 and 1990, when HIV was engulfing eastern and southern Africa, there were only 835 cases reported in all of Asia. In the early 1990s epidemics emerged in Thailand and India, followed in the middle of the decade by Vietnam, Myanmar, and Cambodia. The Asian pandemic had shifted into early takeoff mode. By 1997, 6.41 million adults and children were infected in all of Asia, increasing to 8.9 million by 2003.[7] The Asian continent now has 22 percent of all the HIV infections in the world and the highest number of infected people outside of Africa, but because Asia's population is much larger only about .03 percent of the population is infected—compared to 4 percent of sub-Saharan Africa's total population.

By 2025, demographic expert Nicholas Eberstadt thinks that AIDS in Asia will exceed sub-Saharan African levels and that 5 percent of China's population, 7 percent of India's, and 10 percent of Russia's population will be HIV positive. Eberstadt projects that China will have more than 100 million new infections and 48 million deaths, India will have 140 million infections and 85 million deaths, and Russia will have 19 million infections and 12 million deaths. He believes that more people will die in China, India, and Russia than have died in all the countries of the world so far. Currently, about 3 million people die from AIDS each year. By 2010 Russia, India, and China will have at least 1.7 million deaths per year, increasing to 6 million by 2025. By 2015, China will have at least 1.2 million new cases each year and India 1 million.

Not only will HIV/AIDS "extract a staggering human toll over the next quarter-century in the region's three pivotal countries," he says, but economic costs will be "vastly larger than they have been in sub-Saharan Africa" because Asia is vastly richer to start with. Eurasia's HIV/AIDS epidemic will not only be a humanitarian tragedy, Eberstadt says, but it "stands to affect, and alter, the economic potential—and by extension, the military power—of the region's major states," and will also change "the relationship between Eurasian states and the rest of the world."

———◆◆◆———

From the microbe's perspective, genetics is not a rigid blueprint but more like a game of Scrabble, where each organism internally manipulates its letters, passing some on to its neighbors while trying to hide what it's doing from opponents.[8] Viruses are alive but will not stay that way for long without help because they cannot "eat" or reproduce by themselves. They manipulate host cells in bacteria, animals, and humans to survive but do not cause cell death, tissue injury, or illness unless an environmental change initiates a different response. Human immunodeficiency virus, or HIV, is a retrovirus and is unlike most other viruses and all other cellular organisms because it carries its genetic information in RNA (ribonucleic acid) instead of DNA (deoxyribonucleic acid). Using a special reverse transcriptase enzyme, it reverses its host cell's normal process of changing DNA into RNA to make the DNA it needs to reproduce. Other retroviruses cause liver cancer and leukemia in humans.

HIV belongs to a subset of retroviruses called lentiviruses that cause slow progressive diseases. Its closest relative, SIV (simian immunodeficiency virus), is found in *Pan troglodytes troglodytes*, a chimp found in equatorial West Africa. HIV has crossed the species barrier more than once, most recently about seventy years ago. Other members of the HIV family are found in cows, sheep, horses, and cats, which have lived with the virus for a longer time and are immune to debilitating infection. One of the common misperceptions about HIV is that it passed from monkeys to humans through sex. Although HIV did jump from monkeys to humans, it made the leap because Africans eat bush meat, hunting monkeys and other wild animals for food just like Americans hunt deer, squirrel, or snakes. In 2002 researchers screening blood from 573 monkeys sold as meat and 215 kept as pets in Cameroon found that one-fifth tested positive for HIV and its relatives. While most cross-species transmissions go nowhere, Beatrice Hahn, the University of Alabama researcher leading the study, now advises locals not to eat monkey meat for fear of another HIV-type crossover.

HIV was discovered in 1983 at a time when only two other retroviruses had been identified. A single HIV particle looks like a rubber ball covered with suction cups that help the virus stick to its host cells through chemical interaction. Thousands of times smaller than the cells they infect, 250,000 HIV particles laid end to end barely make an inch. HIV has enormous adaptive ability but is extremely fragile outside of the human body. Compared to cold viruses, for instance, that can linger for days on doorknobs and other surfaces, HIV dies within hours when it hits the air; is rendered inactive by bleach, alcohol, or soap and water; and is vulnerable to the stomach acids that also protect us from a whole array of other germs. HIV is virulent and crafty when inside the body, however. After sneaking into cell nuclei and cloning itself, it mutates rapidly to avoid recognition by the immune system and reproduces on a massive scale. When an HIV-positive person gets a disease like tuberculosis or pneumonia, HIV overwhelms the immune system and the patient dies.

There are three main strains of HIV and eleven subtypes identified by letters from A to K. When HIV first appeared, different subtypes were clearly associated with the major modes of transmission, but since HIV mutates freely, new combinations of the basic subtypes are still occurring. When HIV was first identified in China, for example, the predominant form of the virus was subtype E, brought into coastal settlements by visiting sailors. Subtype C arrived from India, then B arrived from Europe and America. In the Golden Triangle, around Ruili in China, it was recently learned that these two strains of HIV have combined to form a new one, B/C, which is spreading along the heroin-trafficking route. New combinations develop within individuals who acquire two types. A drug user, for example, can get the B subtype from sharing needles and C from a sexual contact. During vaccine trials in Thailand, the dominant subtype, B, was almost completely replaced by subtype E in the test group in only a few years.

In only twenty years, since the first autoimmune deficiency disease, or AIDS, case was diagnosed in 1981, scientists identified the human immunodeficiency virus (HIV) responsible for it, developed blood tests to diagnose the disease, and engineered treatments to extend the life of infected people. This is the first time we have had the capacity to watch a massive, global disease event unfold before our very eyes and the first time we had the means to change an epidemic's course before it became a global scourge. Although repeated waves of many other diseases—plague, influenza, tuberculosis, cholera, syphilis—have swept the world since the turn of the twentieth century, HIV/AIDS is the first epidemic of *a totally new disease* since the 1400s. It is the first global epidemic to begin after medicine crossed the threshold to modernity in the 1950s, gaining the laboratory capability to identify a disease and its causes quickly, the field capacity to prevent its spread, and the data systems needed to track epidemic growth virtually as it occurs.

Although people are living longer with HIV than they were when the disease was first identified in the 1980s, death from AIDS is usually a difficult and prolonged affair. "As I traveled from orphanages in Africa to hospices in Russia to clinics in Thailand," one reporter wrote, "I saw the tortured face of AIDS. It grimaced with the pain of fever and nausea. It gasped with fluid-filled lungs. It wore huge, open sores that emerged from deep in the throat and spread over the lips, neck, and torso. In advanced stages of the disease, the central nervous system can begin to deteriorate, leaving some victims powerless even to close their eyes and mouths. Nerve endings in the extremities go numb or tingle as if pricked by thousands of needles. AIDS robs the brain of its cognitive functions, leaving patients raving with dementia. It saps the body's protein, wasting muscles to the bone. Even the release of death can lie weeks or months away." AIDS has created millions of twenty- to thirty-year-olds who turn old overnight and waste away rapidly, skeletons draped in nothing but skin. HIV erodes the body's defense system, exposing the infected person to a range of lung diseases, cancers, fungal infections, diarrhea, wasting, rashes, sores, and other painful and debilitating conditions. Eventually these AIDS-related illnesses overpower the body's ability to fight back, causing physical—and sometimes mental—ruin and death. There is no cure for AIDS, but antiretrovirals extend life by slowing the progression of HIV. Opportunistic infections that kill nine of ten AIDS sufferers also can be treated, but most developing countries cannot afford the necessary drugs.

The picture of a society suffering from AIDS is just as disturbing as its individual face. In some countries of Africa, the Black Death is repeating itself. Hospitals in Swaziland, a tiny county of less than 1 million people where 38.6 percent of adults are infected (the highest HIV prevalence in the world), are bulging with the near dead. In less than ten years, the infection rate increased 900 percent because Swazi officials denied the growing rates and failed to inform the public of how to protect themselves. On returning from a visit to Swaziland in March 2004, Stephen Lewis, UN Secretary General Kofi Annan's special envoy for HIV/AIDS in Africa, said "Death is so pervasive . . . it's a scene out of Kafka." The dying fill the beds and floors of the capital city's hospital, and close to 60 percent are women, 87 percent of whom are younger than thirty. "You can see the virus on people's faces in the street," Lewis said, "you can see the virus on the faces in a crowd, you can see the virus on faces of rural villagers. HIV/AIDS has reached into the viscera of Swaziland and is tearing it apart." Crop production has declined precipitously because "so many farmers—almost all women—have died of AIDS or are ill that the fields are shriveling from neglect . . . if it weren't for the World Food Programme, a large part of the population would be starving." In a society that was prosperous and buzzing five years ago, Lewis said that people begged for food wherever he went. Orphans were everywhere already and will make up 10 to 15 percent of the total population by 2010. Fully 10 percent of all households are headed by children, some as young as eight. "A lot of the children are HIV positive, and their faces and bodies are marked by scars and rashes and lesions. It's simply awful," Lewis said, "to think how much pain they endure."

As a pathogenic agent, HIV is ideal because it has virtually no external symptoms for seven to ten years. Ninety-five percent of HIV-positive people around the world feel healthy, do not get tested, and easily and unwittingly pass the virus on to wives, husbands, partners, and friends. Of the five ways HIV is usually contracted, ordinary heterosexual intercourse is the most common, with homosexual or bisexual intercourse and injecting drug use in second and third place. HIV generally starts in a core group of people with a high infection rate—such as sex workers or drug users sharing needles—and quickly fans out to the wider group of people with whom they have contact—customers, spouses, children: people with ordinary lifestyles and no high-risk behavior of their own. The fourth transmission route, from mother to child in utero and during birth and breastfeeding, means that 30 percent of the babies born to HIV-positive mothers will be positive unless a brief, easy, and cheap preventive therapy with antiretrovirals is provided. The last transmission route is through infected blood transfusions or blood products, such as those used by hemophiliacs. Since the first blood bank scare in the United States in the early 1980s, countries have tried to protect, with varying degrees of success, the safety of their blood supply. Many developing countries have trouble doing so because they are too poor to purchase enough test kits or because they do not perceive HIV as a threat.

When it was first discovered in the mid-1980s that HIV was transmitted in bodily fluids, five ways to prevent HIV transmission were immediately obvious: safe sex through condom use (male or female); abstinence; reduction in the number of sexual partners; testing the blood supply and blood products; and use of clean injecting equipment by drug users. Transmission can also be prevented from mother to child in the womb or during the birthing process (called vertical transmission); treating sexually transmitted diseases (STDs); through male circumcision; and by providing treatment to people with the virus. Issues surrounding prevention through blood safety, vertical transmission, and clean injecting equipment are discussed later in this book; other prevention methods are discussed below.

The oldest form of birth control, the male condom, is still one of the most effective ways to prevent HIV transmission. Gabrielle Fallopius first described the condom in 1564 and demonstrated its use for prevention of sexually transmitted diseases in syphilis prevention trials on 1,100 men who donned linen sheaths, which were sometimes treated with honey, alum, or lactic acid to increase their effectiveness as spermicidal barriers.[9] The condom had been in use for at least 4,000 years before his experiment, depicted on the walls of a 3,000-year-old Egyptian tomb and in early European cave paintings. "Dr. Condom" supplied King Charles II with animal-tissue sheaths to slow his production of illegitimate children and protect him from syphilis. The oldest actual condoms found date from 1640; they were discovered in the foundations of Dudley Castle near Birmingham, England, and were made of animal or fish intestines.

In 1826 Pope Leo XII banned condoms, believing that the debauched should suffer the consequences of their revels. Public demand did not decline noticeably as a result, and by 1844 Goodyear Rubber was mass-producing condoms from vulcanized rubber. Although latex condoms were invented in the 1880s, they did not come into widespread use until the early 1930s. By 1935, 1.5 million condoms were being manufactured each year in the United States. Condoms were scoffed at then as they are now; "real" men claimed they were "an armor against pleasure, a cobweb against infection." In 2001, World Health Organization (WHO) spokeswoman, Fadela Chaib, reported results of an official review of condom effectiveness showing that "condoms are 90 percent effective against HIV/AIDS infection, and the other 10 percent is when they were used wrongly." Condoms that have expired or are used with other chemicals or with petroleum-based instead of water-based lubricants can break.

Over the past three years, the effectiveness of condoms has been attacked by politically-motivated policymakers eager to please the religious right. In these arguments, condom effectiveness is often confused with failures resulting from misuse or lack of a regular supply.[10] In October 2003 Catholic cardinal Alfonso Lopez Trujillo, a Colombian who is president of the Vatican's Pontifical Council for the Family, was roundly criticized by public health experts for preaching that condoms were so unreliable that their use "is like betting on your own death." Arguing for total abstinence from sex, Trujillo so wrongfully exaggerated the problems of condom use that other high-ranking cardinals attacked his claims as "dangerous." Belgian cardinal Godfried Danneels, favored to become the next pope, said he "deplored" Trujillo's comments and advocated condom use as moral protection from a lethal infection. Condom use, he said, "comes down to protecting yourself in a preventive manner against disease or death." The World Health Organization (WHO), concerned because other Catholic authorities were repeating Trujillo's claim—Nairobi's archbishop Raphael Nzeki and other priests and nuns in Kenya were telling their parishioners that AIDS has spread so fast because condoms are laced with HIV—attacked the cardinal, saying that "these incorrect statements on condoms and HIV are dangerous when we are facing a global pandemic which has already killed more than 20 million people."

The Vatican's anticondom stance has also been adopted in Catholic countries outside of Africa. The 2003 Catholic Bishop's Conference in the Philippines blocked legislation that would have provided national funding for condoms. The government awarded the money to an organization called Couples for Christ that provides "natural family planning" advice that discouraged condom use. Nurses in government clinics teach that condoms have holes in them, and police use possession of condoms as evidence to prosecute prostitution, despite the fact that sex workers rarely use condoms. Human Rights Watch said that the Philippine government's inadequate prevention policies are putting large numbers of men, women, and children at risk and that its actions are "courting" a severe AIDS epidemic.

U.S. funding for condoms declined in the 1990s, just when AIDS was becoming worse in Africa and taking off in Asia. Condom supplies dropped everywhere just when education programs had succeeded in creating a demand for protection. The U.S. government suddenly stopped condom donations in 2002, causing an unprecedented supply crisis worldwide. Accusing the UN Population Fund (UNFPA) of supporting forced abortions in China, it also cut their funding, which cut condom supplies even more. U.S.-funded "abstinence until marriage" programs became a staple of American foreign policy on HIV/AIDS. The United States also opposed a reference to "consistent condom use" for HIV/AIDS prevention at the 2002 Asian and Pacific Population conference, despite the fact that there is simply no other prevention approach available for those who have sex. In 2003 the UNFPA warned that condom scarcity in the Pacific Islands, including Hawaii, was contributing to rapid spread of HIV.

STD treatment also reduces HIV transmission by almost half, even in the absence of other protective measures. STDs increase the amount of HIV virus, or the "viral load," present in ejaculations and other bodily fluids, and STDs can cause genital ulcers which provide easy entrance for the HIV virus. In both men and women, STDs are strongly correlated with high HIV rates. In addition to HIV, seven major sexually transmitted diseases (also called venereal diseases, or VD, and sexually transmitted infections, or STIs) have been identified since 1837. Three are caused by bacteria (gonorrhea, syphilis, and chlamydia) and most of the others by viruses. Three are ulcerous (chancroid, genital herpes, and syphilis) and four nonulcerous (chlamydia, papillomavirus, trichomoniasis, and gonorrhea). In addition to the seven major types, there are many other milder types of STDs resulting from bacterial or yeast infection, such as vaginitis and urethritis, and several skin conditions transmitted by lice, such as scabies. The first seven are the most dangerous, however, because they are systemic; that is, like syphilis, they infect other body systems and processes, and cause extensive but silent damage to their human hosts, including the slow destruction of nerves, brain, organs, and bones. They cause pelvic inflammatory disease in women, and can be passed to newborns at birth, just like HIV. STDs, even HIV/AIDS, are old diseases, and have played an important role in human evolution.[11]

HIV is spreading just as quickly as other STD epidemics have in the past. Syphilis and gonorrhea made their way from Europe to China in only ten years in the early 1500s during the age of sailing ships. Both were widespread in Asia and the Pacific, and remained so despite the fact that condoms, vaginal diaphragms and caps, and spermicides have been widely available since the early 1800s. They were circulated by sailors, soldiers, colonial authorities, and other travelers, and moved from sex workers into the general population just as quickly as HIV does. The hundredth anniversary of French painter Paul Gauguin's death in 2003 occasioned a spate of research revealing that his interludes in Tahiti after 1891 were far from idyllic returns to innocence. Riddled with syphilis, Gauguin was happy to share his disease with island girls and men, much like French writer Gustave Flaubert, who gloried in the madness it created. STDs are still one of the world's top killers in developing countries where antibiotic treatment is not available. In 2001 syphilis caused 197,000 deaths worldwide, chlamydia caused 7,000, and gonorrhea caused 4,000; 101,000 of these deaths were in Africa and 96,000 in Southeast Asia.[12] One in four Americans has an STD, and they are on the rise in other developed countries.

STD prevalence has been increasing worldwide over the last forty years since the introduction of birth control methods that do not require a condom or other barrier to transmission. Biologist Paul Ewald thinks that as "people start having sex with more people or with less protection, venereal pathogens will not only spread but evolve to become more harmful." Infections that are detected will not lead to death or advanced symptoms if treatment is available, but undetected infections can cause a host of severe biological and mental problems. Public education campaigns are not informative enough to inspire caution, and most people still do not know that untreated STDs contribute to cervical and penile cancer, paralysis, infertility, congenital birth defects, arthritis, arteriosclerosis, and Alzheimer's disease.

Treatment is also an effective form of prevention. In 1998 it was learned that an inexpensive antiretroviral drug (azydothymidine [AZT], marketed as Zidovudine or Retrovir) could almost completely block mother-to-child transmission. By 2002 Brazil proved conclusively that antiretroviral treatment (ART) not only makes HIV-positive adults feel better, but reduces their viral load. By providing ART to all infected Brazilians who needed it, the Brazilian government prevented at last half of the new infections projected for 2002, turning that nation's epidemic clock back to 1995. Treatment averted 146,000 hospitalizations between 1997 and 1999 because it dramatically reduced opportunistic infections. Best of all, the savings realized by the Brazilian government from treatment more than covered the cost of the drugs because Brazil manufactures its own low-cost antiretrovirals. Fixed-dose combination antiretrovirals manufactured in developing countries are now making it possible to treat HIV with one or two pills a day for under $200 a year.

Two methods of prevention that can be controlled by women, female condoms and use of microbicides (gels and creams that act as chemical condoms, killing the virus and bacteria that cause sexually transmitted diseases), have never gotten off the ground because they are too expensive or ineffective for widespread use. Feminist protests regarding the failure to find prevention methods that can be controlled by women in an epidemic fueled by their disempowerment have had little effect on international policy.

Over the past fifteen years, thirty-eight studies from ten countries have demonstrated that circumcised men are less than half as likely to be infected by HIV as uncircumcised men. The tissue of the inner foreskin has very high numbers of HIV target cells so that its uptake of HIV cells is much more efficient than female cervical tissue or other parts of the penis. Exposure to an STD increases the growth of target cells for HIV-1 on the women's cervix and a man's penis and, in uncircumcised men, on the foreskin. Uncircumcised men whose wives or regular partners are HIV positive are much more likely than circumcised men to contract HIV, and uncircumcised men are also much more efficient at passing the virus to their uninfected partners. Circumcision also lowers the risk for genital herpes, chancroid, syphilis, and penile cancer, and reduces the risk of cervical cancer in female partners.[13]

The debate over male circumcision has been raging since the early 1990s, when Australian demographers Jack and Pat Caldwell and Nigerian demographer I. O. Orubuloye first recognized the coincidence of male circumcision and lower HIV rates, identifying a "non-circumcision belt" traversing the countries of eastern and southern Africa that coincides with high rates of HIV prevalence. HIV infection rates in the Muslim countries of northern Africa and in Muslim populations within highly infected African countries are low, even when the groups are living side-by-side and interacting with uncircumcised groups. Despite the effectiveness of male circumcision, adopting it as a national prevention strategy is still political suicide because only 40 percent of the world's men are circumcised. All Jews, Coptic Christians, and Muslims are circumcised, as are about three-quarters of all males in the United States and Canada; rates are much lower in Europe.[14] Most Asian men are not circumcised.

HIV can be prevented with less radical measures, such as consistent and correct use of a condom, but knowing the biological mechanisms of prevention is only a start. Moving from theory to practice, from small-scale applications to large ones, creates an entirely different set of problems, although Uganda, Thailand, Cambodia, and Senegal have proven it can be done. Mid-2000 the infection rate in Uganda dropped to 6.6 percent from 15 percent in the early 1990s, and the number of new cases had been halved. Large-scale prevention demands a huge investment of time, money, and commitment by individuals, communities, businesses, and government. Take condom use, the simplest and cheapest form of intervention, as an example. Informing people susceptible to infection how to use a condom and persuading them to do so require extensive public education, especially for largely illiterate populations with limited media contact. Buying and supplying a sufficient number of condoms and distributing them is costly, especially if road and retail systems are not in place. Of the 24 billion condoms needed worldwide to prevent HIV, only 6 to 9 billion are distributed annually. The cost of closing the gap was $239 million in 2000 and will increase to $557 million by 2015, minus the costs of distribution and education.

———•◆•———

With so many prevention methods available, why do the world's demographic experts believe the HIV/AIDS epidemic in Asia is going to be so bad? How do we get from .03 percent of Asia's population to headlines like "HIV/AIDS: China's Titanic Peril," "The Emptying of Russia," or "Stalking a Killer (in the time it takes the average person to read this story, 40 Asians will die of AIDS. *Time* traces its murderous path)"? According to Eberstadt, "The prospect of tens of millions of Eurasian HIV cases—and AIDS deaths—in the decades ahead is by no means fanciful."[15] Others agree. U.S. National Intelligence Council (NIC) projections say that China will have 10 to 15 million HIV/AIDS cases by 2010; Human Rights Watch estimates there were at least 16 million cases in 2002. The NIC assessment says that "Asia alone is likely to outstrip sub-Saharan Africa in the absolute number of HIV carriers by 2010."[16] There are four reasons why scientists are predicting more than a hundred million new infections and close to 100 million deaths in Asia by 2025: HIV/AIDS numbers are notoriously difficult to interpret and project; many people living with HIV/AIDS are invisible; governments are in denial; and little is being done to prevent HIV's spread.

Official numbers in most countries in Asia (except Thailand) reflect only the tip of the iceberg for a number of reasons. As in Africa, many Asian countries deliberately minimized their HIV/AIDS data out of fear that overly adverse reports would deter millions of tourists and international business investment. Businesses do not want to be stuck with losses from high health and death benefits or the constant hassle of recruiting and training replacement workers. As in Africa, most Asian countries turned their backs on HIV/AIDS for the first ten years, assuming that the disease was someone else's problem or was restricted to small groups of sex workers or drug users. HIV's spread far outdistances any means of detecting it in the early years of a country's epidemic. Surges can be delayed for years or hidden within national averages. Epidemics grow exponentially; that is, they grow slowly at first and then take off once they hit a certain level. Like multiplying 2 times 2, 4 times 4, 16 times 16, the number of infected people starts small but mushrooms quickly. It took less than a decade for the number of HIV-positive Asians to increase from 835 cases to 8.9 million, and the number is at the point where it could double every few years. For most diseases, actual cases are usually 10 to 100 times higher than reported cases because people have no symptoms or seek no care.[17] Even in the United States, where reporting AIDS is mandatory and care is provided, a study in South Carolina showed that 40 percent of HIV/AIDS cases had gone unreported in their early stages.

International HIV/AIDS statistics are prepared by UNAIDS, an eight-year-old coalition of nine United Nations agencies[18] established in 1996. On the tenth World AIDS Day, December 1, 1997, experts from UNAIDS revealed they had been significantly underestimating HIV and AIDS worldwide for at least five years, according to their director, Dr. Peter Piot, and it is likely that official AIDS estimates still understate the actual numbers by one-quarter to one-third. One reason, it seems, is to avoid panic, not to mention the embarrassment that comes with being wrong. In the mid-1980s, the world's first AIDS modelers were reprimanded when they predicted a much more vigorous epidemic in England than actually occurred. Politicians control the availability of data from many countries, and more than a few careers have been broken by bad statistics or by the release of accurate statistics from countries interested in maintaining their global profile and investment base. UNAIDS can only advise countries; it is at the mercy of internal political factors that dictate how good data actually are. More than one UNAIDS country director has been dismissed by an angry government uncomfortable with being pressed for information or criticized for lack of concern.

"HIV's toll has vastly exceeded the most pessimistic reports issued earlier in the epidemic," said *New York Times*'s medical correspondent, Lawrence Altman, M.D., in 2001, "and the misjudgment largely reflects gaps in knowledge about HIV and AIDS." Because AIDS epidemics take off rapidly, in their early stages a few years between surveillance reports can lead to unwitting misinterpretation of the actual growth of the epidemic. The gap between countries' reported HIV/AIDS cases and HIV prevalence (the actual cases in the population) can be very significant. For example, Vietnam now has several thousand AIDS cases, but experts estimate that at least 150,000 Vietnamese are HIV positive. The former figure, along with outdated prevalence data, were reported to UNAIDS for aggregation into the 2002 international report, so the official global estimate for Vietnam is off by at least a factor of ten. These numbers will not be corrected until new estimates are prepared in early 2004. India, Russia, and China are all underreporting and are unable or unwilling to monitor their epidemics closely or devise national responses to confront the devastation and death that is coming.

In a region as big and populous as Asia, epidemics vary widely between and within national borders and also change over time.[19] In China, for example, there are serious localized epidemics among drug users in at least seven provinces; another nine provinces are on the brink of serious HIV epidemics because of widespread needle sharing. Along the coast, outbreaks among commercial sex workers are spreading into the general population because of unprotected sex with nonmonogamous partners. Over the past twenty years, China has undergone a sexual revolution, and the overall incidence of sexually transmitted diseases has increased significantly.[20] In some of the central provinces, China's practice of harvesting blood for commercial purposes has left up to 70 percent of poor farmers infected. Not only was contaminated blood used in China, it was also shipped abroad to neighboring countries for transfusions and development of other biologic products.

A second reason country statistics are off is because many people living with HIV/AIDS "go underground" because of stigma or ignorance, especially in Asia, where many people are getting the virus from injecting drug use and sex work, which is banned in most countries. Under the best of circumstances, many AIDS deaths are falsely attributed to tuberculosis, pneumonia, or other opportunistic infections. Families do not want the true cause of a loved one's death known, and even if they did, there are not enough HIV test kits to confirm diagnoses in most developing countries. The poverty of healthcare systems leaves 90 percent of those who are HIV positive unaware of their status and 40 to 50 percent of AIDS sufferers without medical attention of any kind. Internationally, less than 7 percent of HIV-positive people in poor countries have access to antiretroviral treatments[21] and less than 10 percent have access to treatment for opportunistic infections (tuberculosis, skin problems, and diarrhea) or pain medication of any kind. For a long time, Chinese farmers who attempted to confront their government and demand clear diagnosis and treatment were jailed. In the early stages of Vietnam's epidemic, people with HIV were classed as "social evils" because they were commercial sex workers or drug users and were incarcerated. The government finally realized in 2002 that this policy of containment was not working and is beginning to change it.

A third reason HIV is spreading rapidly is because most Asian governments are in denial. Officials refuse to talk about sex or the many social and economic inequalities that contribute to the infection's spread. Nils Daulaire, who heads the Global Health Council in Washington, DC, returned from a 2004 trip to India discouraged because he saw "the looming devastation of the second great wave of AIDS. Many Indian politicians are saying, 'It can't happen here. We are a deeply moral society.' Then they point fingers at [infected] people for bringing it on themselves." Richard Holbrooke, president of the Global Business Council on HIV/AIDS, says that Indians and Chinese believe "we're different, our culture's different, it can't spread here the way it did in Africa." Holbrooke found that top-level officials were more inhibited by cultural taboos limiting frank talk about sex than the working women he visited, who were "surprisingly open." He told officials, "Your culture is unique but your vulnerability is not, and this disease does not respect cultures. The life-and-death realities trump any individual cultural taboos because the culture itself will be destroyed if the cultural taboos are not lifted."

In the last five years, growing numbers of HIV-infected individuals and AIDS sufferers have succeeded in bringing AIDS to their national agendas, but few governments are equipped to tackle the deep social and economic causes behind the spread of infections. Results of a 2002 UNAIDS survey of Asian governments showed that "political support for the fight against the epidemic remains weak in many countries in the region" and that "few, if any, national resources are directed toward HIV/AIDS efforts, leaving programs almost wholly dependent on external assistance." Of 8.9 million infected Asians, only 30,000 were getting antiretroviral drugs although they are manufactured in the region. Eastern Europe and Central Asia, the UNAIDS region that includes Russia and all the constituent states of the former Union of Soviet Socialist Republics, has the fastest-growing HIV/AIDS epidemic but the slowest governments to respond outside of the Middle East. Only eighteen of thirty countries in the region have a national plan; one-third had not even discussed HIV/AIDS. Surveillance is limited and relatively poor and "few resources have yet to be directed toward the fight against the epidemic, even in ministries of health," the UNAIDS survey found. According to Eberstadt, "The highest authorities in Moscow, New Delhi, and Beijing are unable (and unwilling) to monitor their respective HIV epidemics closely and continuously." From a strategic perspective, this negligence is horrifying, countries with concentrated epidemics that have high rates of HIV in injecting drug users and sex workers are missing their vital window of opportunity to prevent its spread to the general population.

Fourth, little is being done to prevent major and rapid epidemic spread in Asia. Prevention programs are languishing in most countries, victims of disinterested and weak and underfunded public health systems. In India and China, prevention messages reach such a small proportion of the population that they might as well be nonexistent. At the fifteenth International AIDS Convention in Bangkok in July 2004, Thai AIDS activists led a march against "the global war on prevention." Most Asian countries' policies are weak and their tiny AIDS budgets are too small to curb HIV spread. Rich countries were not donating enough to help; worse still were U.S. government-led efforts to hinder access to affordable drugs and condoms. Repeating earlier calls to action, UNAIDS's 2003 global report says that "the current pace and scope of the world's response to HIV/AIDS falls far short of what is required."

Some common denominators are contributing to rapid epidemic spread across Asia: condom use is rare among brothel-based and independent prostitutes; injecting drugs are cheap and drug users share needles; young people are not told how to protect themselves; and ignorance of the disease and its causes is rampant. Tragically, one of the major causes for the rapid spread of AIDS is ignorance. A 2002 UNAIDS survey in three dozen countries found that even where infection rates were high, 66 percent of women and 80 percent of men said they were either at no risk or low risk for AIDS. Half the respondents to 2000 and 2002 surveys in twenty-eight countries say they are unconcerned about getting STDs and 38 percent take no measures to protect themselves.[22] Indian AIDS expert Siddhartha Dube argues that prevention campaigns centered on slogans like "Love Carefully" do not provide the detailed information sexually active people need to protect themselves.

The HIV/AIDS epidemic is also spreading in Asia for reasons that have little to do with individual drug use or sexual behavior. Russia and China, Eberstadt says, "have special potential 'epidemiological pumps' for exposing broad segments of their populations to HIV risk—in the former, the national prison system, and in the latter, the prevalence of HIV-tainted blood transfusions." The economic insecurity and social freedom created by Russia's transition from communism to capitalism was accompanied by a growth in small-scale crime, such as drug use and prostitution. Large-scale crime also grew, linked to growing separatist movements led by gangsters in the Crimean region and Central Asia, who deal in illicit drugs, arms, and sex workers. Russia incarcerates more than a million people at any given time, and prisons are overflowing. Public health is "notably absent in the Russian penal system; prison camps are consequently virtual incubation dishes for diseases such as drug-resistant tuberculosis and HIV." Several hundred thousand prisoners are released every year, a significant proportion of them HIV positive. Eberstadt says that Russia's prison system "functions like a carburetor for HIV—pumping a highly concentrated variant of the infection back through the general population."

In China's case, 60 percent of the blood supply comes from paid donors. Old needles were used to draw blood, donations were mixed, and after plasma was extracted, the remaining fluid was re-injected into donors so they could give blood again more quickly. An international survey in 2002 found that a minimum of 10 percent of all new HIV infections in developing countries are from tainted blood transfusions. The blood safety of the developing world is still badly compromised because more than 45 percent of all blood donations are not screened for HIV, HCV, or hepatitis B or C. Dr. Charles Bennett, who led the study, says that as recently as 1996, 95 percent of India's blood supply was unsafe. Paid donors supply a major portion of the blood pool, which leads high-risk individuals to donate frequently, even when they are ill. According to Bennett, blood supplies will not be cleaned up unless richer nations help countries improve their infrastructure,[23] but even rich Asian nations have had problems. In September 2001 a Japanese court convicted the Ministry of Health bureaucrat responsible for the integrity of that country's blood supply of professional negligence in a blood screening scandal that has caused more than 500 deaths. The pharmaceutical company responsible for blood imports was also implicated.

There are two other epidemiological pumps at work: a multicountry drug industry that spans most of the states in the region, supplying low-grade, injectable heroin at irresistible prices, and the sex sector. The region is home to the top three heroin- and opium-producing countries in the world, so drugs are cheap and plentiful. Drug trafficking is linked with illicit arms deals and trafficking in women and other laborers by gangster bands that operate across the heart of the region. In some countries, the trade in drugs finances rebel groups and radical Islamic movements as well as the government itself. In Eastern Europe and many parts of Asia, the epidemic is spreading rapidly from core groups of injecting drug users. Moscow alone has more than 1 million drug users, including 150,000 needle-using cocaine and heroin addicts. Coupled with a flourishing sex trade, where many addicts work, HIV growth is explosive.

Lin Lean Lim, a researcher from the International Labor Organization (ILO), brought the sex trade in Indonesia, Malaysia, Thailand, and the Philippines out of the shadows in a 1998 study. She says that "the scale of prostitution has been enlarged to such an extent where we can justifiably speak of a commercial sex sector."[24] The sex industry is fully entrenched in other Asian economies as well. Indian researcher Laxmi Murthy says that "far from being a shadowy, brothel-based activity, prostitution has become a global business integrated into economic, social and political life."[25] "Illegal" sex work is a growth industry linked to employment, national income, and overall economic growth. Lim says that "the growing scale of prostitution raises alarming questions, not only about public health, morality and gender discrimination, but about the basic human rights of ever-increasing numbers of commercial sex workers," many of whom are forced or trafficked into the trade.

Asia is not the only continent with a rampant sex industry. Some experts believe it is one of the largest industries in the United States. Americans have sex more often and have a higher number of lifetime partners than any other developed country (124 times per year, a lifetime average of 14.3 partners). Japanese respondents reported an average of 37 times a year, the lowest of any country surveyed, although the country has an enormous sex industry, too. Although 60 percent of Americans polled in 2000 said they are concerned about contracting sexually transmitted diseases, 30 percent take no protective measures. Most still blamed people with HIV/AIDS for getting it, although they did not know how the disease is actually transmitted. More than half of all U.S. adults do not know if they are HIV positive. Although it is easy to get a free HIV test, 41 percent of people diagnosed with AIDS did not get a test until they fell sick, either at the same time as their AIDS diagnosis or within the year before they were diagnosed, giving them more than seven years to infect their partners.

———◦◦◦———

Two things are clear in international HIV/AIDS statistics: the pandemic is becoming younger and more female. Half of all new infections are among females, and UNAIDS executive director Peter Piot says that "HIV prevention is failing women and girls." Because women are much less well informed about sex than men, the virus is spreading rapidly among females everywhere. Globally, 54 percent of all HIV-positive people are female; in Africa the statistic is 57 percent. In Asia, it's only 30 percent, but the infection rate is increasing faster among women than men. In New Guinea, HIV is already infecting men and women equally, and among 15- to 29-year-olds there, female infections outnumber male. "Lack of attention to women's rights is fueling the epidemic," according to Dr. Kathleen Cravero, UNAIDS deputy executive director. "More young women are becoming infected due to a failure to encourage sex education or condom use." Ignorance, especially among women, is abysmal. Asian officials argue that sex education violates cultural taboos, but Richard Holbrooke says that in China and India, all the discussions of cultural taboos "were really about the fact that men felt uncomfortable talking about empowering women."

Lack of employment for women in the region drives many into sex work, where they cannot negotiate condom use. It is commonly accepted that men have more than one partner; as a result, the fastest-growing infection rate is among wives who are infected by their husbands. Most STDs occur among women and girls inside marriage or in a relationship the women believe is monogamous. In a world where women and girls "lack social and economic power," even teaching girls the ABCs (abstinence, behavior change, and condom use) of HIV/AIDS prevention "misses the point," says Cravero. Urging women to abstain from sex in a world where rape and forced sex are common, to be faithful when their partners are not, and to use condoms when they are powerless to negotiate safe sex is "nothing less than cynical." Women and girls in Asia who discover they are HIV positive are often beaten, abandoned, or killed by their husbands and families, and suffer discrimination in housing, employment, and inheritance. Misogyny is so prevalent that sex ratios at birth are wildly skewed in favor of males, promising a huge and problematical gender imbalance that is already affecting women in the region. Vietnam struggles to control illicit cross-border trafficking of young girls sold as brides to Chinese men.

Because most young women in every culture have their first sexual experience with an older male, far more young women than young men are infected in most countries. These trends are part of a worldwide pattern. More than one-third of African girls and boys surveyed had given or received gifts or money in exchange for sex. Japan's *puchi-iede*, schoolgirls who use their cell phones to hook up with men twice their age for "compensated dating," trade pictures of prospective customers through high-tech video displays. In Africa, females between ages fifteen and nineteen are five or six times more likely to be infected than men in the same age group. In many cases, older men are enticing younger girls into sex by offering them marriage, desperately needed money, or promises of favors.

Young people are not alone in taking sexual risks. AIDS has thrown wide-open the window on human sexual behavior. Experience in country after country has shown that scientists and politicians who thought that infection could be confined to "high risk" groups like sex workers, homosexuals, injecting drug users, and soldiers were wrong. As AIDS epidemics have become increasingly heterosexual everywhere, scientists learned that "ordinary" people network high-risk individuals, who also interact with one another. Many homosexual and bisexual men have sex with wives and other female partners in Latin America, Asia, and the Middle East. African men and women were thought to be exclusively heterosexual, but same-sex behavior has been documented among men confined in mining camps or prisons. Anal sex is a common heterosexual practice in many cultures, and pedophilia is more common than was believed. A significant minority of men and women around the world engage in bestiality, or sex with animals. In 1948 sex researcher Alfred Kinsey found that 8 percent of American males and 3.6 percent of females had had sex with animals some time in their lives, including half of all men living in rural areas. By the 1970s the overall proportion had dropped to 5 percent as more farms disappeared, but proponents claim that interest is again on the rise in urban populations.[26] "The presumption that most people are heterosexual and the idea that heterosexuality and homosexuality represent sharply distinct behaviors seem reasonable to most of us. But human behavior is far more complex than that," says human sexuality expert Anne Fausto-Sterling.

———————— ·•◦•· ————————

Among the risk takers are members of huge migratory populations circulating within and between China, India, and other countries of the region, marginal people who move from mines to construction projects to agricultural, seafaring, and fishing jobs as the market demands. In China alone, more than 100 million men and women move from place to place for work as part of a giant floating population. Migration is a key factor in the spread of all global epidemics and has played a huge role in spreading HIV. Canadian air steward Gaetan Dugas, HIV/AIDS's "Patient 0," infected at least 40 of the first 248 gay men diagnosed with the disease in the United States. Dugas had at least 2,500 sexual partners in the ten years he crisscrossed the United States and Canada.[27]

Official and illegal migrants cross borders, grab planes, and jump on ferries to get to desperately needed work. People also move within and between countries to trade, travel to markets and festivals, for government and private business, and as tourists. Unlike Dugas, most of the migrants spreading HIV—men traveling to large job sites in construction, manufacturing or mining, and the women who follow them, as well as teachers, doctors, nurses, nannies, and computer consultants—are not anywhere near as sexually active. They do not have to be rigorously sexually active to catch HIV, which typically infects 50 to 90 percent of a developing country's sex workers unless they are registered and treated by the government. Infected migrants, who receive little if any HIV/AIDS information or education, take HIV home to their entire families with no partner the wiser until one gets sick or a baby is born who does not thrive. Migrants show the highest infection rates in the early stages of epidemics in many countries. In 2002 UNAIDS reported that 28 percent of HIV-infected Filipinos are returning migrants and 41 percent of HIV-infected Bangladeshis have been migrant workers. In Nepal, 17 percent of sex workers returning from India are infected, accounting for three-quarters of all HIV cases; studies in 2001 showed that 10 percent of men returning from work in India were infected.

Thailand's million-plus migrant workers come mostly from Myanmar and Laos, and it sends over 1 million workers abroad each year. Hundreds of thousands of Vietnamese work in Cambodia and abroad; Cambodia sends thousands of workers to Thailand and Malaysia. Laos hosts tens of thousands of Chinese and Vietnamese workers, and sends as many as 100,000 undocumented migrants annually to Thailand. Philippine and Indonesian maids are drawn to Malaysia, Singapore, and Thailand. The region's four socialist republics (Myanmar, Laos, Vietnam, and China) tried to restrict urban-rural migration by denying migrants health and accommodation subsidies, but these have been cut over the past few years, freeing people to move.

Waiting in emigration lines at Hanoi's airport to board a flight from Vietnam to the United States, I learn from the man behind me that he is headed for Perth, Australia, to join an uncle with an established laundry business. "No work Vietnam," he says with a grin, what few teeth he has left gleaming black in his skinny face. Although he is typical of the more than 170 million people around the globe who do not live in the country of their birth, migrants in general are "highly atypical," more adventurous and less fearful than those who do not migrate. Even more people migrate within their own countries each year, but their movements are less well documented. Developed countries, where one of every ten people is a migrant, receive 2.3 million newcomers from less developed regions each year, accounting for more than two-thirds of their annual population growth. Developed countries bar less-skilled immigrants, but welcome third world countries' doctors, nurses, engineers, and scientists. The outlook for teachers is very bright; over the next ten years more than half the teachers in the United States will retire, keeping foreign recruiting firms busy finding 2 million replacements to meet rising student enrollments. The economic value of these mass movements is an extraordinary $73 billion in remittances each year, money sent home to waiting families that amounts to 10 percent or more of the gross domestic product of at least nine countries. Migrant laborers keep their rural families and sometimes their small national economies afloat.

Male and female labor migrants in developing countries leave their families behind for months and years at a time in order to feed and provide for them, but labor migration leads ordinary people into behavior that places them at risk for HIV infection. In sophisticated karaoke bars in Dongguan, China—a hub of global manufacturing just inland from Hong Kong—tall, sleek Mongolian girls bounce on the laps of squat Taiwanese businessmen. At the low end of the scale, sleepy village bars surrounding Lao gold and copper mines and the truck stops en route from Yunnan to Xinjiang turn into steamy hot spots at night.[28] A large proportion of female migrants are kidnapped or lured into the sex trade on the promise of a better-paying job in the city or work for predatory employers even farther away from home to provide their children the essentials. Thousands of mobile and migrant people meet at border-crossing points where transport workers, traders, tourists and visitors, border police and soldiers, service and entertainment workers mingle. Destinations for some migrant workers and transit points for others, many border-crossing points have emerged as special zones where law enforcement is lax and behavior is less tempered by social norms. Entertainment facilities that thrive on commercial migrants also attract tourists and fun-seekers. Asian migration expert Supang Chantavanich says that Poipet, on the Thai-Cambodia border, has seven luxury casinos patronized by foreigners, surrounded by a squalid town of 70,000 poor people. In Muse and Mong La, near the Yunnan border of Myanmar, "Chinese flock to the casinos and transvestite shows, as well as other sex and entertainment venues" which provide shabby glamour amid prevailing poverty.

Other modern travelers are the predatory sex tourists well known in many Asian countries who are interested in more unusual sexual encounters, which are illegal in their home countries but can be purchased from bribe-paying mafias in well-known tourist destinations. Tourism is an even bigger income generator than migration for work; close to 700 million tourists spent $463.6

billion on jaunts outside their home countries in 2001 according to the World Tourism Organization. The United States is the leading sending and receiving country, grossing $72 billion annually, or 8 percent of its gross domestic product. Tourism, like migration, involves powerful financial incentives for countries as well as for individuals, constituting the first or second largest income producer for many developing countries. Tourists are curious enough to pursue a one-time encounter but too foolish to use protection, and high HIV rates are no longer frightening people away. Over the past several years, African tourism has recovered and is increasing dramatically. The Bahamas has a national HIV rate of 3.5 percent, second highest in the Caribbean, but hosts upward of 3 million tourists each year, more than any other country in the region because crime rates there are relatively low and facilities are excellent. Worried tourists need only consider that HIV rates in some boroughs of New York City and even in some rural areas of the United States are higher than rates in the Bahamas.

Another type of migrant—working on short-term maneuvers, stationed for longer periods at border outposts, fighting full-fledged wars, or manning peacekeeping missions—is the soldier. Throughout recorded history, soldiers have been an enormously potent "vector" in the transmission of disease, and many of the world's armies have HIV infection rates two to five times higher than the general population.[29] In Cambodia, for example, 12 to 17 percent of the nation's armed forces were HIV positive in 1999, compared to 3.7 percent of the general population. Countries at war, contested borders, and areas with rebellions or civil unrest are "lethally perfect Petri dishes for HIV." Many countries conscript young men in their late teens and twenties for short periods of military service but only a few countries, like Eritrea and Isreal, conscript large numbers of women.

More than 22 million people, largely young men under thirty years of age, serve in armies around the world. Asia has four of the world's five largest armies of more than 1 million men. Armed forces are important sources of employment and education for young men, and can socialize potentially rebellious youth. "My family is proud of me being a soldier," says a Filipino officer. "I can provide them all of their needs as well as education for my children." Besides protecting national security, many countries' soldiers provide the only source of internal security. In several states the army dominates politics, suppresses dissent, and controls rebellious ethnic minorities. In Myanmar, for example, soldiers have been repeatedly accused of ruthlessly displacing and exploiting the Rohingyas, a Muslim ethnic minority living in northern Rakhine state on the border with Bangladesh. Other ethnic minorities in Myanmar complain of the same type of treatment.

The threat of HIV in armies and peacekeeping forces is so large—in sub-Saharan Africa, 20 to 60 percent of the armies are HIV positive and the risk of dying from AIDS is higher than the risk of combat death[30]—that in 2000 UN-AIDS established an Office on AIDS, Security and Humanitarian Response. STDs flourish among soldiers, especially those in units stationed away from home. In the 1830s, more than one-third of the British soldiers stationed in India were hospitalized for an STD, where British soldiers were twice as likely to have an STD as soldiers stationed in Britain; rates for Indian soldiers, typically married and living with their wives and children, were much lower. In the 1960s, American troops in Vietnam were nine times more likely to have an STD than soldiers stationed in the United States, while rates among American troops in Thailand were 15 times as high. In 1998 men in the U.S. marines, army, and navy had syphilis rates two to three times higher than the general population and women soldiers had three to six times the rate of chlamydia as the general population.

Officers, typically career soldiers in their late twenties, generally have lower STD rates than soldiers because they are more likely to be married, have casual sex less frequently, and are more likely to have some education about STDs. In most armies, the link between the military and masculinity is strong, and physical strength, aggression, courage, and risk-taking are valued along with sexual prowess. A 2002 international study of HIV occurrence in armies says that "the emphasis on promiscuous sex dramatically increases a soldier's chance of contracting HIV." If women are not available, soldiers may have sex among themselves. In Slovakia, for example, men earn half a month's pay from a single encounter. The same survey found that Filipino officers were aware of HIV/AIDS but soldiers had received little information about it. Only a few army-run HIV education programs are effective. The Indonesian Ministry of Health reported that soldiers are supplied with condoms and educated about the risk of unprotected sex. "In the past," says a military peer educator from Cambodia, "police and soldiers were always present at brothels or bars and nightclubs, but now it is rare to see them there."

An infected military drastically increases the chance of civilian infection. Young women find soldiers enormously attractive because they have social position, employment, and in some cases, education. "Because of our uniforms, we are being sought after by women," says a Filipino officer. "If the woman shows the motive and desire, then the soldier will definitely grab the opportunity." Where soldiers are less disciplined, rape and coercion of civilian women is common. Soldiers are often bored and lonely and spend a lot of time in local bars. "When we drink," says one Filipino career soldier, "everything is included in it. When we say we drink in the beer house, it is a given that there is a woman with us on the table." Drug abuse is not uncommon, including use of liquid heroin among soldiers in the Ukraine, where many have been infected by sharing needles. Soldiers are eventually demobilized or return to civilian life. Demobilization of Ethiopian troops after the war with Eritrea spread HIV across the country, where 10 percent of the adults are now infected.

Soldiers serving in Asia's many conflict zones and counter-insurgency actions—Myanmar, southern Thailand, Indonesia, Jammu and Kashmir, Pakistan, Afghanistan, Chechnya, and the former Soviet states in Central Asia—live separated from their families in particularly difficult situations, battling ruthless guerrillas among hostile civilian populations. Indian soldiers stationed in Jammu and Kashmir, all two-year volunteers, have frequent sexual contact with wives, girlfriends, and sex workers when on month-long leave every three to six months. The *jawans*, or ordinary soldiers, are lectured about HIV and STDs, told to use condoms, and given a medical checkup when they return. Military regulations prohibit casual sex but some have sex with other soldiers, and those stationed in the northeastern part of the country have casual sex with local women who are allowed by custom to mix freely with soldiers. In 1999 only 1,400 soldiers in India's 1.1 million-man army tested HIV-positive.

Over the last ten years, soldiers from the U.S. and Thai armies have participated in trials for HIV vaccines and diagnostic techniques and in studies of risk behavior, HIV and STD prevalence, and the effectiveness of prevention programs. Twenty-seven militaries reported mandatory testing of new recruits in a 1995 survey by the Civil-Military Alliance to Combat HIV and AIDS, the most recent international military study. Only one of twenty-three European countries tested recruits, compared to seven of nine American countries and ten of seventeen countries in Africa. Not all armies rejected HIV-positive recruits. The UN provides only voluntary counseling and testing for international peacekeeping personnel, and some countries that deploy peacekeepers do not have mandatory testing.

The poverty that drives migration is so fundamental that it turns life into a constant struggle to survive. "Poverty means working for more than eighteen hours a day, but still not earning enough to feed myself, my husband, and my two children," says a poor woman in Cambodia.[31] Poverty means loss of freedom, loss of dignity, loss of control over the fundamental course of your life. The poor in Brazil call it "living like a dog," because it makes you so hungry you scavenge, so thirsty you foam at the mouth, so needy you'll do anything to make a buck, even sell your body in prostitution. Poverty equates not only with physical suffering and lack of services but with loss of economic and social opportunities and continuous insecurity and anxiety. When drought hit the Punjab in 2000, there was an epidemic of farmer suicides. In debt and despair, farmers in Andhra Pradesh were choosing the same solution. A woman from the Kyrgyz Republic says that "Because of unemployment, young people drink to excess, commit crime, rape, steal livestock. Criminality is the result of poverty. When you're hungry, you have to find a way. Hunger doesn't ask." The poor are denied their rights to services, victimized by public officials, and brutalized by police. In developing countries without basic social welfare systems, local institutions and communities are the most reliable source of support. "We do not go to the hospital," says a young Uzbeki, "because it is necessary to bring out own bed linen, dishes, sometimes even a bed."

Poverty and disease are closely interrelated. The most common reason for descent into poverty is the illness, injury, or death of a close family member. When a family member becomes sick with AIDS, the family is rapidly impoverished. They sell their capital goods, land, and livestock, and then their small belongings, and have no cushion if other problems arise. The climb out of poverty is slow because disposable income is so small and could be lost by chance to natural disasters, poor crops, loss of employment, or another family illness. "Poor people cannot improve their health status because they live day by day," says a woman in Tra Vinh, Vietnam. "If they get sick they are in trouble because they have to borrow money and pay interest." Sex is a major part of the economy of poor women, who "form steady, sometimes clandestine, relationships with relatively wealthy men in the hope that it will bring them some material benefit, the occasional chicken perhaps, school fees for the children, or favorable deals for a few cabbages. [Sex is] practically the only currency they have."[32] In 2002 a study found that the relationship between poverty and HIV is growing stronger over time, and that HIV/AIDS is increasingly concentrated in impoverished populations.[33] HIV victims in developed countries account for only 4 percent of the global total.

More than one-quarter of the developing world's people still live in poverty, one-sixth on incomes of less than $1 a day, and it is in poor countries that HIV/AIDS is the worst. The poorest 20 percent of the world's population

(4.4 billion people in developing countries) share only 1.1 percent of the world's total income, down from 1.4 percent in 1991 and 2.3 percent in 1960. More than 1 billion are deprived of basic needs, three-fifths lack basic sanitation, one-third are without clean water, one-quarter are without adequate housing, and one-fifth have no access to modern health facilities and schooling. One-fifth of the very poor consume too little energy and protein, and 2 billion are anemic. Studies in Cambodia, Vietnam, Nicaragua, and Tanzania show that poor people are less likely to know how HIV/AIDS is transmitted or prevented, more likely to have sex at an early age, less likely to use condoms, and more likely, if female, to turn to sex work for support.[34] Studies from Africa, Haiti, and Brazil have demonstrated that poor women are more easily forced into sex work and are less likely to insist on condom use. In Asia, the number of adult women engaging in either full- or part-time "survival sex" is high, and their lives often include many episodes of physical abuse and sexual violence.

Three-quarters of the world's poor living on less than $2 a day—more than 2 billion people—live in Asia. Over the last decade, poverty fell most rapidly in China, but in other East Asian countries, poverty increased after the 1997–1998 financial crisis. In South Asia the share of the population living in poverty declined slightly, but not enough to reduce the absolute number of poor. Bangladesh still has the world's third largest poor population after China and India. If poverty reduction programs in China and India are as successful as World Bank projections predict, the proportion of people living on less than $1 per day will drop from 28 percent today to 12 percent by 2015. Right now the biggest variable in those economic growth equations is HIV/AIDS. If Eberstadt is right, infections and deaths in Asia will reduce overall growth on the entire continent and markedly increase the number of poor, as they have in sub-Saharan Africa. Poverty plays a fundamental role in the rapid growth of Asia's AIDS epidemics, driving individuals like Phet and Rageena into desperate strategies for survival where they are easy prey for ruthless criminals. The next chapter will explore reasons for the persistence of deep, widespread poverty and other factors contributing to epidemic spread that are rooted in the region's history.

THREE

THE ORIGIN OF ASIA'S STATES OF AIDS

Empire and Overthrow

MOLLY'S DESCRIPTION OF THE SELF-HELP GROUPS she helped start in the Rakai District in Uganda with her friends Robina and Pauline prompted many comparisons with community groups in Thailand, India, Nepal, and Vietnam. "Where people are poor, they learn to fend for themselves," Molly concluded. "We got some international help for a while, but it disappeared when the epidemics in other African countries became worse than Uganda's and the donors started sending money to them instead. But our group in Rakai is still helping people, and it's become part of a local government network all across the county."[1]

"But what happened to Pauline and Robina?" the Japanese woman asked.

Molly cleared her throat. "Robina went to Mityana District. She was such a good district administrator that our president, Yoweri Museveni, kept sending her to straighten out other districts that weren't running well. Then she began to rise in central government. She's headed the Ministry of Labour and Social Affairs since 2002."

"And Pauline?"

Molly drew in a deep breath, thinking for a second that she just might not tell them the truth. They were all HIV-positive and so young; she didn't want them to give up hope. But she knew the truth was always better than any lie, so she composed herself and went on. "Back in those days, when Pauline first got the disease—it must have been 1985 or so—no one even knew what HIV/AIDS was. The virus wasn't identified until 1983, and the first diagnostic test came out in 1985, and then only in the United States. By 1988 or 1989 there were a few test kits in Uganda, but most of them were being used for testing at the blood bank and in hospitals. So Pauline was in a fairly advanced stage of AIDS before she even knew she had it. She got Ka-posi's Sarcoma—you know, those skin cancers—on her face. One day she came back from a trip to Kampala—getting to the capital in those days meant a four-hour ride on very bad roads—and I could see that she'd been crying. 'Slim,' she said to me. 'I've got the Slim disease.' That's what we called it back then because it made everyone so thin. 'The doctors say I probably don't have long to live.'

"Well, I knew Pauline well enough to know that the last thing she needed to do was think about it, so I put her right to work that evening on another project we had for the orphans. The Tanzanians across the border told us about how they had organized day care centers so women could share the care of children and get more done in their fields. Children were also getting nutri-tion supplements and immunizations, and the caregivers could also make sure they were getting enough food if their grannies were too old to feed them. I told Pauline about it, and she started right in. Before she died, we organized ten day care centers in Rakai District. The biggest one was in Kyotera, the largest town, and we named that one after her. The Mama Pauline Mother's Love Next Best Thing Center. I don't think I've ever seen her so happy. It kept her alive for another six years. By then her own children had all grown up, and the day after we wrapped Pauline's body in bark cloth, the youngest, Bernadette, graduated from college. She'd studied social work and came back to Rakai to take over her mother's work."

Molly had visited Pauline's grave the day before she left for Bangkok. "Pauline is still with us," she told the young people. "Her courage made her become the kind of person who never dies. Somehow I feel that she is always with me, laughing at me and helping me all in one."

The group was still for a minute and then Phet blew his nose. "This is the only way I can find meaning in this disease," he told the group. "By helping. I hope that by telling other young people like me about it, maybe I can prevent at least one case. We are starting a community project in our village, and I'm helping to set it up. We have volunteers that visit AIDS patients in their home, and we've raised enough money to keep three orphans in school. I only hope they'll stay there, and not do what I've done."

Rageena took her hands out of the pockets of her jeans and pulled her long dark hair back from her face. "For me, helping others is good, but it is not enough. I am still very angry about what has happened to me. I blame my family and I blame my society. But most of all I blame my government, which has never taken any action to help women and girls live a better life." Rageena adjusted the narrow green scarf draped over her shoulders. "When you are young, there is no way to defend yourself, especially if you are a woman. And now," she said with a nod toward Phet, "I see that even being male is not protection enough. Our parents are too ignorant to know what happens when their daughters are bought by a stranger, who calls herself a *didi*, a sister, an aunt. Maybe they don't want to know. What good is a girl to a family, to a poor family who cannot afford a dowry? They think it is just as well when you go away and they can finally afford a new roof or a cow."

Gita nodded. "It is the same in India, but no politician will take on the rights of women and girls. In our country, children are subject to the worst slavery. There are national laws against it, but they are not enforced because businessmen pay off local authorities. And AIDS is worse, because our politicians are denying it is serious. It is moving from sex workers and drug users to farmers and petty businessmen, who punish their wives for giving them the disease and push them out in the street with their children."

"The life of one who gets AIDS is *khattam*, finished," Rageena said. "It is a terrible disease, a *bideshi* disease associated with foreigners and prostitutes, people who are outside the community. They say you get it from being *randi*, sexually active, so when you are rejected, it is according to the accepted Nepal custom of *chhi chhi durdur*, an ancient form of quarantine. Anyone with a serious illness is separated, sent Yuk, yuk. Far Far, so they will not infect others. It's just a form of social control over bad behavior. These Hindus!"

Gita laughed. "Do you think it is any better for women under Islam?"

Patwani looked up. The shy young Pakistani woman had kept to herself until then. "In Karachi, we are able to uncover our heads. But in Pashtun, it is a terrible thing to be a Muslim woman. You are used for sex, for work, and as collateral to settle the debts of your brothers. My best friend was stoned to death because her brother raped another girl. The families agreed she should be sacrificed for his transgressions. He was not even reprimanded."

"The militancy of men through all the centuries has drenched the world with blood," Emmeline Pankhurst declared. "The militancy of women has harmed no human life save the lives of those who fought the battle of righteousness." The militancy of women from all walks of life who joined her in the furious and passionate battle for equal rights with men convulsed Britain from 1905 to 1914. Resistance organized by the all-female Women's Social and Political Union (WSPU), founded by Pankhurst and her daughter, Christabel, in 1903 provoked a shocking response from male authorities. Women were battered in demonstrations and brutally force fed when they staged hunger strikes in prison. Emmeline was arrested for the first time in February 1908 when she led a deputation to Parliament to deliver a resolution for women's suffrage, armed only with a few lilies of the valley. She would see the Equal Rights Act passed, but not until 1917, although she would return to prison for innumerable acts of resistance against the regime men had created.

Loud crowds of supporters aside, what intimidated the government most was the bad press they got when police jailed, assaulted, and battered the women who taunted them. After 400 women who were marching from the first "Women's Parliament" to Britain's "Men's Parliament" in February 1907 to protest the king's failure to support women's suffrage were beaten to their knees by mounted policemen and arrested, front-page newspaper headlines stirred public outrage. "Raid by 400 Suffragettes . . . Charge by Mounted Police, Women Trampled Upon and Injured, Free Fight in Palace Yard," screamed the *Daily News*, bringing more sympathizers and money into the WSPU fold.

Suffragettes reveled in the publicity. "We shall never rest or falter," Emmeline declared when she was released on bail after her first arrest, "till the long weary struggle for enfranchisement is won." Florence Miller, who had worked with Emmeline on women's suffrage since they were in their teens, wrote how "proud and thankful" they were when their daughters were arrested for the first time in 1906 and chose the discomforts of jail rather than promise to keep the peace for six months. Their daughters were "willing to give their youth, their rare talents, their prospects, without reserve" to the cause that had consumed their mothers' lives.

Fifty years later, one suffragette recalled how Emmeline's ability to maintain her dignity in the midst of the crowds while defying brutal police retaliation was key to her triumph. "A small slender woman who wore kid shoes of size three and a half," the friend recalled, "Emmeline would stand on the platform looking poised and elegant in a dress of dark purple or black. She had an air of authority and although no longer young was still beautiful." Emmeline had honed her ability to mesmerize crowds through thirty years of practice. Her forcefulness and driving energy enabled this fragile-looking, middle-class, law-abiding widow to hold audiences in the palm of her hand.

What brought Emmeline to such extreme blows with Victorian sensibilities in order to win the rights of women? There were two proximate causes. The sudden death of her beloved husband, Richard, in 1898—which she learned about from the black-bordered newspaper opened up by a fellow passenger on a train as she was returning home—left her to bring up her son and three daughters alone. Her father had cut her out of his will, angered when the radical campaigns of his daughter and her husband cost him business. Well-wishers and supporters of Richard Pankhurst's struggle for women's rights, socialism, and anti-imperialism had set up a small trust fund for the family when he died, but Emmeline was shamed by the male trustees several years later into begging for the stipend that was rightfully hers. For a year they refused her the money she needed for the education of her daughters—although they were happy to allow her the money she needed to educate her son—until she threatened to make the matter public.

Through her work over the next few years, Emmeline learned clearly that she was not alone as a single woman in her struggle for her family's survival. The trust fund stipend was minimal, so Emmeline resigned her position as Manchester's Poor Law Guardian after six years of volunteer service to take a paying job as Registrar of Births and Deaths in Manchester's poor district of Openshaw. The working-class women were pleased to have a woman registrar and often told her long stories about their difficulties. "Even after my experience on the Board of Guardians," she said, "I was shocked to be reminded over and over again of the little respect there was in the world for women and children." Dreadful stories of suffering were the daily bread of her job. "I have had little girls of thirteen come to my office to register the births of their babies, illegitimate, of course. In many of these cases I found that the child's own father or some near male relative was responsible for her state." Because women had no rights, "there was nothing that could be done in most cases. The age of consent in England is sixteen years, but a man can always claim that he thought the girl was over sixteen."

The final blow came in February 1906, when the Labour Party chose to support a bill ensuring working men's wages instead of championing a bill for women's suffrage. Emmeline was furious that after the years of support she and her husband had provided, the boycotts and hardships they had endured promoting its liberal agenda, Labour proved itself so steadfastly resistant to championing women's rights. At her urging, the WSPU declared its independence from the Labour Party so they could give precedence to female enfranchisement. To the party's paper, the *Labour Leader*, she reaffirmed WSPU commitment to socialism. "We realize that Socialism is even more necessary for women than it is for men," she wrote, but "the immediate enfranchisement of women must take precedence for us over all other questions." She closed her letter with the wish that it would not be long before "we have secured the emancipation of our sex, and so end the need for a separate women's movement." Little could she imagine how long it would take to secure women's rights in Britain, viewed as one of the most advanced countries of its time.

————◦◦————

With close to 60 percent of the world's population and half of its land area, Asia is emerging as a premier world economic zone. Its leading countries are posting some of the highest and most sustained economic growth rates in the world. This achievement is the result of a thirty-year modernization process so rapid that it has no precedent in human history. In the process of modernization, some traditional values and relationships were maintained but others collided forcefully with modern values. AIDS, which threatens the region's growth and stability, travels on fault lines created by that collision. Phet's difficulties, for example, are shaped by the economic subordination of Laos to one of Asia's economic tigers, Thailand, a historic position developed over many centuries. After independence and the Vietnam War, poverty in Laos was reinforced by stagnant socialist rule, poor economic growth, and pervasive unemployment, conditions which improved only in the last decade when the country opened itself to the outside. Most recently, Phet's life has been shaped by the region's burgeoning sex trade, a modern force that thrives on unemployment and poverty, the low position of women and young people, and ancient subordination of the peasantry to the whims of the elite.

Each of the young people living with HIV/AIDS who tell his or her story in this book is a victim of the collision of deep-set tradition and rapid modernization. Each of them has been victimized by social forces as different as the countries from which they come. Yet as different as they are, Asian nations share many modern problems stemming from rapid change, such as burgeoning population growth, rural underdevelopment and urban overcrowding, poverty, malnutrition, and poor health, including the growing HIV/AIDS epidemics. Many of these problems began during the colonial period in the 1800s, but others have much deeper roots in traditional civilization and social systems. To understand them, we must take a look at the vast complexity of Asian history, which on too close a reading can degenerate into an endless muddle of family dynasties. Seven centuries ago, 2,000 Chinese scholars were able to condense China's history into 11,000 volumes; other countries have histories of equal depth. Since this book is comparatively short, the history it includes is only a selective reflection of Asia's great history. Before we start into some of the details, however, a few key themes can be identified that have particular relevance to the growth of HIV/AIDS.

First, history and tradition are important to Asians themselves, especially the years before colonial domination, when Asia led the world in economic, political, scientific, and artistic achievement. The Chinese, for example, still believe that non-Han peoples have little to teach them, a xenophobia shared by other Asians. Colonialism and its aftermath created few friends, so there is strong skepticism across the continent about the democratic ideals of the West. As in Africa, colonial administrators established arbitrary national boundaries in Asia for convenience, dividing peoples with shared faiths and shared languages across borders. The Tamil Tigers perpetuate a rebellion against the Sri Lankan government that has lasted for centuries, and Indonesian schoolchildren still believe their country has a historic right to Papua New Guinea, parts of the Philippines, and north Australia. In 2003 the Cambodian press caused riots in Phnom Penh when they reported that a Thai actress had casually remarked that Angkor Wat really belongs to Thailand. The Cambodian government eventually paid restitution to Thailand for damages to its embassy caused by the reporter's mistake (although one of the treasures of the Thai national palace is a scale model of that Cambodian temple complex).

Second, Asian ideas of governance are still influenced by a tradition of a near-divine central authority ruling in collusion with a highly privileged aristocracy.[2] In 1997 China's premier, Li Peng, attacked the "Western world order" and supported Indonesia's call to review the UN Human Rights Charter to deemphasize individual human rights relative to collective needs. Non-Asians see the problem differently. "A pattern of economically and social elite exploiting the majority of the people ruthlessly and with often self-defeating avarice, using the backing of armed force," is still a problem, says Asian expert Colin Mason. Brutal exploitation of slaves, peasants, and conscripts was at the heart of the glorious wealth of all historic Asian empires. Major cities existed by the third century B.C. in Asia. Ensuring the agriculture surplus necessary to support them required control of vast water canals, dams, levies, and irrigation and drainage systems, giving birth to a brand of authoritarian government once known by historians as oriental despotism. After consolidating their grip on the peasantry, few of these despots could resist the temptation to bleed the populace mercilessly. This tendency, of course, was not limited to Asia. However, European kings were much less sophisticated in their approaches to extraction, and until colonial times were more synonymous with Asia's petty feudal lords than with the emperors of their great kingdoms.

Third, in Shang China (770 to 221 B.C.), rulers developed a professional bureaucracy, the mandarinate, which was perfected by the Han and adopted by other countries. This meritocracy was used primarily to collect taxes from the peasantry with as little corruption as possible. In good times, it acted as a counterweight to the avarice of the emperors against the survival needs of their peasant workforce. In bad times, when emperors squeezed too hard and lost control of their administrations, the mandarinate's corruption made them indistinguishable from the self-serving aristocracy. Weakness was inherent in the aggressive accumulation of imperial wealth that ignored the needs of the poor, who suffered, starved, and sold their children into slavery to survive. Underpinning the showy and opulent life of the imperial court was the debasement and everyday drudgery of the ordinary peasant's life.

Fourth, when the bureaucracy failed, three social forces emerged to oppose the abuses of absolute rule: nomadic invasion, peasant uprisings, and religious reform. Peoples of the steppes and deserts of Mongolia and Central Asia periodically toppled the emperors of settled and complex societies weakened by their own avarice. Emperors also were toppled by disenfranchised peasants happy to end their ruler's mandate from heaven so they could get something to eat. Finally, each of Asia's major religions and ethical systems arose to counter the worst abuses of power. Their early adherents were the world's first human rights advocates, arguing for moderation, community, compassion, and the unity of human kind. Natural disasters and disease aided all three groups— nomads, peasants and believers—in bringing about the collapse of avaricious states. Asia is and always has been an area of vast unrest, and its cultures, peoples, economies, and political systems are still far from stable. All of the ancient actors and processes still play themselves out in Asian society, most recently in the spread of HIV/AIDS.

Fifth, the continent was united by all of its great nomadic empires— Hun, Muslim, Mongol, Mogul, and Manchu—which also kept most Europeans out of Asia until the 1600s. The continent's history was radically changed when Asia's nomads thundered eastward and westward across the steppes and deserts and bounced off settled populations in China, India, and Europe. Although Asia's national histories have created unique and identifiable peoples, they have been so linked by conquest culturally and genetically that it is possible to speak of Asia and Asian history in a continent-wide perspective. Finally, to understand Asian history, it is as important to keep a topographical map handy because these waves of conquest swept along natural geological and ecological boundaries, which defined the settlement and movement of people.

The Asian continent and Pacific Islands stretch across twelve time zones, or half the circumference of the earth, and sweep all the way from the North Pole to ten degrees south of the equator. The world's highest mountains, the Himalayas and their foothills, sit like a belt beneath a fat man's belly, dividing South and Southeast Asia, largely tropical, from the northern two-thirds of the continent, largely temperate except for the deep Arctic fringe. The land beneath the "belt" breaks into two large promontories separated by the Bay of Bengal: South Asia (India, Pakistan, and Bangladesh), and Southeast Asia (Myanmar, Thailand, Laos, Cambodia, and Vietnam). These overgrown peninsulas extend 1,000 miles or more southward into the Indian Ocean and the South China Sea. Extending even farther southward, the Malay Peninsula ends in an almost continuous chain of islands swinging eastward through the China Sea. The islands range in size from tiny specs to the huge islands of Kalimantan (Borneo) and Sumatra, among the largest in the world. By themselves, the 3,000 islands south of Malaysia known as Indonesia spread 3,000 miles to the east. At their end, they swing northward to the Philippines and Japan and out into the tiny states of the Pacific.

The big rivers of Asia—the Indus, the Ganges, and the Mekong—plunge from their source in the perpetual snows and glaciers of the wild and sparsely populated Himalayas southward through South and Southeast Asia to sea-level deltas. Behind the deltas and their miles of swamps and mangrove forests are flat fertile plains flooded and enriched yearly by alluvial soil. These are the major food-producing areas of South and Southeast Asia and home to the most concentrated populations. In the east, the Himalayas taper down to the coast as mountainous stretches of forbidding jungle separating China from its smaller southern neighbors. These mountains extend southward, acting as partial boundaries among the states of the region. In the west, the "belt" separates India and Nepal from China and the states of Central Asia (Kazakhstan, Kyrgyzstan, Tajikistan, Turkmenistan, and Uzbekistan). These states are further separated by a rib of mountains running up Pakistan's back and into Afghanistan. Here, food production is limited to the Punjab region of eastern Pakistan, to high, fertile valleys like the Kashmir and Fergana, and to carefully irrigated oases maintained from historic times. Nomadic peoples still move their herds across these high, arid plains to fertile valleys in seasonal migrations.

North of the "belt," Asia's great mountains settle gradually into the vast plains, deserts, deep forests, and icy reaches of the Siberian Arctic. To the east and north of the Himalayas are the high, desolate, cold plateaus of the Pamirs and northern Tibet. They continue into the forbidding Taklamakan region of China, where temperatures reach the boldest extremes on earth, then rise again into the Tian Shan and Altai mountains, the western boundary of modern China. Farther east, the mountains give way to the loose sands of the Gobi Desert, defining the boundary of Mongolia and China. Past the Gobi are the fertile loess soils of northwestern China and Manchuria's grasslands. To the south sweeps China's heartland, where, in the valley of the Yangtse and along other rivers like it, Asia's third great concentration of people are found.

The most forbidding features of Asia's topography define its chief cultural areas: South Asia (India, Nepal, Bhutan, Bangladesh, and Pakistan); Southeast Asia (Myanmar, Thailand, Laos, Vietnam, Cambodia, Singapore, Malaysia, Indonesia, Papua New Guinea, and the Philippines); Central Asia (the "Stans"); Eastern Europe and Russia; East Asia (China, Mongolia, North and South Korea, and Japan); and the Pacific Islands.[3] The continent encompasses some of the highest, wettest, driest and coldest lands on earth, physical extremes matched by extremes in human cultural and social organization. It includes Russia, still the largest country on earth; China, India, and Indonesia, three of the most populous countries on earth; and Bhutan, Fiji, Brunei, some of the world's smallest states. A continent that is home to ancient bodies of literature is also a place with massive illiteracy, home to some of the world's poorest and richest people. Speaking a huge number of languages from most of the world's major language families and practicing all of the world's major religions, Asians live in some of the densest and most sparsely populated settlements on the planet. Their cultures range from sophisticated high-tech societies to forest-dwelling hunter-gatherers and nomads. Asia, which birthed three of the world's major religions, includes large numbers of people who still believe in natural spirits and fast-paced gangsters who have forgotten their gods entirely.

In front of this panoramic backdrop, the stage of Asian history is set. On it, the play of development forces that contribute to HIV's current spread in the region is about to take place. As you follow its complex and convoluted plot, take careful note of the forces behind the rise and fall of each of the empires described, because the reasons behind nomadic wrath and peasant rebellion still play a critical role in explaining Asia's AIDS epidemics today. Asia's history is not an easy subject but it is critical to understanding its present, so have patience with the drama that unfolds in the sections that follow below.

———◆———

"I am the flail of God," thundered Genghis Khan at the refugees huddled before him in the shadow of Bukhara's central mosque in February of 1220. "If you had not committed great sins, God would not have sent a punishment like me upon you." The "falcon with the sun and moon in its two claws," as a shaman called the Great Khan when he was only eight years old,[4] had burned the outer city, and his horsemen drove its inhabitants before them as a human shield in their assault on the citadel. All was destroyed. When the great West African traveler Ibn Battuta passed through the city a century later, he praised the gardens but mourned "its mosques, colleges, and bazaars [all] in ruins."[5] Thirty thousand of the city's defenders were slaughtered, and the survivors were stripped of their possessions and herded before the Mongol armies intent on subduing all of Khwarazm, whose shah had seized a Mongol caravan competing for trade with the West and provoked the great Khan by beheading his chief envoy and burning the beards off his lieutenants.[6]

The battle was the first round in a clash of two great nomadic empires that played major roles in shaping Asia's history: Dar al-Islam, the Peace of Islam, the world's largest empire from the mid-600s until 1220 when the Khan struck, and the Mongol empire which he founded, which lasted until 1600. The Muslim empire had been born six centuries before the Khan's coming when Muhammad persuaded warring Arabian nomads to end their murderous cycle of vendettas. Like the warring Mongol tribes brought together by Genghis Khan's vision, "the Arabs had found themselves for the first time members of a united community, free from the burden of constant, debilitating warfare," says religious scholar Karen Armstrong.[7] But the peace of *ummah*, the community, created its own problems. Raiding had been the chief occupation for tribal bands in their barren homeland. Dar al-Islam meant warring tribes could no longer prey on one another, so they turned outward, preserving their unity and livelihoods by preying on neighboring states to bring new lands under tribute.

Umar, Muhammad's second successor, or *caliph*, led the desert horde forth from the Arabian Peninsula to conquer Palestine, Iraq, Syria, Egypt, and the north African coast. They swept over the Persian army in 637, and by 732, only a century after the Prophet's death, Muslims controlled all the territory between the Pyrenees and the Himalayas. A despised out group like the Mongols, the Arabs inflicted major defeats upon the Persian and Byzantine empires, exhausted from fighting with one another. "There was nothing religious about these campaigns," says Armstrong. Umar and his successors plundered to preserve the unity of Islam. To Islam's first raiders, Europe was remarkably unattractive prey, a primitive backwater with few opportunities for trade, little booty, and a very bad climate. They had headed east instead, across Persia and through Central Asia to India, and remarkably rich city-states fell to their sway all along the way.

The Muslims also pushed their way steadily across Iranian and Turkic lands into the China's sphere of influence in Central Asia, but "neither of these medieval colossi really wanted war with one another"[8] that would disrupt the Silk Road trade and prompt rebellions in their subject states. The Tang dynasty's control of eastern Silk Road trade routes had been continually threatened by Tibetan bandits, so it sent a large army westward into Central Asia in 747. A petty quarrel between two princes in the Fergana Valley prompted a showdown, and after five days the Muslims had completely destroyed the Chinese army. "God cast terror into the hearts of the Chinese," wrote a contemporary Arab historian. "Victory descended, and the unbelievers were put to flight." China's few thousand survivors were pushed back to the Tarim Basin, which marked the extent of Chinese rule thereafter. The Khwarazm became solidly Muslim, and Chinese prisoners of war were put to work making paper in Samarkand. This fertile, well-irrigated region south of the Aral Sea was a flourishing agricultural and urban civilization rivaled only by contemporary China, the last outpost of the Muslim federation boasting huge cities that hosted caravans the size of small armies.

The Arabian horsemen never forced conversions or disturbed farmers, who paid rent to their Muslim overlords. Occupying troops sequestered themselves in strategically located garrison towns centered on a mosque for Friday prayers and were given lessons in civic responsibility. The Muslims found that "ruling an empire seized by force was very different from ruling a desert kingdom inspired by religion," says historian John Man, and the ideals of *ummah* were soon sacrificed to empire building. By the early tenth century, conflict among the emerging caliphates had split the empire into five loosely connected sections (Spain, North Africa, Cairo, the Near East, and Transoxania), but the Muslim world preserved its economic unity. Dar al-Islam drew much of its staggering wealth from a trading empire that linked North and East Africa, Europe, Russia, the Middle East, India, and China, including trade in slaves. Gold was seized from the pharaohs' tombs and mined by slaves in the Caucasus, Armenia, Nubia, and sub-Saharan Africa.

Far greater than any European states, Islam's rich capitals in Cordoba, Damascus, Cairo, and the Silk Road entrepots of Samarkand and Bukhara in Khwarazm (present-day Uzbekistan) were the wonders of their day. Baghdad was one of the largest and wealthiest cities in the world, the hub of a federated empire larger than Rome's. The most advanced civilization of its day, Baghdad's "court scientists were perfecting algebra (from an Arabic word for calculating—*al-jabr*) and the measurement of degrees of latitude while . . . Charlemagne and his lords were . . . dabbling in the art of writing their names."[9] Destroyed by the Mongols, Bukhara's library had housed a collection of 45,000 volumes. Man says that "medieval Islam, assured of its superiority, was innovative, curious, and surprisingly tolerant of other cultures and faiths,"[10] building on Greek scientific and philosophic foundations to create its own body of medical and mathematical knowledge, rediscovered by Europeans only in the Renaissance.

It took three centuries for Chang'an, the capital of China's Tang dynasty, to finally reach 2 million people by 907; Baghdad's population skyrocketed in less than a century to almost 2 million by 800. Half a million people lived in Samarkhand at this time, and Cairo became that large less than a century later. European cities were not that big until the nineteenth century or later. During the Renaissance, Milan, Venice, Naples, Florence, Ghent, Cologne, London, and Paris had only 50,000 to 100,000 people each. A Florentine who visited in 1384 said Cairo was big enough to contain Persia's ten largest towns, that one of its streets had more people than the entirety of Florence, and that three times the number of ships were docked on the city's Nile port of Bulaq than in all of Venice, Genoa, and Ancona combined. For 750 years, Islam "was the central civilization of the Old World," says historian Philip Curtin, "and transmitted innovations across its empire.[11]

But as great as Islam was, in fifty years the Mongols built an even larger empire that covered all of the Eurasian landmass except India. Before Genghis Khan united them, the Mongols had been an illiterate group of nomadic, shamanistic people about 2 million strong who could barely support their herds of cattle, sheep, and goats on the desert and grassy steppes of their northeast China homeland. Intertribal warfare was frequent and brutal until the Great Khan organized a tribal confederation like Muhammad's. In 1206 he took the title of Genghis Khan, Ocean Wide Lord, the chosen one, rightful master not only of the "peoples of the felt tent" but also of the entire world. Like the Muslims, Mongol stability depended on outward expansion, and so their conquests began. They subdued the eastern Tartars in 1202, the Siberian tribes in 1205, the Buddhist Tanguts of Xixia in northwestern China in 1209, the Ruzhen of northeastern China in 1211, and China's Sung and Jin rulers in 1215. When Genghis Khan returned to Mongolia in 1217, among his captives was a Jin mandarin of Mongolian ancestry, Yehlu Chutsai, who convinced the Khan that he should tax his subjects and reap the bounties of food, salt, gems, and precious metals rather than destroy them.

Only 10 percent of subjugated men were conscripted, and subjugated peoples were allowed to worship as they chose. The Mongol language was committed to writing, and a record-keeping and court system was introduced. Fast, efficient communication over the 5,000-mile relay system known as the orto made the huge empire governable.[12]

In 1220 when Khwarazm's Shah Muhammad insulted his emissaries, the great Khan headed west and defeated twenty nations on a 5,000-mile circuit of conquest around the Caspian Sea. As grand as they were, Islam's capital cities fell one after another before the Khan's horsemen of doom, who humiliated their enemies by desecrating ancient mausoleums and diverted the Syr Darya river to flush out the crumbling ruins of Urganj. The Mongol reputation for ruthlessness and savagery was enhanced when they poured molten silver into the eyes and throat of Otrar's defeated governor and collected sacks of their victims' ears to meet their deadly quotas. Skulls of the vanquished were piled into pyramids; even dogs and cats were killed. Thriving cities ceased to exist, and death tolls were extraordinary: 700,000 at Merv; 1.7 million at Nishapur. Only skilled craftsmen were spared and sent back to the Mongol heartland.

The Khan ravaged a good part of northern India in the spring of 1222, and when Herat in modern Afghanistan rebelled, 1.6 million people were massacred. While the Khan consolidated his victories in Persia, 40,000 of his horsemen pushed through Azerbaijan and Armenia. They crushed the Teutonic knights, who had been clearing the southern Baltic coastlands of pagan inhabitants and had created a rich military state encompassing Prussia, Livonia, and Estonia. The Mongols captured a Genoese trading fortress on the Crimea, wintered on the Black Sea, then occupied the Volga, Georgia, and Armenia. "The Mongols have done things utterly unparalleled in ancient or modern times," said thirteenth-century Arab historian Ibn alAthir. "May God send a defender to the Muslims for never since the Prophet have they suffered such disasters." The largest empire the world had ever known was a territory where "not a dog might bark without Mongol leave." The Mongol's yak-tail banner was a demon "with a devil face and long gray beard" to Muslims and Christians alike.

Returning to Mongolia, Genghis Khan died in 1227 after a fall from his horse while hunting. The five khanates of his empire were led by his sons and grandsons, subordinate to his favorite son and successor, Ogudai, who subjugated Korea and rode through northern Persia. Ogudai's son, Batu, threatened Eastern Europe with an army of 150,000 men. "Piercing the solid rocks of the Caucasus, they poured forth like devils from the hell of Tartarus," said the chronicler Matthew Paris. "They swarmed locust-like over the face of the earth and brought terrible devastation to the eastern part of Europe, laying it waste with fire and carnage." Batu's horsemen swept up the frozen Volga 1238, invading Christian Russia in a lightning winter campaign. They took Rostov, Moscow, Vladimir, and captured Kiev in 1240, suffocating Prince Mstislav in a pile of carpets. After defeating the Polish army and devastating Moravia and Silesia, the Mongols took Hungary and by 1241 had reached the outskirts of Vienna.

Europe was spared when Ogudai died following a bout of binge drinking in December 1241. Batu had to return quickly to Karakorum, the Mongol capital, to vote for a new leader at the tribal gathering known as kuriltai. Pope Innocent IV took advantage of the Europe's temporary reprieve to send an envoy to the Great Khan begging him not to invade Europe and to convert to Roman Catholicism. Although the new Khan, Guyuk, was not a Christian, Sorkaktani, his wife—and the mother of the Khans Mongke, Hulegu, Arik-Boge, and Kublai—had converted to Nestorian Christianity along with Hulegu's wife before Pope Innocent's envoy had even left Rome. An aging and overweight Franciscan friar, John of Plano Carpini, set out from Rome with the pope's blessing on Easter Day in 1245 and returned two years later with bad news. Guyuk, as ruler of the world, demanded the pope's submission. Unchastened, the pope sent the Dominican friar Ascelin to demand the cessation of Mongol hostilities. Although Ascelin's boorish manners nearly got him killed, Aljigiday, the Mongol's western leader, sent him back to Rome in 1248 accompanied by two Mongol envoys and a proposition for alliance. Aljigiday also sent word to King Louis IX of France, who was on a Crusade in Cyprus, that the Mongols would help Christendom reclaim the Holy Land and destroy Islam. On May 7, 1253, William Rubruck, a Flemish Franciscan monk fresh from King Louis' crusade to Palestine, set out to firm up the arrangements.

Attacks on Europe had been furthur delayed by a second *kuriltai* in 1251 naming Mongke, Genghis's grandson, to succeed Guyuk. Mongke sent Hulegu to finish the conquest of western Asia while his other brother, Kublai, advanced deep into Sung China. Hulegu massacred the Ismailis, an extreme Shia Islamic sect that controlled the mountains south of the Caspian Sea. Too frightened to fight, the Seljuk Turk dynasty surrendered. In Baghdad, Hulegu locked Islam's world leader, the caliph, in a tower with his treasure to starve to death when he refused to eat his own gold. Baghdad's refugees poured into Syria, Egypt, and India, but the city's Christians were spared and the Nestorian patriarch, Makikha, was installed in one of the caliph's palaces. Shia Muslims, who had joined the Mongol invaders, rejoiced at the fall of the Sunni caliphate, and Muslim leaders from northern Iraq, Syria and Anatolia rendered fealty to Hulegu. In Syria, Aleppo fell in a week. The Christians of

Damascus were spared by the Mongol general Kit-Buqa, a Nestorian Christian, after the city surrendered in April 1259.

Preparing for his conquest of Egypt, Hulegu hurried east after learning that Mongke had died while invading China's Sichuan Province. The force of 10,000 men he left behind continued to Palestine to fight Egypt's Mamluk army. Professional fighters, the Mamluks were Turkish Kipchaks enslaved by earlier Muslim conquerors and were horse warriors as fierce as the Mongols themselves. They defeated the Mongols at the battle of Ayn Jalut; and although the Mongols returned five times over the next fifty years and eventually destroyed Damascus, their westward expansion had ended. The Delhi Sultanate stopped a Mongol invasion of northern India, and in Japan the Mongols were defeated by the shogun, ending the Mongol's eastward expansion. But the rest of Asia, from Korea to Russia to Damascus, was theirs.

Gaining ascendancy over the rich eastern khanate in 1264 after a minor war with one of his brothers, Kublai crowned himself Son of Heaven and Emperor of China. Although he was raised in China and educated by a Confucian scholar, his war against the Sung Chinese was so thorough it has "seldom been equaled before or since," says Mason. Beijing was burned and plundered, along with cities in China's northwest that "have never again been populated, remaining desolate to this day." Plague carried by the raiders reduced China's population from 100 to 70 million in a few decades.

During the first part of his reign, Kublai tried to repair some of the damage by returning to the Confucian ideals of his youth. He promoted education, transport, trade, and famine relief. But the empire began to sag as he blended swashbuckling Mongol appetites for women, hunting, drink, and excessive display—he brought 200 elephants back to China from his campaigns in Burma, where their performance in battle had almost undone his cavalrymen—with ultra-refined tastes in art, clothes, music, literature, and theater. Supplying the emperor's bed kept the imperial commissioners busy round the clock rating eligible virgins. A team of six concubines attended him at all times, working in three-day shifts. Among the Europeans drawn by his reputation were Marco Polo's father and uncle, Nicollo and Maffeo, whom the Khan instructed to return to China with "a hundred men of learning, thoroughly acquainted with the principles of the Christian religion" and oil from the lamp above the sepulcher of God in Jerusalem. The Vatican—buzzing with rumors of the fabled empire of Prester John, a Christian lord who would swoop from the East to free them from Muslim domination—was quick to comply. On their return, the Polos also brought 17-year-old Marco.

The khan's capital of Zhongdu (Xanadu) dazzled the young Polo, who was used to a still poor and thinly populated Europe. As an official emissary, he had his pick of the khan's concubines, who paid their taxes by providing free services to special guests.[13] Polo saw porcelain, asbestos, coal, the world's biggest ironworks powered by hydraulic machinery, gunpowder, grenades, and repeating crossbows, all unknown in Europe. He saw Sung books that had been printed in five colors three centuries before the Gutenberg Bible. Private libraries were common, and the royal library housed a 1,000-chapter encyclopedia and anthologized political texts, folk stories and fables. Kublai had inherited Sung paper money and credit banking, streetlights, city sanitation, and fire protection, hospitals, orphanages and homes for the poor and aged financed by inalienable trusts, smallpox variolation, and textbooks in medicine, forensics, architecture, mathematics, geography, horticulture, and archaeology. Million-strong cities lined rivers, canals, and seacoasts and were centers of trade, industry, and maritime commerce with playhouses, shadow theaters, acrobats, and performing monkey shows. Pleasure-seekers had their choice of wine shops and brothels open twenty-four hours a day. The Chinese navy was the world's largest merchant marine, with crank-operated paddlewheel boats and five-masted ships with drop-keels and watertight compartments that could carry 1,000 people. Naval maps and charts had detailed depth soundings. Canton was one of the world's biggest ports, controlling trade across the East and South China seas to the straits of Melaka in Malaysia.

The co-opted Confucian elite of China saw the khan as a righteous up-holder of their ideals. To Muslim subjects, he was a wise and respectful protector and patron; to Buddhists in Tibet and other parts of his realm he was *Manjusri*, a Boddhisattva (living Buddha) replete with wisdom. But as his reign dragged on, the khan progressively impoverished the Chinese peasantry and eroded China's efficient bureaucracy by larding it with Mongols and tax-exempt foreigners. To make his kingdom the center of the world, Kublai waged costly land wars for suzerainty over the kingdoms of Southeast Asia and equally expensive but less successful naval wars against Japan, the Philippines, Java, and Malaysia. The difficulties the Mongols had faced while conquering southern China—large scale death from unfamiliar diseases, heat and terrain unsuitable for cavalry—multiplied when he attacked the four kingdoms of Southeast Asia: Annam in northern Vietnam, Champa in southern Vietnam, Khmer in Cambodia, and the Burmese in Myanmar. After a four-year land and sea war, the Annam and Champa agreed to pay tribute in 1285. The Burmese king resisted. He stopped paying tribute, executed the Mongol delegation, and attacked China, provoking Kublai into a war of retribution that lasted until 1297, when the Mongols reached Pagan and the king surrendered.

Kublai brought Korea into his orbit in 1273. Earlier it had been ruled by a succession of ruthless and efficient Koryo oligarchs who lived off the land's sturdy but rebellious peasants while fending off northern nomads and the Japanese invaders. They exported raw copper, silk, paper, furs, and horses to China in exchange for tea, lacquer ware, dyes, cosmetics, and medicine. Warlordism and banditry had weakened the Koryo, which fell to a succession of savage Mongol invasions. "The walled cities resisted bravely," Mason says, "attracting praise even from the Mongol generals, but in the end fell to the relentless professional assaults." The Mongols had adopted Chinese siege machinery and used "firecarts fueled with human fat made from boiling down prisoners." Predatory Mongol rule brought "fresh horrors of starvation and disruption to a society already on its knees."

Kublai then set off to subdue Japan, whose rulers also enjoyed fabulous wealth gained on the backs of miserable peasants. In 1257, after a massive earthquake in Kamakura accompanied by plague and famine left dead peasants lying the field, graffiti on Kyoto's palace walls said it all: "In the land, disasters. In the capital, soldiers. In the palace, favoritism. In the provinces, famine. In the shrines, conflagrations. In the riverbed, skeletons." Kublai demanded submission and would have been successful had his two expeditionary fleets not been mysteriously destroyed by sudden typhoons. The Mongols, annihilated twice by the divine wind—or *kamikaze*—troubled Japan no more after 1281.

Tibet acknowledged Kublai's suzerainty, and he retained control of the western khanates. In 1287 when he was seventy-two, Kublai personally subdued a rebellion in Manchuria led by Nayan, a Nestorian Christian descended from one of Genghis Khan's half-brothers. After a forced march of twenty-five days, Kublai supervised the battle from a wooden tower perched on the backs of four elephants. It was a rare triumph in a sad old age, marked by the death of his beloved chief wife, Chabi, in 1281, and of his son and chosen heir, Chen-chin, in 1285. Kublai, depressed and grossly fat, died on February 18, 1294. He was buried near the tombs of his grandfather, Genghis Khan, and his brother Mongke on a hill known as Burdan-kaldum, soon overgrown by dense forest and lost to history forever.

Rife with quarreling factions after the khan's death, Mongol armies were unable to maintain control of China in the face of natural disasters. The Yellow River burst its levees and swept hundreds of villages to the sea, and paper money became valueless as the financial system collapsed. In 1368 the Mongols were pushed out of China, and their control over the rest of their empire rapidly evaporated. They were driven out of Korea in 1361, replaced by a dynasty that functioned like a police state. One hundred thousand or more conscripted laborers built palaces for a bureaucracy whose tentacles embraced the nation. All Koreans wore identity tags, the land was carefully mapped, and movement was closely monitored. Taxes were squeezed from the peasantry by policemen who got no pay except what they could skim from their jobs. Household batches of 5,000 policed themselves and provided conscripts for military service and public works, including thousands of water storage dams. The state's hundreds of thousands of slaves were so much better off that freeman tried to join them. Soon the peasant guerrillas joined rebellious bands of slaves who took over the ruling class, turning Korea's old social order upside down.

In the rougher cultures of Russia and Central Asia where governments were not as well developed, the Mongol's lack of administrative experience was less of a handicap and their rule was more enduring. Their sword continued to harvest tribute and taxes for another 130 years in the north until they were overthrown by the Russians in the late eighteenth century. The Persian khanate had already been absorbed into Islam, and Il-Khan's rule in Iran and Central Asia had degenerated although Bukhara and Samarkand still flourished as trade centers under a figurehead khan. But by 1360, warring tribes had destroyed the surrounding agricultural lands, and a militia of craftsmen, merchants, and teachers known as *sarbadars* arose within the great cities to throw off Mongol oppression.

Another character had emerged in the drama for power. Starting in the late fourteenth century, recurrent waves of plague rolled from China to Europe, killing one-quarter to one-third of the continent's population. Historian William McNeill speculates that the Black Death, rampant on the steppes of Asia, was a major factor in the spread of the Mongol empire[14] but also fostered its decline and that of Dar al-Islam. In nomadic khanates like the Golden Horde, the loss of one-third of their military was a disaster. In areas where the khans had settled their armies were smaller, and slaves eager for military advancement replaced those who died from the plague. Muslims accepted the plague as God's will and made no move to protect themselves through the system of quarantine being used in Europe.[15] Natural birth control further reduced their populations. The medieval Muslim belief that "love is kissing and the touching of hand—going beyond is asking for a child," created "a vicious spiral . . . linking drastic population reductions to economic decline and contracting agriculture," says historian David Nicolle.

Genghis Khan's direct descendent Timur-i-Lenk—"Timur the Lame" or Tamerlane—seized power in Samarkand in 1369 and sent the Chagatai Mongols, weakened by plague, into retreat just as the Ming Chinese were overthrowing Kublai's successors.[16] Timur vanquished Herat and built his first "minaret" from the heads of its defenders and encased 2,000 individuals in wet cement to create a living tower in Sabzawar. In 1395 he turned back from an attack on Moscow when he saw that the Russian principalities were too poor to warrant occupation. Instead, he cut the northern trade route and forced all trade between China and Europe to pass through his lands, collecting enormous tolls and taxes. The carnage continued as Timur suppressed one rebellion after another until he controlled everything from Central Asia to the Black Sea. He returned to Samarkand in 1396 with the plundered wealth of western Asia and most of its skilled artists and scholars, who built the monuments that still adorn his favorite city.

In 1398 Timur began his assault on the rich Delhi sultanate of northern India, angered by the ruling Muslims' excessive toleration of Hindus. He first massacred the *Siyal-push*, Afghanistan's "black-robed pagans," succeeding where Alexander the Great, Muslim invaders, and even the modern Soviet army failed. On a ridge five miles north of Delhi, he slaughtered 100,000 prisoners taken en route, slitting Muslims throats and flaying Hindus alive. After Delhi fell and the usual towers of severed heads had been created, Timur headed home with the booty of his conquest, leaving Delhi destroyed and rent by civil war between his administrator and the old Sultan. In the winter of 1399–1400 he laid waste to Christian Georgia in a march on the Ottoman empire in Anatolia, fought his way to the Aegean, and ravaged Georgia again on his way home in 1404. Insulted by an embassy from Ming China whose emperor called him a vassal, Timur set off in December 1404 at the head of an army of Mongols, Turks, Iranians, and Afghans to bring the banner of Islam to the continent's most populous country. His army was soon mired in unusually bad snows, and the sixty-six-year-old emperor caught a cold and died. The invasion of China was called off, and he was buried in Samarkand's Gur-Emir Mausoleum.

———◆———

With Timur's death, the balance of power shifted for the last time away from nomads to the settled, urbanized agricultural states that bordered the steppes. The great nomadic empires were the last, long gasp of a disappearing way of life that had emerged when humans first domesticated animals in 12,000 B.C. It was the life-way of "a cavalry force of nomadic tribesmen who were still a law unto themselves and moved with their herds wherever they wished," says Karen Armstrong, a life-way followed to this day by small groups of nomads in

Mongolia and Central Asia. Armstrong suggests that the Mongols' ferocity "expressed the nomad's pent-up resentment against urban culture." Nomads had been enslaved to build the extravagant cultures they attacked, and they had watched the lavish wealth of neighbors grow while the suffering of the peasants increased.

Inherently more egalitarian than their complex neighbors, their simpler societies even allowed for the full participation of females. Nomads have a harsh life, living simply and close to the bone. "They do not use table cloths or napkins," Carpini reported, never cleaned their cooking utensils or pots, and would happily eat dogs, wolves, foxes, and even body lice—but rarely vegetables. "I have even seen them eat mice. They consider it a great sin if any food or drink is allowed to be wasted in any way," Carpini wrote. Mongolia, the papal emissary told his audience when he returned to Europe, "is large but otherwise—as we saw it with our own eyes during the five and a half months we traveled about it—it is more wretched than I can possibly say." Social organization in egalitarian tribal societies remained simple because the people were busy scratching out a living from the marginal steppes and deserts in which they lived. Yet eventually, once they conquered and became settled themselves, they grew accustomed to the life of the elite emperors they had once scorned. Genghis Khan had predicted that "after us the people of our race will wear garments of gold, eat sweet greasy food, ride decorated horses, hold the loveliest of women and forget the things they owe to us." He remained on the steppe, telling a visiting Chinese sage that "Heaven is weary of the luxury of China. I shall remain in the wilderness of the north. I shall return to simplicity and moderation once again. I shall have the same clothes and food as the cowherds and grooms, and I shall treat my soldiers as brothers."

The great khan's vision eventually came true as the nomadic empires gave way to settled civilizations with more hierarchical forms of social organization. But each left an indelible mark on Asia and the world. Timur's empire, fragile even during his lifetime, fell apart soon after he died, but by moving the chess pieces of central and western Asia around, he changed the course of Asian history like Genghis Khan and the Muslims before him. He saved Europe, vulnerable and distracted by the Hundred Years' War, from Turkish conquest and crushed the northern khanates, freeing Russia. Timur's accomplishments were dwarfed by those of Dar al-Islam and the Mongol khans.

The Mongols and Muslims, like the Huns before them, had kept Europe in the primitive distance of the Dark Ages from which Marco Polo admired China and the other Asian kingdoms that shine with exceptional brilliance from the pages of his memoirs. In the fifth century, the Huns had severed Europe from its Greek and Roman heritage and Europe was kept in a perpetual backwater by later waves nomads and the plagues they brought. Crusades against the Muslims continued to drain energy and money from the West thereafter, so when Europeans finally came to the east in the 1500s in larger numbers, what they saw dazzled their imaginations and excited their greed. But hostile Islam's presence in the Middle East forced the Europeans to find sea routes around Africa, delaying European colonization of Asia for another hundred years while they developed their maritime skills.

The Islamic empire had lasted for 500 years and the Mongol Empire for 300 years in some parts of Asia, longer than the empires built by Alexander the Great or Charlemagne. Mason says that "the Mongol subjugation of China, then ruled by the cultured, refined and broad-minded Sung emperors, must be recognized as one of the major events of history," and profoundly affected China's future development. China diverged from Sung ideals of refinement under its Mongol overlords, and the last native dynasty, the Ming, was powerful but "bigoted, inward-looking and conservative. In the Mongol conquest, then, was the seed of the great Chinese disasters of the nineteenth and twentieth centuries."

The Mongol and Muslim conquests had far-reaching consequences beyond the political. They fought hard for control over the Silk Road but kept it open, spreading new developments from Cordoba to Beijing, spurring the development of technology, and bringing countries and cultures into contact. Silk is but one example of how technologies spread. For 2,000 years, the Chinese jealously guarded the secret weaving of silk, discovered by an Empress in 2640 B.C. They summarily executed anyone who tried to export mulberry tree seeds or silk worms, eggs, and cocoons. Travelers were searched at border crossings, but immigrants from China established Korea's silk industry in 200 B.C. and Japan and India began production 100 years later. The ancient Persians unraveled Chinese silks to reweave them into their own designs, and when Darius III surrendered to Alexander the Great, he was wearing splendid robes of silk. Alexander was so jealous that he demanded the equivalent of $20 million in silk included in the spoils of war. Gauis Julius Caesar restricted silk to his exclusive use and for the purple stripes on favorites' togas, but silk became so popular in Rome Tiberius had to ban its import. Finally, Emperor Justinian sent two Nestorian monks to China in 550 who returned to Byzantium with silk worm eggs and mulberry seeds hidden it their walking sticks. This ended the Chinese monopoly. Muslims carried silk culture to Central Asia, North Africa, Spain, and Sicily in the eighth century. By the thirteenth century looms were established in Lucca, Florence, Venice, and Genoa, whose velvet silk was the envy of the Renaissance.

However, "the most significant commodity carried along this route" says historian Oliver Wild, "was not silk, but religion."[17] The Mongols promoted religious tolerance so Islam, Buddhism, and Christianity easily spread throughout their empire. Although they disappeared to Asia's high steppes, Islam survived and was diffused by merchants and missionaries to China, India, and the islands of Southeast Asia. In many cases, its adherents were at the core of powerful resistance movements against European colonial incursions in Asia.

Muslim and Mongol conquests also had far-reaching ecological consequences. In Turpan, China, the first oasis town on the northern Silk Road, 400 subterranean irrigation channels up to ten miles in length still bring water from the nearby Flame Mountains, feeding a sudden burst of sown land in a desert so hot an egg can be cooked by burying it. This ancient irrigation system and the fields of grain and orchards it nourishes are reminders of the bounty of Central Asia's Samarkand region before Genghis Khan's conquest. Developed in ancient Persia, the irrigation technology spread through Dar al-Islam and was brought to China's oases in the twelfth century by Uighurs, Turkic Muslims from Central Asia. Genghis Khan deliberately destroyed these life-giving irrigation systems along his southwestern border, creating "dead lands" to act as a buffer zone where only rudimentary nomadic populations could survive. Once the cities were reduced to rubble and their inhabitants murdered or scattered, the ancient underground irrigation canals crumbled. Settled agriculture permanently declined, the land returned to desert or steppe, and remaining populations moved away. The flourishing farmlands of Central Asia, which once supported fabulously wealthy cities like Bukhara and Samarkhand, never recovered. Central Asia's desolation was perpetuated by the Soviet occupation and agricultural policies, and western attacks on Afghanistan and Pakistan have prohibited ecological recovery there. In historic times, Timur devastated the Sistan region, transforming its irrigated farmland into the desert it is today, and Kublai devastated northeastern China.

Perhaps most important, the nomads blended peoples. Dar al-Islam's slaves were its backbone. Early in its conquests, slaves were captured wholesale—100,000 netted in a single eighth-century North African campaign, for example—and later the supply was sustained by trade. Freemen in countries bordering the Muslim empire, including in Western European and Byzantine Christians, European Jews, Vikings, and the frontier tribes of Eastern Europe, Central Asia, and Africa, supplied the Arabs with slave labor. There were three main categories of slaves—eastern European Slavs, Central Asian Turks, and blacks from Sub-Saharan Africa—with lesser streams of Indians and Anglo-Saxons. Slavs captured by European Christians were shipped through France via Verdun and Lyons to Cordoba and Cairo, or to the castration center at Prague and then to Venice, the Mediterranean hub of the trade. From Kiev, the Rus shipped captives to Constantinople. Slavs shipped through Khazar lands were castrated in an Armenian center and sent to Baghdad. Central Asian Turks came through the cities of Bukhara, Samarkand, and Urgench, all castration centers for domestic slaves, but since they were favored as soldiers they were spared the treatment. Slaves from West Africa were sent north to Morocco and Spain, and Nubians from the Upper Nile were castrated at Aswan before being sent north and east. Ethiopians and east African slaves came through Aden for onward shipping to Egypt or Persia. In India many Ethiopian slaves rose to positions of power and influence in armies and governments.

Medieval Islam believed slavery was ethical, as long as the slaves were not Muslim. Freeing a slave was a "good work" for Muslims, who believed it would be rewarded in the next life, and slaves could convert. Slavery was a way up the social ladder for domestic slaves and concubines who became wives, scholars, bureaucrats, and ministers. The soldier slave could rise to become an officer, general, commander, or even a sultan. A concubine who had a child could not be sold and was freed when her master died. Many of the Abassid caliphs were sons of slave women, and the Mamluk slave army was key in Egyptian history. Turks eventually took charge of much of the Persian and Mongol empires. "For centuries," John Man says, "slavery was a door through which uncounted hundreds of thousands entered the Islamic world, and influenced it profoundly." Dar as Islam was undermined when the trade began drying up and "old trade routes . . . became warpaths" for Turks, Crusaders, and Mongols.

Genghis Khan's strategy of conquest altered ethnic boundaries, erased ethnic allegiances, and shifted entire populations. He moved whole populations; for example, the Iranian and Christian Alans of the northern Caucasus were herded to the eastern steppes. The Mongol army had been drawn from a confederation of Turco-Mongol (Ural-Altaic) tribes to which Uighurs, Krighiz and others were gradually added. Soldiers were conscripted from subjugated states and intermarried and moved to new areas of the empire. By the time Genghis Khan died in 1227, Turkish warriors outnumbered their Mongol officers, and the Mongol elite who remained abroad to administer the empire had been absorbed through intermarriage with their numerically greater subjects.

Genghis Khan also managed, according to a recent genetic study, to leave another lasting mark on the world. Eight percent of men living in the former

Mongol empire carry his y chromosomes, meaning that 0.5 percent of the world's male population, or 16 million men, are his confirmed descendants. According to geneticist Spencer Wells, "It's the first documented case when human culture has caused a single genetic lineage to increase to such an enormous extent in just a few hundred years."[18] The Khan, his sons, and other male relatives got the first pick of captured women and maintained enormous harems. His eldest son, Tushi, had forty legitimate sons. Kublai had twenty-two, plus countless sons and daughters from the concubines he kept. The oral tradition of at least one group, the Hazaras of Pakistan, maintains that they are the khan's direct descendants. A khan in the Crimea who claimed descent from Genghis was deposed by the Russians in 1783; the khan of Khiva in Central Asia boasted the same blood line until 1920, when the Russians forced him to abdicate.

The north route of the Silk Road passed just south of the Gobi desert and Mongolia through the great Ming fort at Jiayuguan, skirting the end of Great Wall in a nearby gray-blue precipice. The land is studded with the remains of battlements, palaces, and pagodas built and abandoned as Chinese power waxed and waned. The northern route passed west of Marco Polo's Sand City, modern-day Dunhuang, where the desert deepens to swallow settlements and caravans. "On many days," says travel writer Colin Thubron, "extended mirages hover all along the horizon."[19] Dunhuang's caves are frescoed with centuries-old Buddhist and Hindu paintings, "but the monks who once thronged the site have all gone, and so has their quietude." It was here, Thubron says, that "traditional China petered out. Han Chinese, who grew up along the great eastern rivers, feared the wilderness and despised nomadism. . . . Beyond [the Great Wall] was only a barbarian dark, haunted by robbers and drifting herdsmen of inexplicable habits." Hans who died in the vast wastelands of the West "would be torn from their desert graves by demons, and Buddhists condemned forever into lowly reincarnations." Even today Chinese who pass west through the Great Wall's final portal say they are going "outside the mouth."

The Mongols were but one of many nomadic warlike tribes that roamed China's borders and threatened the tranquility of the serene empire as early as 400 B.C. The Chinese hated and mistrusted them, claiming that they raided frontier villages and carried young Chinese women off for breeding purposes. Although they were reviled, the conquering nomads founded two of China's major dynasties: the Mongols, whose Yuan dynasty lasted 90 years and succeeded in unifying all of China and extending its influence and reputation over much of the globe; and the Manchus, whose Qing dynasty lasted 270 years until 1911 and carried China through its colonial period and into the modern world.

While the Mongol and Manchus adopted strict separatism, looking down on their subjects as much as the Han looked down on them, in China as in other Asian states, the dominant "pure," or majority populations have inter-married with the outsiders despite rules against mixing. Battles and migrations brought about large-scale merging of ethnic groups, and marginal peoples in one setting became dominant in another. In the mid-seventh century A.D., the T'ang dynasty encouraged the growth of the ancient Nanchao state in what is now China's southern Yunnan Province. They called the Thai inhabitants of Nanchao *man*, or southern barbarians, but found them useful in fending off powerful western neighbors like Tibet. Nanchao blocked Chinese influence on Southeast Asia's civilizations while gradually extending its own rule into Burma and northern Vietnam. In 751, two months before the Central Asian battle of Talas against the Muslims, Nanchao won its independence from the T'ang. It remained independent until 1253, when Kublai Khan's forces drove the Thais from Yunnan into the valleys of modern-day Thailand, Laos, and Burma, where they started Southeast Asia's most brilliant kingdoms. Rem-nants of nomadic and forest-dwelling groups who were not as successful as the Thais were forced into Asia's arid, mountainous, and highland regions. A thir-teenth-century Chinese ambassador to Cambodia described how tribesmen from the neighboring hills were caught and sold en masse to ruling families who owned more than a hundred apiece and treated them as animals. "They bow the head and dare not make the least movement," he said, because they were beaten for the smallest fault."

Reflecting the historical threat they have constituted, "tribal peoples" are still viewed as slightly uncivilized, potential threats to settled groups, and are persecuted even today in China, India, and other Asian states, often because they occupy strategic and valuable land. Living in remote locations where pro-vision of basic services like health and education is difficult and costly, their development often lags that of majority populations.

The Yunnan Institute of the Minorities in Kunming and the Thai Hill Tribes Research Center in Chiang Mai identify forty or more ethnic minority peoples in the states of Southeast Asia and southern China. Most belong to the Tibeto-Burman linguistic group with much smaller numbers of Tai, Miao-Yao, Karenic, and Mon-Khmer speakers, and also have different cultures and reli-gions than the majority populations. Their numbers are substantial: ethnic mi-norities constitute one-third of Myanmar's, one-quarter of Thailand's, one-third of Laos', and one-tenth of Cambodia's and Vietnam's populations. The official policy of Southeast Asian governments is to integrate "Hill Tribes" into modern life through cultural assimilation. But they are denigrated and stigmatized, in part because marginalization leaves them poor and unable to integrate into mainstream cultural life. In China, Thailand, Laos, Myanmar, and Vietnam, the hill tribes—marginalized by their locations and by education and environmental policies that limit traditional forms of food production and access to modern forms of employment—play an important role in illegal drug production. Less peaceful minorities in Myanmar have rebelled against the central government, which suppresses them with strong-arm tactics in the same way most forms of dissent and difference are dealt with by the military regime.

China recognizes fifty-five ethnic minorities and officially encourages them to maintain their cultures, but some of these groups suffer systematic discrimination. Although together they make up only 8 percent of China's 1.3 billion people, they occupy over 60 percent of the land, much of it strategically important or rich in natural resources. One of their poorest provinces, Yunnan, where a third of the people are minorities, borders Southeast Asia and has some of China's largest timber reserves. Most of their minorities live in China's five autonomous regions (Guangxi, Xinjiang, Tibet, Inner Mongolia, and Ningxia), which ring the country's borders on the north, west, and south. Predominantly Muslim Xinjiang, for example, bordering Russia, Mongolia, Afghanistan, Pakistan, and India, is rich in oil and minerals. As border provinces, they host relatively large numbers of Chinese troops.

It is in China's minority provinces that the HIV/AIDS epidemic gained its initial foothold. AIDS first hit in Yunnan and Sichuan, bordering Yunnan on the north, and in the Guangxi and Xinjiang Autonomous Regions. The prefectures of Tibet bordering Yunnan are also thought to have high HIV rates, but Tibet has so few testing sites it is difficult to confirm. Because China has spent only $2.75 million on AIDS prevention annually until recently—compared to $4.5 million in Vietnam and $74 million in Thailand—few services exist in these poorer and more remote areas. Minorities argue that the government's apathy about HIV surveillance and failure to provide services are part of a deliberate policy of genocide.

Muslims make up one of China's largest minority groups. The Prophet told believers to "seek knowledge even unto China" and eighteen years after Muhammad's death, the third caliph sent a deputation under the Prophet's maternal uncle to invite the Chinese emperor to embrace Islam. Arab and Persian traders established a permanent outpost in Canton, and Muslims virtually dominated China's export/import business under the Sung dynasty (960–1279).

Under the Ming dynasty (1368 to 1644), Muslims were forbidden to speak Arabic or wear Islamic dress and were forced to marry non-Muslims. The Manchus (1644 to 1911) incited anti-Muslim sentiment throughout China. The armed conflict developed into rebellion against the Manchus in Lauchou, northwest China's Islamic center, from 1862 to 1877. A second rebellion racked Yunnan under Tu Wenshui, who established a separate Muslim state for sixteen years (1856 to 1873). Manchu reprisals took the lives of more than four million Muslim rebels in these regions. When the rebellions were suppressed and Yunnan had been recaptured, the Muslim Hui escaped across the border to Kazakhstan and Kyrgyzstan, but slowly returned and are now China's largest group of Muslims at 8.6 million-strong.

The fortunes of Islam rose under Sun Yat Sen but fell again under the communists, who discouraged the formation of an independent Islamic republic and systematically repressed Muslims. During the 1970s Cultural Revolution, thousands of mosques were destroyed and millions of Islamic holy books were burned. When China declared religious freedom in 1978, an Islamic revival began. Today, there are at least 20 million Muslims living in China, concentrated in Xinjiang. Of the roughly 33,000 mosques, 23,000 are in Xinjiang. Sixty percent Muslim and Turkic, Xinjiang has the strongest economy of any province outside of China's southeast coast because it has the country's largest oil, gas, and mineral deposits. The threat of rebellion in Xinjiang haunts Chinese authorities. In 2001 Xinjiang's top university was forced to stop teaching courses in the local language, Uighur, and begin teaching exclusively in Mandarin, ending fifty years of bilingual education. Xinjiang's Muslims accused the government of using the terrorist attacks of September 11, 2001, as an excuse to suppress dissent.

In China, India, and other Asian countries, policymakers are scrambling to address the issues of poverty and underdevelopment in their ethnic minority areas. In 1999 the Chinese government issued a white paper on its national minorities policy stating that it "is well aware of the fact that, due to the restrictions and influence of historical, physical geographical and other factors, central and western China where most minority people live lags far behind the eastern coastal areas in development."[20] The paper acknowledged that the majority Han population, who comprise 92 percent of the population, "treat non-Han-Chinese as outsiders, although the complexity of multiethnic relations is in constant flux."[21] The government has adopted measures to promote economic development among minorities to enable them to "catch up with the Han," including the Great West Development Campaign. This 2001 economic tourist development program aims to attract Han migrants to

Xingjiang to "realize social stability and the great national solidarity of our country [impossible] without overall revitalization of the Western region." Chinese first settled there during the Han dynasty and have been resettled in this region ever since, "creating ugly, periodic riots. For the two people are deeply unalike. The Chinese are conventional, bureaucratic and collective, the Uighur are relaxed, sensuous and individualistic," says Thubron.

"The whole world is mine," gloated the first Han emperor, Lui Bang, as he claimed the Chinese throne in 202 B.C. at the head of a peasant army after a brutal six-year civil war. Known for his ruthlessness, when a rival threatened to boil his father alive if he did not surrender he replied, "Send me a cup of the soup!"[22] He showed little of the promise of what was to come, because as it grew, the Han empire he founded exceeded its contemporary, Rome, in territory, people, and wealth. Just as the West inherited Roman and Greek traditions, contemporary Hans—Chinese—identify with this dynasty as the source of Chinese culture. The Han period—206 B.C. to A.D.220—was a Golden Age when porcelain and paper were invented, Chang Hen calculated the value of pi and invented the world's first seismograph, and the wheelbarrow was first used to speed up public works, deliver military supplies, and carry injured soldiers off the field—a modest but valuable tool that made its first European appearance 1,000 years later, when it revolutionized medieval cathedral building. But most important, Han emperors reconstructed the five Confucian classics in order to systematize the mandarin's education.

The mandarinate was the balance on the flywheel of Chinese power that reduced the emperors' vulnerability to their own excesses and to the ravages of nomadic invasion and peasant rebellion. Developed by philosophers of government well before the Han realized the ideal in their rule, the idea that Chinese emperors were "sons of heaven" who had the "mandate of heaven" or divine right to rule if they ruled reasonably and well was articulated during one of China's earliest dynasties, the Shang (1700–1027 B.C.) by a court advisor named Yi Yin. Instructing the youthful second king, Tai Jia, on the duties of kingship, Yi Yin said that there had been no "calamities from heaven" during his father's reign because "he displayed his sagely prowess; for oppression he substituted his gentleness, and the millions of people gave him their hearts." Emperors could be dethroned, he told Tai Jia, if they were cruel, unjust, or proved otherwise unable to intercede with the forces of heaven to produce prosperity. Emperors must seek out wise men and avoid "constant dancing in your palaces, and drunken singing in your chambers." Ruination will come to emperors who "dare to set their hearts on wealth and women, and abandon themselves to wandering about or to the chase;" or who "dare to despise sage words, to resist the loyal and upright, and put far from you the aged and virtuous, and to seek the company of . . . youths." A state run by a prince addicted to such fashions "will surely come to ruin," Yi Yin told the young man.[23]

The five Confucian *Classics of History* including the emperor's instructions were ancient by the time Confucius taught from them during the Zhou dynasty (1027–221 B.C.). By then, China's kings had evolved from being heads of ancestor- and spirit-worshipping cults to lords of amalgamated city-states under centralized, impersonal rule supported by routinized agricultural taxation. The mandarinate, or civil service, had grown, education had spread, and a merchant class had emerged. Several Zhou cities had more than a quarter of a million people and the emperors controlled huge public irrigation projects. Confucius preached the limits of self-interest, and his ethics were clear and uncompromising: love others and treat them like you would be treated, honor your parents, and do what is right, not what is advantageous. The best rule is by moral example, not force, he said; "A ruler who resorts to force has already failed." According to Mason, "If the scholar-teacher lived today, he could probably [be] considered a dangerous radical" who believed that the welfare of ordinary people was more important than ruling class privilege. Confucius was tolerated, but it is telling that he led an itinerant life, moving frequently to new places with his teachings.

Confucian ideals had been out of favor in the preceding dynasty, the Qin (Ch'in is the anglicized version from which modern China gets its name), who had taken control from the Zhou in 221 B.C. Shi Huang Ti, who called himself First Emperor, a title that had been reserved for deities and mythological ages, was also Qin's last emperor because he failed to behave like one. To reduce the potential for rebellion and minimize Confucian dissent, he ordered that all books be destroyed and that 460 scholars be buried alive. An army of 8,000 terra-cotta archers, infantry, and cavalry was built to protect him after death. Although he called in all weapons and melted them down for statuary, he so feared assassination that he slept in a different place every night. When he died while touring his empire, his courtiers hid his body under a load of rotten fish until they could get it back to the capital, but rebellion broke out immediately and all seven of his children were murdered. He had abused his mandate roundly by demanding enormous levies of labor and taxes for public works, including an early version of the Great Wall, and by imposing rigid laws and horrifying punishments. Construction of his summer palace alone required a labor force of three-quarters of a million men. Technological development had been ongoing; blast furnaces discovered near his cache of ceramic soldiers produced steel that would not be matched in Europe for another century.

To forestall rebellion, the Han emperor Wen reinstated Confucian social ideals, especially filial piety. Respect for the elderly was sternly enforced—even slander of old people was a capital offense—although wife beating was allowed. Excessive monopolies, food speculation, and private coinage were curbed, and the iron and salt industries were nationalized. Armies were sent in every direction, conquering most of present-day China, Vietnam, Korea, and western Central Asia beyond Samarkand and Bukhara. Like their Roman contemporaries, the Han's powerful armies kept the "barbarians" on their flanks subdued. Ironically, the Han drove the nomadic Hsiung-nu (the Huns) west and south in the first century B.C., laying the seeds of Rome's destruction by later Hun invasions. Trade flourished after the Han emperors subdued Tibetan and nomadic bandits and established settlements of soldiers and peasants along the Silk Road, gradually taking control of the west's far flung oases from their primarily Caucasian settlers.

Like the Roman empire, the Han dynasty lasted for nearly five centuries before it collapsed under the weight of its own corruption, degeneracy, and weak leadership. The Han's granaries and treasury overflowed, but wealth was siphoned into official pockets and Confucian ideals were forgotten. Peasants were impoverished, interest rates soared, and many freemen sold their children into slavery to survive. While profiteers enslaved the peasantry, the nobility were "extravagant in clothing, excessive in food and drink," wrote a first-century historian. Even slaves, servants, and concubines wore the finest brocades, gems, and silks. Peace had brought a burgeoning population, but the government was unable to curb corruption and "the widening gap between rich and poor became the dynasty's most explosive problem," says historian Mike Edwards. Although students from the capital's Confucian academy protested corruption, disgust with the excesses and deprivation created a "mass revulsion from Confucianism," says Mason.

Many turned to the newly arrived faith of Mahayana Buddhism, brought to the capital in A.D. 67 by two monks leading a white horse loaded with scriptures and statues who had entered China via the Silk Road. Taoism inspired the second-century Revolt of the Yellow Turbans, when millions of peasants were killed. Peasant uprisings, said a contemporary historian, rolled through the provinces "like a billowing sea." When the Yellow River flooded thousands of villages, mobs of fleeing peasants and hungry looters called the Red Eyebrows, for their painted foreheads, sacked the capital and separated the son of heaven's head from his shoulders. Hsiung Nu tribesmen invaded from the north, and for the next sixty years, during the Three Kingdoms period, the Wei, Shu, and Wu dynasties overlapped and fought with one another while fending off barbarians and exploiting peasants. Gunpowder was invented during this period and found its way to Europe, and where it was first applied to weaponry. China's power pendulum swung back toward unity in 581, but the cruel and short-lived Sui dynasty fell in 617 after popular revolts against its crushing taxation and forced labor and a very ill-advised incursion into Korean territory. The Tang dynasty (618–907) reinstated order and Confucian ideals and perfected the mandarinate. Military defeat by the Muslims at Talas in 751 was followed by thrashings from the Tibetans, the Uighur Turks in Mongolia, and the Khitan in Manchuria, setting off peasant rebellions that lasted until the T'ang fragmented into five northern dynasties and ten southern kingdoms. The Song dynasty provided a brief period of unity (960–1279) until Kublai Kahn and the Mongols arrived to establish the Yuan Dynasty.

The Mongol dynasty lasted seventy years until the Mongols fled before the orphaned, illiterate peasant Chu Yuan-chang and his White Lotus rebels, who founded the Ming dynasty (1368–1644). Ming China was larger and more populous than the whole of Europe with far greater wealth and resources, and Chu succeeded in balancing the military against the mandarinate so neither would dominate the government. But the balancing act lasted only until the second Ming emperor, Yung Lo, was crowned. He sent Chinese ships throughout Asia and by 1425 claimed tribute and token fealty from scores of Asian principalities. Expeditions under Admiral Zheng He, China's Christopher Columbus—the brilliant and tenacious son of Muslim rebels who survived radical castration to build a fleet that would not be rivaled in size until World War I—visited Indonesia, India, the Persian Gulf, and the Red Sea, skirted the east coast of Africa, and reached North America.[24] After excesses that would have made the Mongols squirm with envy, Yung's newly built Imperial City in Beijing was struck by balls of lightning in a spectacular loss of mandate that reduced his throne to cinders and killed his favorite concubine. The treasury had been drained, imperial taxation reduced the peasants to eating grass, and plague took 174,000 lives in one district alone. The bodies lay rotting in the fields, and twenty-six mandarins rode out to "calm and soothe" the outraged people. Yung Lo came around to the way of moderation, but it was too late. Although his fat, studious, and religious son proclaimed that "relieving people's poverty ought to be handled as though one were rescuing them from a fire or saving them from drowning," China's mandarinate had been co-opted by the palace's 70,000-strong band of eunuchs, who were very far from the Confucian ideal.

The Manchus took advantage of the chaos to invade the capital unopposed. Trained by the Ming to farm and build forts, they had traversed hundreds of years of development in a single century. After deposing a young Ming prince and exiling him to Burma, where he was strangled with the string of a Manchu crossbow, they proclaimed their own child emperor as they first of a dynasty named Qing, or "Pure." Although they prohibited intermarriage and enforced strict separation from the Chinese, whose men were forced to shave the front of their heads and wear their hair in a queue, by the nineteenth century the Manchu language survived only in the court because the invaders had been thoroughly sinified. Despite that, they were always viewed as a foreign dynasty by the Han Chinese. One of Sun Yat-sen's first acts after founding the Chinese republic in 1911 and ending Manchu rule was to pray at the Ming imperial tombs.

The Manchus conquered Outer Mongolia, defeated the Uighurs and annexed Xinjiang, gained control of central Asia to the Pamirs, and renewed suzerainty over Korea, Burma, Nepal, and much of Vietnam. When the Tibetans protested the installation of a Chinese nominee as the Dalai Lama in 1720, the Manchus invaded and established garrisons, maintaining nominal control until 1911. During the reign of the second Manchu emperor, Kang Hsi (1622–1723), the last outpost of Manchu resistance, Taiwan, was annexed. China's population grew to 300 million by 1790. Cultivation intensified but in the absence of agricultural innovations the land was exhausted and destroyed by erosion. "Rural poverty gradually developed to its full horrors," Mason says, including "the exposure of newborn girl babies in the fields at night to die, the selling of children into slavery, the growing rapacity of officials and landlords, themselves struggling on the edge of the abyss." The mandarinate devolved into a cruel aristocracy that expected groveling obedience and for whom "death was not enough," Mason says. "Men were whipped on the soles of their feet until gangrene set in, or their heads confined in the cangue, a heavy wooden square which made it impossible for them to feed or care for themselves, then left to die slowly and painfully."

For the last 120 years of Manchu reign, the country was in chaos. In 1795 the White Lotus rebellion began as a tax protest in Shensi, Hupei, and Szechuan provinces, led by a secret religious society that forecast the Buddha's advent and restoration of the Ming. The Manchus resettled rebellious populations in stockaded villages and after nine years crushed the guerrillas, but rebellions broke out in other parts of the country. An assassination attempt on the emperor in 1812 led to harsh reprisals, but bandits and warlords "marched through the unhappy countryside, raiding and destroying crops, burning villages, and pressing conscripts into their service," Mason says. Twenty to thirty million were killed during the Taiping Rebellion (1851–1864), a messianic Christian movement to establish the Kingdom of Heavenly Peace. Four million Muslims lost their lives in the Xinjiang and Yunnan rebellions and more than 40 million others died between 1840 to 1873 from famine and plague.

The collapse of economic and social order had other terrible consequences beside the deaths of 60 or more million peasants. New barbarians—Europeans—were poised at the gates. Although the Manchus believed they had secured China's borders, "the chief threat to China's integrity did not come overland, as it had so often in the past, but by sea, reaching the southern coastal area first," says University of Maryland Asia expert Leon Poon. The trickle of Western traders, missionaries, and soldiers of fortune that began arriving in the sixteenth century turned into a flood. In response, the Manchus banned all foreign trade except from Canton and did little to control the pirates terrorizing their coasts. An epidemic of opium addiction was draining China's silver reserves and enervating its people.

After several wars with the British, opium imports were legalized in 1856 and foreigners, including Christian missionaries, were allowed to travel freely in China. France took control of the Chinese tribute states of Cambodia, Cochin China (southern Vietnam), and Annam (northern Vietnam); Japan took Korea and Taiwan; and Russia took Xinjiang. "Only jealousy between the powers, carefully cultivated by the Chinese, prevented complete partition of the country," Mason says. General "Fighting Charles" Gordon, who later died in the Sudan, is often credited with saving the Manchus from the Taiping Rebellion. The British also helped the Manchus as they hurriedly tried to adopt western political and social institutions, but change was not quick enough. Unrest continued as more Chinese joined the nationalist movement and by 1900 thousands of "Boxers"—rebels who practiced the martial arts—were slaughtering foreign missionaries in the countryside. When they advanced on the capital to lay siege to the foreign missions, they were repelled by an international force but mass violence continued until the Manchus allowed a parliamentary election in 1913. After Manchu assassins killed enough democratic leaders to ensure that a Manchu sympathizer was elected president, he suspended parliament and re-established the monarchy in 1915.

Peasant rebellions roiled the countryside. Warlords took control of independent provinces, opening the way for the Japanese invasion of Manchuria. Sun Yat Sen became president of the nationalist southern government. When the West ignored his request for help, he signed a deal with the Soviet Union, which also allied itself with the new Chinese Communist Party (CCP) at the same time. Sun's general, Chiang Kai-shek, regained nominal control of most of China by 1928 after quieting an insurrection in Hunan Province led by Mao Zedong. In 1935 and 1936 the 100,000-man Red Army made its heroic "Long March" of escape under Mao, tramping 6,000 miles through eleven provinces in western China, over eighteen mountain ranges and twenty-four rivers, to land in Shaanxi Province. In the meantime, the nationalist government modernized the legal and penal system, built railroads and highways, stabilized prices, reformed banking and currency, augmented agricultural and industrial production, and expanded education. But war with Japan undermined nationalist control, and most of the nationalist army surrendered, deserted, or were killed. After the end of World War II, the Red Army defeated the Nationalists in 1949, but the prize it won, China, was at its lowest point in history.

In their battle with chaos, illiteracy, and famine, the communists were ruthless. By 1954, they had purged 830,000 "enemies of the people" and redistributed their land to the peasants, who were then collectivized when private ownership of land and real property was abolished. The Yellow River was dammed and electrified, ancient forests in the Northwest were re-created by planting tens of millions of trees, and millions of children were immunized by "barefoot doctors." China helped North Korea turn back a UN force and annexed Tibet. In 1957, 300,000 intellectuals were sent to labor camps; in 1958, Chinese society was organized into communes to further counter private property and family loyalties. Droughts and resistance brought severe food shortages, aggravated by diversion of labor to infrastructural development in the "Great Leap Forward." Deaths from malnutrition probably ran into the tens of millions and China's population had declined by 1960. By 1963, riots forced a complete retreat from communes and the "Great Leap Forward." In 1966, Mao, crippled by Parkinson's disease, encouraged the "Cultural Revolution," a violent campaign by thousands of Red Guards against traditional Chinese culture that annihilated another million or so Chinese. Continued worker and peasant unrest forced the "correction" of these and other of Mao's "leftist errors" after his death in 1976.

At the Eleventh Central Committee meeting of the CCP in 1978, Long March veteran Deng Xiaoping led party members toward "socialist capitalism" and economic liberalization. Private enterprises, collectives (employee-owned businesses), and joint enterprise with foreign investors were legalized. To stem population growth, China's famous "one child" policy was introduced. Farms were returned to family ownership and specialized production was allowed, increasing agricultural productivity. The economic results have been extraordinary. The gross national product has grown 10 percent per year since 1978 and there has been a massive inflow of foreign capital. By 1997 China was one of the world's top exporters, coming from the twenty-ninth position in 1980. Jerry Chen, a Taiwanese businessman in the Chinese special economic zone of Dongguan, inland of Hong Kong, says that the Chinese are now enjoying the last laugh. "A hundred and fifty years ago the Westerners flooded China with opium. Now China is flooding the West with the opium of cheap goods."[25] But the cost has been high. China has a "floating population" of unemployed numbering over 100 million. The disparities between rich and poor have widened, and inflation, financial corruption, and food insecurity are growing. The "social evils"—drug use, commercial sex, and crime—have increased. Peasants are impoverished and while tens of millions have deserted the land for better-paying jobs in the cities, there is a huge labor surplus in agriculture. And despite its liberalization in other areas, the CCP allows no contenders in the political arena.

———◦—

Throughout their history, the settled hierarchical aristocracies of Asia's great empires have been threatened by the massive labor forces that underlaid their wealth. "From early times," Mason says, "the peasant revolt had been China's natural answer to tyrannical or inefficient government and also, grimly enough, to pressures of population." Peasants resented their rulers' extreme exploitation abetted by a corrupt mandarinate and religious authorities who justified the hierarchical regimes and kept slaves themselves. While nominally free, peasants' lives were squeezed by aristocratic taxation and they often became slaves through debt bondage. Peasants were taxed to the verge of starvation, conscripted into armies, and exploited for countless large-scale public works. When their food supply and very lives were threatened by the floods, famines, and pestilence so frequent in Chinese history and the ruling class ignored their plight, peasants turned to insurrection. Emperors and warlords who never learned to take the mandate of heaven seriously took their turn until 1949, when the peasant-won Communist Revolution attempted to redress the balance for good.

There have been two peasant rebellions in China every century since the beginning of this era except in the 1800s, when there were at least seventeen.[26] Rebellion became more frequent because Manchu policy aggravated growing structural problems. The population had more than doubled in the late 1700s and early 1800s while the amount of cultivated land and the food supply diminished. Ruinous taxation forced many small farmers to sell, concentrating land in the hands of the rich. As the tax base shrank, more people lost their land, increasing unemployment and banditry. The government's poor management of a succession of floods and droughts exacerbated the plight of millions of peasants. Official corruption was rife, especially in the coastal areas, where immense profits were to be had by facilitating or participating in the opium trade. Four to ten million Chinese were addicts, including 20 to 30 percent of the government's officials. Throughout the nineteenth century, Manchu rule created a series of mutually reinforcing disasters and foreign invasion was just the last blow.

Millions of dislocated peasants and laborers were on the prowl, looking for work or something to steal. "The militiamen are bandits and the local people are bandits too," remarked a local official in Fukien. "They start as militiamen and end up as bandits." Peasant mutual assistance societies, *yishi*, originated in the eighth century during the Tang dynasty. *Yishi* pooled capital for purchases, weddings, funerals, and childbirth expenses, acted as mutual protection societies during times of internecine violence, and provided a base for cults, rebellion, and criminal gangs. During unsettled times, youths migrated in search of work, banded together for survival and protection, adopting the feudal tradition of blood oaths. Yuan-chung's secret society, the White Lotus, consolidated dissatisfied peasantry into a fighting machine that brought down the Mongol empire in the 1279. "These societies," Mason says, "were so firmly based even the mandarins hesitated to tamper with them." Nevertheless the Qing cracked down in 1646, making membership in a blood oath society punishable with 100 lashes. When this deterrent proved ineffective, they instituted the death penalty. Forced underground, the societies emerged with a vengeance in the nineteenth century.

Outraged peasants, pushed to the brink of extermination by excessive aristocracies, are a force shaping modern China's history even today. In 1998, local officials expropriated relief money sent from Beijing to rebuild ruined rice terraces after a Yangtze River flood and then tried to tax the villagers for the repair work. Villagers from Yuntang in Jiangxi Province refused to pay and rallied to prevent tax collectors and police from entering their village in 1999 and 2000. The revolt spread through the Yangtze River provinces, and in August 2000, 20,000 peasants from five villages clashed with police sent to collect taxes. In April 2001 local authorities declared the villagers "criminal gangs" and sent armed riot police and paramilitary forces, who killed two peasants and wounded twenty in the ensuing conflict. "Farmer heroes" who did not flee were jailed, but when the peasants sued the local government, police barred the peasants' lawyers from the courtroom. One leader told the press, "These officials don't believe in communism, they just want power and money."

Beijing was unsympathetic. Its free-market agenda included central budget cuts, so it had transferred responsibility for health, education, and other services to local governments in 1994. When local leaders raised taxes, the farmers could not pay them. With farm income stagnating, the average farmer made $125 a year. Of that, $81 went to fertilizer, pesticides and seed, netting the farmer $44. In 1996, when farm households were asked to pay $36 in taxes—leaving them $8 to live on for the entire year—the tax revolt began. In March 2001 the Communist Party abolished local levies, charging county governments with collection and redistribution of tax revenues to localities. The central government also allocated $2.5 billion to help villages finance infrastructure, education, and health. "These measures," says reporter John Chan, "only paper over the growing tensions in the countryside. China's townships currently owe $36.5 billion in loans and debts," making it impossible for local governments to meet payrolls, service their outstanding debt, and continue to provide education and health services.[27]

Since the 1978 market liberalization, many of the conditions that created peasant unrest in classical China have reemerged. Poverty is up, employment is down, and the social safety net is fraying, increasing disparities between rich and poor. The central government has failed to address widespread corruption, major drug problems, environmental degradation, and crime. Human rights incidents against dissidents, labor activists, and alleged separatists in Xinjiang and Tibet have increased. Over 100 hundred million young and poorly educated internal labor migrants are moving from the countryside to the city in search of jobs, repeating a pattern often seen in Chinese history. All of these problems create a situation in which China's growing HIV/AIDS epidemics can thrive.

———•◦•———

China now has three AIDS epidemics. The first is circling the western perimeter of the country, moving rapidly through the minority provinces on the backs of drug dealers and truck drivers. The second is moving along the coast, carried by sex workers, drug addicts, and migrant workers. The third originates in China's heartland, among the marginalized peasants of China's interior. UNAIDS says China is facing a "titanic peril' and is "on the verge of a catastrophe that could result in unimaginable human suffering, economic loss and social devastation."[28] A 2003 survey found that 17 percent of China's population had never heard of HIV/AIDS and 77 percent did not know that condom use could prevent transmission. HIV is seen as a "foreign disease" brought to China from the West in the 1980s. Carriers are stigmatized by homophobic, anti-drug user, and xenophobic attitudes. Growth of the epidemic among Yunnan's drug users in the early 1990s coupled with "the growing prevalence of HIV in areas dominated by ethnic minorities only bolstered the impression of many in China that AIDS was a problem for stigmatized tribal peoples, and that it was linked to moral corruption and 'backwardness,'" says Human Rights Watch.[29] After "centuries of imperial relationships" with the autonomous regions' ethnic minorities many Han Chinese think that "ethnic minorities are morally 'loose' and sexually promiscuous." Migrant workers are also viewed askance; after the Guangdong Federation of Trade Unions distributed 1 million condoms to female migrant workers in 2002, they protested the implicit message that they were promiscuous.

The epidemic was first seen in China's Yunnan provinc in 1989, carried there by gem traders and heroin dealers from Myanmar. "From all around Asia," say reporters Tim McGirk and Susan Jakes, "men gravitate to Ruili [in Yunnan] for jade, heroin, and sex. Then they move on. This has turned Ruili into a confluence of HIV, a main artery where various strains flow together and mutate in lethal ways before racing up into China's bloodstream."[30] Yunnan's growing sex tourism industry is crowded with young Burmese prostitutes and enlivened by gambling and "eroticized ethnic song and dance reviews staged in hotels and restaurants," says Human Rights Watch. The virus "hitchhiked" north to Urumqi in Xinjiang along the transportation corridor through Sichuan and Gansu provinces with truckers carrying Burmese heroin in their flatbeds, providing drugs and the disease to farmers along the way. Poor teenagers working as waitresses in roadside truck stops sell sex, often without a condom, and many truckers have gonorrhea, increasing their chances of HIV infection. China's highest HIV rates are in the western drug route provinces (Yunnan, Sichuan, Gansu, Shaanxi, and Xinjiang), where between 60 and 70 percent of the drug users are HIV-positive.

"The disease's traveling companions are a familiar crew," say McGirk and Jakes. "Drug users and traffickers, prostitutes and truckers, itinerant workers and salesmen. And wherever AIDS visits, it finds familiar accomplices to help it jump to the next town: official denial, public ignorance, discrimination, and poverty." In 1996 researchers discovered that HIV in the western corridor is a new mix of HIV's B and C strains, the first from Thailand (originally from the United States and Europe) and the second from Indian sailors along China's seacoast. The B/C strain swept through the Dai minority on the Myanmar border, and struck the tribal Yi in Sichuan, the Muslim Hui in Gansu, and the Uighurs in Xinjiang, where it soon came to account for all new cases. Between 1998 and 2000 when reported cases in Xinjiang doubled, public health officials were initially panicked because they thought B/C was an HIV "superstrain."

Heroin is also trafficked eastward from Ruili into China's crowded coastal provinces and port cities, where sex work and needle sharing by drug users is common. According to UNAIDS, seven provinces have serious epidemics among their drug users, and nine are on the verge. Millions of young Chinese, who migrate to these provinces to work as unskilled labor in the factories visit sex workers and carry the infection back to their villages. Asian correspondent Arthur Kroeber says that "this part of South China has transformed from a subtropical backwater into a hub of global manufacturing."[31] Its population of 40 million, 3 percent of China's total, produces one-third of China's exports, 7 percent of its gross domestic product, and absorbs one-quarter of its foreign direct investment. In this freewheeling business environment, police collude to enforce contracts with strong-arm tactics in the absence of a legal system. Official corruption is rife, and Chinese labor and residency laws are not enforced so cheap labor can easily move through. "As long as the taxes and payoffs keep rolling in, local officials don't care whether plants obey the rules," Kroeber says, so firms typically meet payroll taxes on less than half of their employees and "often, the township party bosses lower those numbers further and pocket some of the tax money."

Kroeber says it is "the world's most extensive and systematic exploitation of transient labor by mobile capital. And the people who oversee this system— and profit handsomely from it—are the officials of the world's largest Communist Party." Taiwanese companies are moving there by the thousands because wages start at 21 cents an hour. With overtime, the average worker makes between $40 and $60 a month and many live right in the factories so they can send most of their earnings home to their families. When China's pioneer personal injury lawyer began winning compensation cases for employees losing arms and fingers to the machinery, he was run out of town. A flourishing sex industry serves Taiwanese businessmen who live with what Kroeber calls "a strange intensity; when they're not compulsively working, it seems, many spend their time drinking and whoring."

A third epidemic is occurring in China's seven central provinces, where, during the 1990s, "local authorities were complicit in the transmission of HIV to hundreds of thousands or even millions of villagers through an unsanitary but highly profitable blood collection industry," says Human Rights Watch.[32]

Infection rates in some villages are as high as 75 percent, and the number of infected in Henan, the only province with an accurate estimate, is 1 million. With official infection rates between 4 and 40 percent in the other provinces, Human Rights Watch estimates that 16 million are now infected. Beijing estimates that 260,000 children will be orphaned by the scandal by 2010, but massive deaths are already starting to occur. The blood drive "was like a poverty-relief program," a Henan peasant said. Through village and school campaigns, the government encouraged farmers and factory workers to sell their plasma for $5 a pint. The provinces affected by the scandal were described in a Chinese application for international AIDS assistance as areas with "increasing unemployment, increases in rural to urban migration, reduced rates of retention in schools, and a dramatic decline in the rural health care system" where poor households affected by HIV are unable to afford care.

To simplify collection and administration, health officials dealt with "blood heads" or "pimps" in charge of donor groups. Pooling unscreened blood from a number of donors, they removed the plasma and returned the cells so people could give several times a day. In some locations, the pimps kept their blood "donors" in locked hotel rooms and gave them traditional medicine to increase blood volume and hide dangerous infections. "Many government officials made a lot of money," says a Henan patient advocate, selling the blood for as much as $40 a pint.[33] In Beijing, blood from paid donors infected the blood supplies in hospitals used by the official elite. Even in official collection centers and hospitals, syringes and lab pipettes are rewashed and reused without being sterilized and low-quality test kits are used.[34]

When HIV-infected farmers in Henan protested, calling for accountability and demanding treatment, their leaders were detained along with a TV crew attempting to cover the scandal. In 2001 the protestors traveled to Beijing but were blocked from attending the first national AIDS conference. By 2003 when protests intensified, the police retaliated with arrests, beatings, and destroyed the homes of local leaders. Local party officials threatened other activists and put their homes under surveillance. Journalists and sympathetic local public health officials were harassed and expelled, or detained and interrogated. Wan Yanhai, a retired Ministry of Health physician turned AIDS advocate, was detained in September 2002 and interrogated for a month, accused of releasing state secrets on the blood-selling scandal in Henan over the Internet. Rather than investigate and punish guilty official officials, Beijing transferred and promoted some of them, continuing "to abet the local cover-up of one of the world's greatest HIV/AIDS scandals," Human Rights Watch says.

Under rising international criticism, the government arrested four officials and charged them with embezzling large sums of public money from the
blood sales. In May 2004 Beijing announced that it would provide treatment
in provinces with high HIV/AIDS rates, but in many rural areas dumped antiretrovirals at health centers with no instructions for their use. The Chinese
manufacture generic versions of the anti-AIDS drugs and were selected by
UNAIDS to participate in an international campaign to increase drug access.
To address the chronic blood shortages that created the lucrative procurement
industry, China is now accepting only voluntary blood donors. A local expert
says that young, educated Chinese may donate, but "older Chinese are likely
to believe that blood is a gift from their ancestors and that losing even a little
bit can be harmful." Work units are encouraged by extravagant paid leaves to
donate and some provinces require donations from their residents.

Chinese law conflicts with international standards by permitting compulsory HIV testing. China's public security officials can consign a suspected drug
user to a detoxification center without trial, where draconian living conditions
and forced labor projects are the primary therapies. Suspects are given compulsory HIV blood tests, but authorities do not have to share the results with
the individual. Hospitals can test without the patient's permission. Quarantine
for testing or treatment is also legal, as are local bans against swimming pool
use and marriage by HIV-positive people. People with HIV/AIDS have no
legal redress against eviction, job loss, discrimination, or slander. Many local
authorities require work units to report suspected HIV carriers for examination, and they are notified if a worker tests HIV-positive. Hospital authorities
have told people with positive tests to "go home and die" and refuse to treat
known carriers. Sex workers and drug users, spurned as spreading "social
evils," are being expelled from their villages and neighborhoods to become
part of the floating population in larger cities. As migrants, they cannot access
state services without residence permits and go underground to avoid forced
detention. A few cities like Suzhou respect human rights and bar discrimination based on HIV status, and authorities in Sichuan Province were consider-
ing regulations that would permit HIV-positive people to marry.

All of China's HIV/AIDS epidemics have been fueled by the government's
failure to set up prevention programs and maintain public health infrastructure.
The cradle-to-grave national health care system created during the first
decades of the Chinese Republic was dismantled after 1978. Healthcare access
is now severely limited, especially for China's rural 70 percent. Out-of-pocket
costs for physicians, hospitals, testing, and drugs are spiraling upward in the
profit-driven system. WHO's Dr. Daniel Chin declared China's public health
program "a shambles" that excludes the poor. Until 2004, HIV/AIDS preven-

tion was grossly underfunded. In 2002, the national government budgeted $12.8 million for HIV/AIDS from a national gross domestic product of $123.2 billion, with provincial governments contributing an additional $60.41 million. In 2003, the western provinces received an additional emergency allocation of $120.9 million to strengthen blood banks and public health infrastructure. The HIV surveillance system is inadequate and Ministry of Health officials deliberately cover up their HIV situation so their cities or regions will not lose external investment. Trained medical personnel are in short supply. In April 2004 China's vice minister said that "in many disease control centers at the county level I have visited about 90 percent of the staff are not professional workers."

Although China began allowing more international NGOs with AIDS and orphan experience to respond to the epidemic in the central provinces, Communist Party members and police "are reluctant to permit the expansion of civil society for fear that it will increase public scrutiny of officials, expose corruption, lead to increase demands on government, and perhaps even lead to civil unrest," says the 2002 Human Rights Watch report. Human Rights Watch notes that "official corruption is a serious hindrance to effective delivery of funds and care to rural persons affected by HIV/AIDS," and peasants in Henan have already protested misuse of AIDS funds. Senior Chinese economists are advocating for public health system reform, arguing that a substandard system impedes economic growth. China has shown that it can respond to a health emergency when it chooses. Faced with a major SARS epidemic, the state-run media was mobilized, social stigma was controlled, and the disease was contained. The central government fired the minister of health, the mayor of Beijing, and more than 100 health officials responsible for covering up the outbreak. International authorities have pressured the government to bring that fervor to AIDS control, fearful that the rapidly spreading epidemic in China will have a serious impact on global public health and world stability. The human rights exposés have sufficiently embarrassed Beijing to respond to the needs of infected peasants and reform its blood supply. But many international experts wonder if the central government has resources to rebuild its public health system quickly enough to contain the epidemic or the strength to deal with the local corruption, denial, and discrimination that continue to fuel it.

China is not alone in its plight. In many countries of Asia, the ancient tensions among ethnic groups and aristocratic disdain for the underclass have increased the disparity between rich and poor and aggravated the HIV/AIDS epidemic, contributing to its spread. But these are not the only problems being faced. In Chapter 4, we will take up the more recent causes of social displacement and epidemic mismanagement, using two South Asian states, India and Bangladesh, and the states of Southeast Asia as examples. In all of Asia, many of the communalities that lead to fast growing epidemics stem from the colonial period and from more recent historical and economic events that stalled Asia's development and heightened the conflict between tradition and modernity.

FOUR

CHAINING THE ELEPHANT

The Impact of Colonialism

RAGEENA TOSSED THE END OF HER LIGHT GREEN SCARF over her left shoulder and shoved her hands defiantly into the back pockets of her jeans. "Shall I tell you my story now?" she asked the group. No one looked as lovely, or as fragile. How utterly and completely brave she is, Molly thought, admiring the girl's strength.

"When you are more mature like we are now," Rageena told the group, "you understand life. You share ideas with your relatives, family, and friends. You idolize the prince that has grown inside you, and you cannot be coaxed into evil deeds by a man who doesn't fit into your ideas." She coughed and cleared her throat. "But it is not the same when you are a little girl and you can become ensnared like a bird in the net of an evil one. My parents were kind and hardworking. I wasn't beaten as long as I did all my chores on time. I resented my little brother going to school, but we were poor and my father said that was our only chance. In Kalena, where I come from, the most often spoken proverb says 'Mutton for the mother of a son, pumpkin for the mother of a daughter.' Our fields were small and never produced enough.

"In Nepal there is so much erosion, and important families have grabbed up all the good land, so we were forced to work very hard, and sometimes we had only the milk of the buffalo to drink. Our king and aristocracy, you must understand, do not have the interests of their poor people at heart. Their greed has sustained us in an underdeveloped state, and this poverty fuels HIV/AIDS. Rural people are badgered by the communists, who say that they will help us but do nothing but increase violence in rural areas and interfere with tourism, harming our livelihoods. Millions of Nepalis are forced to migrate within the country or to India to find work each year, and many women and children are trafficked for labor or sex. In 2000, the government got a jolt when it learned that ten percent of returning migrants are HIV positive.

"My oldest brother migrated to India when he was sixteen to look for work." She shook back her thick long hair, the bangles on her slim wrists rattling. "He too came back with the AIDS *rog*. He had no help like me, and after giving it to his wife, he died two years later on the eve of Tihar. I was very sad during that Festival of Lights. Tihar lasts a week in late November, and on Bhaitika day, brothers and sisters give and receive *tika*, the colored spot of powder we sometimes wear on our foreheads. There was only my little brother left that year." She dabbed at a tear in the corner of her left eye.

Oh, my, Molly thought, preparing to intervene again. There is no end to the suffering these children have endured. But after a moment, Rageena lifted her shoulders proudly.

"I was only twelve years old, and the day my future husband came was like every day before it but no day after. Each day I woke when the first cock crowed, swept the room of our house and the courtyard, went to the stream three times for enough clean drinking water to fill our two storage pots, milked the buffalos, and headed off to the nearby town at a run. It took an hour to reach there if I walked fast. The townspeople always nagged me if I was late and complained that the milk was mixed with too much water, trying to get a better price. If I was late and could not sell the milk at all, my parents would punish me. When I sold the milk and could bring home a notebook or pencil for my brother, I would be very glad.

"It is funny," Rageena said, "but now I would give anything to get that life back, as hard as it seemed as a little girl. My life was like endless drudgery to me then. After the milk was sold, I would run back home to take the buffalos to pasture and collect food for them in the forest. My chores would never be finished until it was time for bed, and all the while I did the work, I would dream of how the rich people lived in the towns. But I was born on Aunsi, the fifteenth day of the Hindu lunar calendar. In the Hindu tradition, this is very inauspicious. It is said that a girl born on this day will cause the early death of her husband, so she must marry someone also born on this day. So when the evil trafficker came," she said with a sigh, "and told me I was beautiful and told my father he would give him enough money to pay off the debt which held my family in bonded labor, I was very happy.

"We were married the following week and he took me off to the Terai right after the wedding. I did not want to leave my home in the highlands. I was afraid of that low and evil place on the border of India where all Nepalis know that the most unfortunate dwell, but my husband was very sweet to me and told me he had to take me to live with his mother. This is customary in our society. My mother took me aside and talked to me. 'A woman is like the earth,' she said. 'She must bear every hardship. The husband is like a god. So no matter how he treats you, you must respect him.' I kissed my mother, brother, and father good-bye and left with him in his truck.

"That first night we drove down from the mountains into Kathmandu. We stayed there for some time, and it seemed each day my new husband grew colder. He was ashamed of me and made fun of me because I was from the village. 'You are a stupid country girl,' he would say to me. 'Here, even in the alleys, I see girls who are ten times more beautiful than you. And they fuss over me when I go to see them.' Even though he seemed to hate me, he would still beat me if I refused to have sex with him. I stayed inside and hid, afraid the neighbors would see my bruises if I ventured out of doors. I was so afraid and confused, and too ashamed to ask for help. I remembered my mother's words, and thought it was all my fault for being bad and stupid. I tried to be cheerful and keep our little house clean and cook for him when he would give me money for the market. And I kept asking him to take me to the Terai to live with his mother, as he had promised.

"Well, one day I woke and there was a strange man in the house. My husband had not come home the night before. The man said his name was Mr. Sharma, and he told me that my husband had sold me to him for 12,000 rupees. He said my husband laughed when Mr. Sharma asked if he would like to say good-bye to me. 'She is a useless thing,' he had told the man, taking the few rupees he offered and leaving in a rush. I often thought about my husband afterward. I am convinced that he only married me to lure me from the village, and that he had probably done the same thing to many other girls. I know that he made a good profit from selling me, and that as the carpet man dragged me to the barracks at his factory, my husband was probably spending some of his profits getting drunk and bedding another woman."

Rageena had slumped in her chair, her face a miniature storm cloud. Phet leaned forward, caught her eye and gently took her hand. Then he looked at Molly. "Maybe someone else could take a turn now."

—◦•◦—

July 1858, the month of Emmeline's birth, saw the birth of a scientific revolution as profound as the revolution in political thought born at the Bastille sixty-nine years earlier. At a July 1 special meeting of London's Linnean Society called just before their summer recess, members listened listlessly in the summer heat as Darwin's 1844 draft of the *Origin of the Species* and related correspondence was presented alongside Alfred Russel Wallace's essay, "On the Tendency of Varieties to Depart Indefinitely from the Original Type." Wallace's essay, received by Darwin in June, so closely anticipated his own work that geologist Charles Lyell and botanist Joseph Hooker rushed the evidence to the Linnean "jury" so that Darwin's claim to the theory of evolution would not be displaced by an itinerant scientific upstart.

Wallace posted his paper to Darwin from Ternate in Asia's Spice Islands on the same day he sent a letter to Henry Walter Bates, a longtime friend with whom he had scoured the Amazon for collectible insects some years earlier. Bates received his letter with its Singapore and Southampton cancellation marks on June 3 and it is likely that Darwin got Wallace's package on the same day, two weeks earlier than June 18 when he claimed to have received it. Five days later, on June 8, Darwin wrote Hooker that despite a furious outbreak of boils, he had finally work out how species develop in nature, the very subject of Wallace's new paper. Having "discovered" survival of the fittest, his evolutionary keystone, Darwin told Hooker he would now rewrite the chapter on species change in his 1844 "big book" on evolution and it could now be published.

Recent investigations suggest that Darwin's sudden "breakthrough" came straight from Wallace's 1858 paper. Wallace had gone to Asia in 1854 to collect specimens to sell to European museums, but the plants and animals he found there inspired his love of biological theorizing, so he put his keen intelligence to work on the theory of evolution. In six years of travel through the Malay Archipelago, the most interesting specimens he collected—and people he met—were in Borneo. Wallace had gone to never intended to visit Borneo but met Sir James Brooke, the white Rajah of Sarawak, in Singapore while he was searching for passage to Java. It was not difficult for Brooke to persuade Wallace to change his plans because it was in Sarawak that he could see the orangutan, which Wallace wrote was "one of my chief objects in coming" to Asia's great islands. Wallace spent 14 months on Borneo's northwest coast, staying with Brooke when he was not collecting specimens in the jungle.

The son of a British East India Company official, Brooke had grown up in India and after school in Britain became a cavalry officer in the British Indian Army. Serious wounds incurred during the first Anglo-Burmese War (1824–1826) sent him back to England, where he resigned his military commission. During the 1830s Brooke toured Asia, stopping by the Straits Settlements (Penang, Malaka, and Singapore) on his way to China, where he met the administrator, Sir Thomas Stamford Raffles, who believed that Britain should contest the Dutch for a greater role in the Malay Archipelago. When

Brooke returned to England in 1838, he wrote a treatise arguing that Britain should possess territories in Asia rather than rely on treaty arrangements. Ignored by the government, which thought such an arrangement would be far too expensive, he bought a 142-ton schooner with his inheritance and headed for the East on a geographical and scientific expedition of his own.

In August 1839, after exploring Maruda Bay at Borneo's northern tip, the Celebes, and New Guinea, and Brooke stopped by Kuching on Borneo's north coast to deliver a thank-you note to the governor, Pengiran Hassim, who had rescued survivors from a British shipwreck. Hassim was struggling to contain rebellions against the Sultan of Brunei, who had controlled the island's northern half since the late 1700s. Harsh treatment of local slaves in the sultanate's antimony and gold mines had incited anti-Brunei uprisings. In desperation, Hassim offered Brooke control of Sarawak (now a province within the Islamic Federation of Malaysia) and the title of rajah if he could quell the rebellions. Brooke successfully intervened and was installed as the rajah of Sarawak on September 24, 1841, founding a dynasty of white rajahs that ruled for 100 years. Brooke enlarged Sarawak's territory, fended off attacks of Chinese gold miners, and exterminated 500 pirates in a single battle, all the while propping up a succession of pro-Brooke sultans in Brunei. The "Brooke tradition" of rule emphasized protection of native interests against large-scale colonial ventures, low taxes, and full local participation in the government. Brooke chose not to enrich himself at native expense, hoping instead "that thousands will be benefited when I am mouldering in dust; that my name will be remembered . . . as one whose actions showed him above the base and sordid motives which so often disgrace men in similar circumstances."[1]

After Wallace's first visit in 1854, Brooke's personal secretary Spenser St. John wrote that "Wallace, who was then elaborating in his mind the theory of the origin of species," was a charming companion. "If he would not convince us that our ugly neighbors, the orangutans, were our ancestors, he pleased, instructed and delighted us by his clever and inexhaustible flow of talk—really good talk." Wallace spent Christmas of 1857 with the rajah and his entourage at Brooke's hill station retreat at the foot of the Santubong Mountains. After the holiday, Brooke left Wallace there with a Malay cook to recover from his latest bout with malaria. It was the rainy season, and Wallace later recalled that "during the evenings and wet days I had nothing to do but look over my books and ponder the problem which was rarely absent from my thoughts." He reviewed his catalogs of insects and plants from the Malay Archipelago and recalled the British Museum collections and his own expeditions in the Amazon, thinking carefully about the geographical distribution of plants and animals.

"It occurred to me that these facts had never been properly utilized as indications of the way in which species had come into existence." When he published the "Sarawak Law" on species evolution, he told the readers that it had been ten years since the idea suggested itself to him, but that it took only three nights to write his essay once his ideas fell into place.

During his ten years of travel, Wallace had meticulously recorded the geographic distribution of known birds and animals in a species registry, to which he added all new findings. He could quickly tell if any of the birds, insects, or animals he collected were new and how they compared in distribution and characteristics to all other known species. After studying his systematized records, he deduced from the patterns that every new species arises "coincident in space and time with a pre-existing closely allied species." In other words, every new species has a closely related ancestor, although sometimes it was obscured by the extinction of intermediate types. Even humans had a close living relative, he said, but never confessed to anyone but Brooke and St. John that he thought it was the orangutan, "the great man-like ape of Borneo" that inspired his trip. In return for all his courtesies, Wallace ensured that his host would always be remembered in the name of Malaysia's most famous butterfly, the magnificent Rajah Brooke's Birdwing.

———◆———

At the time of Wallace's stay with Brooke, the impact of European colonial exploitation on Asia was beginning to show. As late as 1750, living standards in Asia had been higher than in Europe.[2] The average Chinese consumed five pounds of sugar compared to two for the average European, and ordinary Chinese were more likely to own jewelry and furniture than were Europeans. South and Southeast Asian countries were only slightly behind China. As late as 1820, Asia accounted for 58 percent of global gross domestic product (GDP), more than the United States today. In that year, Asia's first economic crisis—colonialism—hit, causing a sustained economic decline that lasted until the 1950s, when its share of the global GDP dropped to the all-time low of 17 percent. After 1820 Asia steadily began losing its advantage over Europe along with the other great colonial continent, Africa. The declines in Asia and Africa had three causes: Europe's greed; the two world wars fought by European powers with the help their colonial possessions; and the struggle of Asian nations to escape from that greed and develop using their own models of growth.

"This enormous decline," Colin Mason says, "was no accident. While the industry and economies of the dominators boomed, those of the colonies were deliberately restrained." The process was not simply extractive. The colonies' raw materials were extracted under trade arrangements favorable to the Europeans, processed into finished goods in Europe, and sold back to the Asia colonies. Half of India's imports were British, and half of Indochina's came from France. India, once the world's major supplier of cotton fabrics, lost its position to the English Midlands. Asia's European masters deliberately exploited agricultural production while they retarded their colonies' industrial development so they could realize the economic rewards. The colonies were netting their European "owners" $3 billion annually by 1930.

Extractive economic policies created major social problems in the colonies that continue to this day. Agricultural land was turned over to export crops, and as population grew, more people starved or suffered from malnutrition. Education was provided the tiny native elites that administered the colonies. According to Mason, "By the end of the colonial era, when virtually the whole world outside of the colonies was literate, the vast majority of the dominated peoples remained illiterate." In 1998 most of the world's billion people who still could not read or write—16 percent of the global community—were located in former Asian and African colonies. Colonial governments perpetuated gross disparities in wealth, colluding with predatory native merchants to impoverish the ignorant majority. Basic infrastructure was developed only where it suited the colonists, so that in 1950 China, India, and Indonesia combined had only 38,000 miles of railroad compared to 217,000 in the United States. Factories, power generation, and other resources needed by modern states were comparably underdeveloped. A 1913 colonial text put it bluntly: "The colonies are countries which have been conquered. They are the property of the country that administers them [and] develops their riches for its own profit . . . They have no right to be put on the same footing as the governing country." The modern Western nation-state did not have an Asian counterpart until after World War II.

Since the 1950s, Asia has gained much lost ground. With growth rates among the highest in the world, by 2025 the region is expected to have between 55 and 60 percent of the global GDP. The presence of AIDS in Asia, however, threatens to substantially limit projected growth. In India, for example, Nicholas Eberstadt estimates that even an "intermediate" epidemic could cut economic growth by three-quarters over the next twenty-five years. Meager improvements in the living standards of the poor would evaporate, causing extraordinary suffering.

Asia's AIDS epidemics are much less severe than Africa's, but many of their underlying causes are similarly rooted in colonial exploitation, wars of independence, the world wars, and experiments with communist government. With few exceptions—Japan, the Philippines, Malaysia, Singapore, and Thailand, all small states that began internally directed, deliberate programs of modernization in the late nineteenth and early twentieth centuries—modern Asian states are relatively new. Most began their process of modern state formation as recently as fifty years ago, their transitions delayed by nineteenth century colonialism and twentieth century conflicts. In some states, like Cambodia where violence finally ended in 1998, modern state formation began only a few years ago. The struggle with socialism in communist states also retarded growth: China did not liberalize until 1978, Vietnam until 1986, and Russia until 1991. Fission and struggle continue in Indonesia, Pakistan, Afghanistan, Nepal, Russia, and Central Asia. In Myanmar, state formation has been frozen by a violent military regime struggling to control drug trade profits.

The process of condensing two centuries of delayed development into a few decades has left most Asian states highly vulnerable. While freedom from colonial political domination and economic subordination was won in the 1950s, many governments are still balancing the extractive agendas of their former colonial masters with the needs of their own people. Internal factions competing over wealth and development agendas are still negotiating state control in many nations, leaving central government structures remarkably weak. Maintaining social order, containing civil unrest, even establishing boundaries with their neighbors continue to present major challenges. Asia's relatively new states have the tremendous responsibility of reordering economies distorted by world events for nearly two centuries. Significant in relation to AIDS, much of this distortion came from the orientation of their cultures, politics, and economies to the production and marketing of drugs by colonial powers, a discussion taken up more fully in the next chapter. Playing catch-up in rebuilding their vital productive infrastructures, Asian states have also had to reorient their economies to the fast-paced demands of economic globalization over the past three decades.

Asian countries struggle with massive unemployment, illiteracy, poor health, and their very conception of social justice—in other words, who should get what. Freed from authoritarian rulers with minimal concern for their mandate from heaven, they came under the thumb of colonial regimes whose only mandate was maintaining the labor productivity of the masses. After World War II Asian states entered a world where entitlements were universally prescribed and their progress was measured by UN agencies. In the 1990s, the game suddenly shifted again to a world where anything goes and the dollar is king. At the same time, governments were called upon to respect and fulfill their citizens' human rights. Including the excluded—be they minorities, farmers, the poor, children, young people, or those socially marginalized by the sex and drugs industries—has now become even more urgent in the face of growing HIV/AIDS epidemics. In postsocialist countries, recent liberalization and market reform have spurred economic growth but left poor and rural populations behind, exposing them to a variety of influences favorable to HIV transmission. The poor in states that chose to defer questions of entitlement, including health, education, unemployment compensation, and old age security, find themselves paying a big price.

Many Asian states have made tremendous strides in improving health, but primary healthcare is still shaky and public health systems responsible for managing infectious diseases, water, sanitation, nutrition, immunizations, protection of blood supplies, and access to hospital services and drugs, including those for HIV/AIDS, have been neglected. The World Health Organization's (WHO) New Delhi office says that "the safety and quality of blood still varies greatly among countries." Thailand, Indonesia, Maldives, Nepal, and Sri Lanka screen almost all donated blood for HIV, but other countries in the region have been less successful, particularly India, Bangladesh, and Myanmar.[3] As in China, traditional beliefs discourage blood donation, so countries have had to pay donors or import blood.

Education is the second entitlement that gravely affects HIV/AIDS. Central, East, and Southeast Asian countries have achieved almost full literacy, but South Asia's literacy levels are as low as 30 percent. Female literacy is almost universally lower than male, reflecting women's lower social status and making them extremely vulnerable to HIV infection. Without literacy, it is not only very difficult to provide HIV/AIDS education so people can protect themselves, it is also difficult to change traditions that foster the epidemic's spread. For example, women in many Asian cultures are obliged to work to support not only themselves but their parents, a tradition that often sends at least one daughter in a family into sex work if other opportunities are lacking. The tradition of filial piety and respect for ancestors makes it extremely difficult to recruit volunteer blood donors. Notions of male sexual potency and appropriate sexual behavior that validate multiple partners and use of sex workers by men is another tradition that is hard to challenge in an uneducated society.

Poor education contributes to unemployment and lowers the overall standards of living for Asia's huge populations in poverty. Blood donation in India and other countries is as much a "poverty reduction" program as it is in China, providing essential income to the poor who must violate traditional and religious laws that the upper classes can afford to observe. Asia's poorest poor are female, who are shuttled into lower-paying jobs or sex work to support themselves and their children. In India and Nepal, Hindu caste-based societies, the lowest caste also incurs the costs of discrimination and economic disadvantages built into the social structure. By ignoring the needs of their poor minorities, many countries suffer ongoing unrest, an ideal condition for HIV transmission. This chapter explores these key themes in colonial and postcolonial Asian development relative to HIV/AIDS, looking principally at South and Southeast Asian states where colonialism played a major role. The first of the countries considered are two of Asia's most populous states, India and Bangladesh, where AIDS epidemics promise to be among the worst outside of China.

———•◆•———

Almost one-quarter of the people living with HIV/AIDS in Asia are Indian. India's HIV infection rate (0.8 percent) is the third highest the region, after Thailand and Cambodia, it has the largest number of infected people because it has the biggest population. During 2002 alone, almost 600,000 new cases were identified—two-thirds of the U.S. total for the entire epidemic. First diagnosed in the mid-1980s, HIV was spread across India from Mumbai (Bombay), Chennai (Madras), and Bangalore by truckers and migrant workers moving along the country's major highways who have unprotected sex while they are away from home. India's unregulated sex industry has more than 2 million male and female commercial sex workers and at least 75,000 brothels. A large proportion of sex workers, like Rageena, are trafficked from other countries; Nepalis called AIDS "Mumbai disease" because so many migrants came home sick. Currently, 28 percent of India's HIV cases are female compared to 72 percent male, but this ratio is likely to shift as the epidemic spreads. Since men are not expected to be sexually faithful, the number of women infected by their husbands is mushrooming, a process facilitated by relatively high rates of sexually transmitted diseases (at any give time, one in ten Indians has an STD). Injecting drug use fuels epidemic growth in a second epidemic epicenter along India's border with Myanmar, connected to Yunnan's illicit narcotics trade. India's third epidemic, emanating from its substandard blood supply, has affected the entire nation.

Many of China's HIV/AIDS-related problems are paralleled in India's epidemic: The blood supply became a national scandal in the early 1990s; despised ethnic minorities and lower-caste Indians have less access to healthcare; the drug trade and human trafficking flourish; sex work is rampant; and large numbers of unemployed people follow seasonal migration patterns. India is "one of the great migration centers of the world," says writer Michael Specter, because it has an excellent system of national highways.[4] More than 100,000 long-haul truckers traverse the subcontinent on a regular basis, and tens of millions of farm workers come to the cities several months a year looking for work when farming is slow. While poverty underlies all of these causes by creating incentives for risky behavior—India has the largest number of extremely poor people in the world—government policies are also to blame. India's public health system is just as weak as China's and government denial as strong. Public education has been weak, and as a result, a 2003 survey found that two-thirds of all Indians had never heard of HIV/AIDS or any other sexually transmitted disease (STD).[5] Seventy percent of women had never heard of AIDS, and three-quarters of India's 750 million-strong rural population, who comprise the second largest "country" in the world, were also ignorant of the disease. Among the few who knew of AIDS, many more men than women (70 percent compared to 48 percent) knew condom use could prevent infection. With the migration of HIV to "rural areas in the heartland of India, [AIDS] is going from bad to worse," said Mumbai AIDS advocate I.S. Gilada.[6]

In addition to Manipur and Nagaland on the Myanmar border, the worst-hit states are Andhra Pradesh, Karnataka, Tamil Nadu, and Maharashtra. These are all of India's southern states with the exception of Kerala, where education and literacy rates are extraordinarily high. Each of these states have populations as big as many countries. By 2001, more than 1 percent of adults in these states were infected, a sign that the epidemic had caught hold and was gearing up. Infections have been reported in people from all walks of life, including farmers, businessmen, hotel and service sector workers, and the unemployed. AIDS deaths are so frequent in southern India that locals erected a shrine to India's new AIDS goddess, Aidsama, at a temple near Mysore.

In 1998 WHO estimated that one-fifth of India's HIV infections were from improperly screened blood and blood products. In 1991 blood was screened only in New Delhi, Calcutta, Chennai, and Mumbai. In 1992 the health ministry reported that only 138 out of the country's 608 blood banks were equipped for HIV screening, and that it was flagrantly intermittent. Thirty percent of the blood supply came from private, unregulated, profit-making blood banks that depended on paid, professional donors. Professional donation dates back to colonial times and was institutionalized during World War II when large quantities of blood were needed. Since few Indians are willing to donate what is traditionally viewed as a precious fluid, most donors were poor drug addicts and sex workers, 86 percent of whom were HIV positive. By 1996 the government had so visibly failed to improve the situation that the Indian Supreme Court ordered an end to paid donations. An international study in 1996 estimated that 95 percent of India's blood supply was unsafe, compared to 60 percent in prescandal China.[7] At particular risk of infection from this source are pregnant women, whose high rates of anemia increase their need for transfusions.

The government, which made no effort to educate the public or develop a voluntary system, aggravated the blood shortage by banning donations from relatives or friends. When large quantities of blood were needed for survivors of Gujarat's 2001 earthquake, the worst in India's history, blood donated by prison inmates was rejected by top government officials who said prisoners were a high-risk group for HIV and hepatitis B. Inmates get a month deducted from their sentence for every two donations they make each year, but the Red Cross had to refuse their blood even though it was screened. By 2003 hospital blood banks were still understaffed and undersupplied; healthcare facilities and blood banks were reusing unsterilized needles. India's $540 million in blood product imports in 2001 were part of a steadily rising trend, but because of the cost, most of it goes to the well-to-do. In 2002 the government gave Rotary International's regional blood bank in Delhi $1 million to expand services even though Rotary blood is twice as expensive as Red Cross blood. "India's notorious social distinctions based on caste and class have spilled into the blood donation sector," said *Asia Times* reporter Ranjit Devraj. "Even reputable blood banks now advertise blood that is guaranteed not to come from the dregs of society."[8] Physicians reportedly look the other way when desperate patients make deals with "vampires" who arrange donations from the old professional donor network, now driven underground.

India's National AIDS Control Program, established in 1987, was sidelined when most of its AIDS budget was spent on unsuccessful efforts to clean up the blood supply. In a country known for computer outsourcing, HIV surveillance has become adequate only in the last few years, and five years passed before the government could bring nationally manufactured condoms up to standard. Oblivious to its failures and blind to increasing HIV rates, the health ministry announced that it will reduce new cases to zero by 2007. HIV/AIDS control by India's states is even worse except in Tamil Nadu, where HIV rose from 1.5 percent in 1995 to 6 percent in 1997, prompting development of the most effective prevention program in India. More typical is Goa's decision in 2004 to target barbers and beauty parlors for infection control instead of its blood supply. Critics charge that during the 1990s India spent more money trying to prove it did not have an HIV/AIDS epidemic then it did on actual prevention, and that unionized sex workers in Calcutta's Sonagachi red-light district did a better job responding to the AIDS threat. Following Thailand's model, they demanded health care and STD treatment, forced customers to use condoms, stopped police harassment, and started education programs for their children and savings programs for themselves. Infection rates topped out at 5 percent in Sonagachi, compared to 70 percent for prostitutes in Mumbai.[9]

In 2001 the government rejected an offer of free neviraprane, a drug that is almost 100 percent effective in preventing mother-to-child HIV infection, from Yusuf Hamied, whose Cipla Pharmaceuticals leads international manufacturing of generic HIV drugs and sponsors the only Indian television commercials that talk about AIDS. When Bill Gates offered $100 million in AIDS money to India's four hardest-hit states in 2004, a central government minister wanted to turn the billionaire down, saying that Gates' predictions of 25 million HIV-positive Indians by 2025 were exaggerated. I.S. Gilada, who leads Mumbai's People's Health Organization and has confronted government apathy for more than a decade, said that "it is a pity to have such ministers . . . from top to bottom, there's no ownership. The government of India has not spent one rupee or one dollar from its coffers on HIV programs." In ceremonies announcing distribution of free anti-AIDS drugs to 100,000 Indians in May 2004, S.P. Agarwal, chief health officer in Delhi, said that "an unmitigated disaster is looming on the horizon."

Health spending is about $10 per person per year for India's population of 1.3 billion. The country has 18 million new mouths to feed every year, more than half the population of Canada added to a country one-third Canada's size. Each year there are more than 1 million cases of malaria and 2 million cases of tuberculosis. The country accounts for 70 percent of the world's leprosy, has endemic encephalitis and yaws, and has the largest remaining pool of polio (although recent outbreaks threaten a rampant epidemic in AIDS-afflicted Africa). Sixty percent of Indian women are anemic and half are illiterate, and they account for a quarter of all the world's deaths in childbirth each year. More than half of all children under four are malnourished, and 30 percent of its newborns are underweight. Although child mortality has been halved since the 1970s, critics charge that achievements in public health are relatively modest for one of the fastest-growing economies on the planet. In 1991, after four decades of state planning, liberal economic reforms introduced a free-market approach that has kept India growing more than 6 percent a year ever since. Rich in mineral wealth, with millions of trained professionals and a growing middle class of at least 250 million people—more than the entire U.S. population—India ranks as one of the world's ten largest emerging markets. Bangalore is a new Silicon Valley. But an ever-richer India lacks compassion for its poor, critics say.

India has one-quarter of the world's absolute poor. Despite an economic growth rate averaging 6 percent per year since 1990, about 25 percent of India's population still live in poverty and are entitled to government assistance and special development schemes. Most are members of the lower or "scheduled" castes and tribes. India has the second largest concentration of tribal peoples in the world next to China, organized into seven major tribes with hundreds of branches. With a literacy rate of 40 percent compared to the national average of 65.2 percent, their settlement areas also have fewer health services and more health problems. Many are forcibly settled nomads who still practice slash-and-burn cultivation. As in China, most of India's mineral wealth is located in an area called the tribal belt, which is more like a shawl draped low on India's shoulders from Myanmar to Pakistan. Instead of protecting the rights of tribal people, the government is aligning with private-sector companies to displace them. It is "like someone asking you to get out of your house so that they can dig for gold while you are being made to beg outside," said one observer.[10] Tribal insurrections by the Zomi Revolutionary Army occur so regularly in Manipur and Nagaland, two of India's most AIDS-affected states, that a local official says "insurgency is an industry here."

Ethnic discrimination in India is compounded by the Hindu caste system, the world's oldest form of social stratification, dating from the Aryan expansion into India in 1500 B.C. The Aryan newcomers were herdsmen and hunters from Persia who subjugated the more advanced Harappans they replaced. To control their new subject people, the Aryans formalized a class system in the religion and culture of Hinduism. There are four castes: the highest, Brahmins or priestly teachers; the soldier-nobles; the merchants; and the lowest, the untouchables, now called *Dalits*, who were darker skinned and did all the work except for cremations, which were carried out by the lowest of the low, the *Chandals*. The caste system is "a pattern of privilege [that] inevitably resulted in discrimination, oppression and harsh laws," aided by a liberally applied death penalty that kept the aristocracy immune from revolt according to Mason. "The mass of people, living in villages similar to those today, were heavily taxed to support their masters" and were often so destitute that minor weather changes could cause major famines. Because caste status is ordained in a past life by karma, the system "has an inevitability that reinforces its acceptance by those who believe in it." Retaliation against any of the 160 million *Dalits*— leather workers, farmers, and other tradesmen—who attempt to assert their rights is still frighteningly harsh. In 2003, for example, Girdharilal Maurya's neighbors beat up his wife and daughter, ruined his farm and tractor, and burned his house down because he demanded to use the new village well.[11] Parliamentary attempts to reform the caste system has always failed because of the tiers of self-interest that maintain it. It flows from the upper classes on down, keeping everyone tightly locked in place.

Despite its failures, India's healthy parliamentary democracy has more than twenty political parties and freedom is preciously guarded. In 1975, when Prime Minister Indira Gandhi defied a High Court judgment and dared invoke emergency rule to suspend civil liberties, within two years the electorate responded by driving her from power. One Indian commentator described India's 2004 election upset as "the modern equivalent of medieval England's peasant revolts." The "wretched of the earth" turned up at the polls to reject an out-of-touch government more concerned with its fleets of Mercedes-Benzes than with the "ragged skeletal creatures whom a brutal capitalist system deals out of the spectrum of a dignified human existence."[12] Neocapitalist economics have turned India's urban-rural gulf into an abyss much like China's, says that commentator—dangerous to the health of governments, "a point not lost on China's command-and-control dictators as they watch the coastal provinces surge to First World per capita/GDP growth levels while a 100 million peasants have nothing in their rice bowls." India's chief minister, dining with Bill Gates at Davos while drought-stricken farmers in Andhra Pradesh committed suicide, was turned out of office in the next election even though farm crops had recovered.

———————◆◆◆◆———————

In India's early history, like China's, a succession of broad-based Hindu and Buddhist kingdoms alternated with periods of disarray when warring princely states carved the subcontinent up into merciless and extortionate feudal domains. Here, too, nomadic invasion played a major role in shaping history, starting with Timur's invasion in 1398, which broke the back of the Delhi sultanate, shaking Muslim control over northern India. When Babur, the last of Timur's dynasty, was evicted from Samarkhand in 1525 he marched through the Khyber gorges and defeated Delhi's army of 100,000 with a force of only 12,500 men. He began the Muslim Mogul Empire, which gradually covered a third of the subcontinent. The Moguls, who built some of India's finest architectural monuments, including the Taj Mahal, drew their wealth from taxes on 150 million Hindu farmers. The third Mogul emperor improved the legal code and established a professional civil service to eliminate official bribery and extortion. But after his death the Moguls began taxing the peasantry to the point of starvation while leaving the responsibility of public works up to local officials, who rarely did much to the peasant's advantage. Banditry was rife, travel was dangerous, and villages were dirty and impoverished. The sixth emperor, Aurangzeb, tipped the balance with a series of costly military campaigns and persecuted the Hindus, prompting a number of rebellions.

Mogul rule declined and in 1739 the Persians attacked Delhi, leaving 30,000 dead and grabbing the gem-encrusted Peacock Throne. Hindu Maratha princes were "too self-seeking and disunited" to grab power, "more interested in plunder than politics," says Mason. The country was too disorganized to oppose the establishment of western trading posts that turned into swelling settlements along the Indian coast. By 1700 England's East India Company had settlements in Bombay and Calcutta, and within another one hundred years gained predominance over the subcontinent through alliances with the weak native rulers. Six years before his death in 1701, Aurangzeb sealed India's fate by granting the British East India Company (the Company) the right to collect revenues from their lands around Calcutta. When raids by Afghan and Maratha warlords "brought cries for protection" from the Hindu princelings, says historian John Keay,[13] India fell into Britain's lap "while she was sleeping, like an over-ripe mango."

Although Bangladesh is now the runt of the litter, as the pivotal state of Bengal it was then the wealthiest part of the subcontinent, and by 1750 the Company's fortified trading post in Calcutta was its busiest port. In 1756, when France began to contest British control over the rest of the subcontinent, the Nawab of Bengal stormed Calcutta to throw the British out. European men, women, and children who had not escaped were stowed for safekeeping overnight in the infamous Black Hole of Calcutta, from which only twenty-three emerged in the morning. Robert Clive, an East India Company junior clerk who had distinguished himself in earlier British-French colonial contests, led a counterattack against the Bengalis and over the course of the famous "Two Hundred Days" conquered Calcutta. The Nawab colluded with the French, giving Britain an excuse to move north into Bengal. Mogul rulers, who by then had only nominal control over Bengal, ceded it to the British, anointing Clive as the *diwan*, or chancellor, in what Keay describes as "a decidedly tacky ceremony." The Company gained virtual sovereignty over the province and monopolies on exports of saltpeter, indigo, opium, and sea salt in exchange for paid protection from fresh waves of marauders. It allied with the feudal lords, or *zamindars*, to collect taxes. Clive alone reaped well over £400,000, the largest fortune made by one Englishman in India. He later told a British parliamentary committee that he had been exceptionally moderate. "A great prince was dependent on my pleasure," he said, "an opulent city lay at my mercy; its richest bankers bid against one another for my smiles; I walked through vaults which were thrown open to me alone, piled on either side with gold and jewels."

From its Bengali stronghold, the East India Company allied with local leaders to "ring fence" the subcontinent against the warlords. Their political, judicial, and financial alliances were "supposedly designed to restore a traditional order [that] while advantageous to the British regime, would bring security and prosperity to all," Keay says. Large areas of agricultural land were forcibly converted to plantations for opium, tea, spices, coffee, indigo, jute, sugarcane, and cotton. Rural industries were suppressed to expand the market for British manufacturers, while Britain's merchant-allies reduced the tribal peasants to debt bondage. Famines caused frequent and widespread peasant rebellions, suppressed by British forces allied with local princes. But no one was content. In 1857, Indian princes took advantage of a mutiny among the British East India Company's Sepoys (soldiers), and joined peasants and disaffected Muslim soldiers to overthrow Company rule. At this point, the British crown stepped in, crushed the rebellion, and assumed direct rule.

Colonial exploitation increased. In rural areas polarized by the commercialization of agriculture, conflicts erupted between peasantry and rich elites as debt bondage and landlessness grew. Britain's failure to develop industry to absorb labor aggravated growing unemployment. To create a civil service for administration of the Raj, Britain expanded educational opportunities for higher-caste Hindus while their censuses and ethnological surveys hardened religious, caste, language and racial stereotypes. Soon, the British-educated teachers, doctors, lawyers, journalists, and businessmen, familiar with contemporary English reform movements, demanded the franchise and home rule. In a concession they hoped would stem growing unrest, the British allowed the first Indian National Congress to meet in 1885. Only two of the seventy-two delegates were Muslim, however, and Muslim disaffection grew as they were marginalized by the reform process, especially in Bengal.

In 1905 Britain's Foreign Office approved Lord Curzon's plan to slice Bengal into Hindu East Bengal and Muslim West Bengal, to reduce the growing violence. "Bengal united is a power. Bengal divided will pull several ways," one of the viceroy's advisors explained. "One of our main objects is to split up and thereby weaken a solid body of opponents to our rule." Muslims in East Bengal "relished their new empowerment," says historian Carl Meyer, and the All India Muslim League was formed in 1906. Infuriated, East Bengali Hindus believed the plan gave undue status to West Bengali Hindu peasants who had only converted to Islam to escape lower-caste status.[14] "It was from the end of 1906 that we became conscious of a new kind of hatred for the Muslims," said Hindu political observer Nirad Chaudhuri, and it "poison[ed] our personal relations with our Muslim neighbors and school-fellows." The Calcutta press urged a boycott against British goods that started the *Svadeshi*, or "buy local" movement, which Gandhi later built into a national protest against British rule. Protests became so impassioned that when George V acceded to the throne in 1911, he abandoned the partition and transferred the British capital from Calcutta to Delhi. Historian Stanley Wolpert says that "*Svadeshi* and boycott, national education and *svaraj* [self-government], the major planks of India's independence movement, assumed national significance for the first time."[15]

During World War I more than a million Indians were conscripted to fight in Europe and immediately after the war, the bubonic plague, raging across India since the turn of the twentieth century, combined with the worldwide influenza epidemic to kill almost 30 million Indians. Worsening social conditions and tightened British antisedition laws caused periodic rioting. In 1920 the drive for independence became a mass movement. Mohandas Gandhi returned from South Africa, assumed leadership of the Indian National Congress, organized urban middle-class reformers into freedom fighters and built a rural following by including farmers' complaints in the Congress platform. In 1930 Gandhi's 240-mile walk to the sea protesting the British salt tax, which had cost millions of lives since it was imposed in the nineteenth century, reopened an old wound. The harshness of British reprisal created worldwide sympathy for India's cause, although the salt tax was not repealed until after the Indians won their independence in 1947. With the handwriting on the wall, the British began planning for the introduction of homerule in 1937.

Under its divide-and-rule policy, Britain educated Hindus for lower-level civil service jobs and isolated Muslims. As nationalism grew, the Hindu-Muslim antagonism this created increased. In 1940, when the Indian National Congress called for the British to "Quit India," the Muslim League, led by Mohammed Ali Jinnah, passed a resolution on calling for them to "Divide and Quit." The dream of an independent Pakistan had been growing. "PAKISTAN is both a Persian and an Urdu word, composed of letters taken from the names of our homelands: Punjab, Afghania (N.-W. Frontier Province), Kashmir, Iran, Sindh, Turkaristan, and Baluchistan. It means the land of the Paks, the spiritually pure and clean," declared a 1933 pamphlet.[16] Gandhi believed that Hindus and Muslims could work out their differences in a united India. "How are the Muslims different from the Hindus and the Sikhs?" he asked. "Are they not all drinking the same water, breathing the same air and deriving sustenance from the same soil?" But the schism between the India's Hindu-dominated National Congress and the Muslim League, the "twin engines" of India's liberation, had grown too wide.

In 1942 Britain's proposal to establish India as a dominion after the war was rejected by National Congress leaders who threatened civil disobedience. Britain threw them all in jail, where they stayed until the end of the war in 1945. The following year famine swept Bengal, squeezed by the military's requisitions and cut off from Burmese rice imports by the Japanese occupation. "In July the walking dead began straggling into Calcutta to expire on the streets," and Heay says that by November, the new British governor knew he was facing "one of the worst disasters that has befallen people under British rule." With the death toll rising over 2 million, Hindus and Muslims accused one another of hoarding. "Out of the famine, as out of other forms of agrarian and industrial distress," Heay says, "communal hatred was born." The three-day "Calcutta Killings" that followed took the lives of 4,000 Muslims, Hindus, and Sikhs, and only ceased when Gandhi sped to the scene to calm the violence.

During the war, India had not only paid off its debts to Britain with its industrial output, but rang up a credit balance of over £1 billion. This ended economic justification for British rule, and the British prepared to grant India its independence. Muslim League demands for a separate state, however, brought India to the brink of civil war in 1947. "We will have a divided India or a destroyed India," Jinnah declared, so partition lines were hastily drawn and India and Pakistan became independent states on August 14, 1947. Pakistan was split into two halves, East Pakistan (formerly Bengal) and West (the Punjab). When Jinnah's demands for a corridor across northern India to unite the two halves were ignored, he bitterly took the reins of a "maimed, mutilated and moth-eaten Pakistan." By the terms of the Partition, 15 million people uprooted themselves in "the most massive transfer of people ever, with Hindus moving out of what would be Pakistan and Muslims moving in."[17] India now has 950 million Hindus, the overwhelming majority of the population, but 100 million Muslims remain—only Indonesia and Pakistan have more—along with 20 million Christians, 18 million Sikhs, 7.5 million Buddhists, 4 million Jains, and millions with other faiths.

In East Pakistan, Bengali Hindus and Muslims, exhausted by earlier rioting, relocated relatively peacefully because Gandhi intervened when tempers flared. In the Punjab, where contesting groups were more militant, trouble broke out even before independence. The Sikhs, who had "provided two-fifths of the entire Indian army and constituted the most militant religious brotherhood on the subcontinent," viewed the Punjab as their empire's core, according to Heay, and demanded the creation of Sikhistan. When they accepted the partition line, they believed they would retain their religious sites and shrines. Instead, one of their most valuable shrines, Lahore, was allocated to Pakistan because the city's population was primarily Muslim. When the actual partition line was announced on August 17, torrents of refugees fled for their lives. The "land of the five rivers" was red with the blood of mass murder, rape, and slaughter; the roads were blocked with "mangled migrants." "Ghost trains" "chuffed silently across the new frontier carrying nothing but corpses." In a few cataclysmic weeks, 1 million people died.

"Outwardly," Meyer says, "partition seems a pragmatic way of splitting the difference, thereby honoring the principle of self-determination and separating antagonistic peoples."[18] But in the long run, "with rare exceptions, the postcolonial and post-Communist division of countries into separate states has uprooted millions of people, fomented internecine wars, degraded the citizenship of trapped minorities and perpetuated ancient grievances, closing both minds and frontiers." Partition prolongs conflict, whether in Pakistan, Kashmir, Ireland, Palestine, or Cyprus. In India's case, partition sped independence, but in the long run it provided a precedent for Muslim separatism and had deleterious consequences for the entire subcontinent. Gandhi foresaw that partition would fire community violence and was planning to visit the newborn Pakistan on a peace mission when he was shot and killed in 1948 by a Hindu fanatic who resented his "partiality" to Muslims.

———◆•◆•◆———

Mohammed Ali Jinnah, Pakistan's *Quaid-e-Azam*, or Great Leader, died of tuberculosis one year after his dream of a sovereign homeland for Muslims came true. As early as 1948, the Pakistan Constituent Assembly's East Pakistan (Bengali) members were complaining because their homeland had the representation of a single province even though it had more people than all of West Pakistan's provinces put together. In the early 1950s, riots broke out in East Pakistan when West Pakistan decreed that Urdu, spoken by only 8 percent of Pakistan's population, would be the national language. Anger cooled during the 1965 India-Pakistan war, but when Bengali leaders demanded autonomy afterward, they were thrown in jail and martial law was imposed. In March 1971, when Bengal's Awami League proclaimed independence for Bangladesh, West Pakistan's tanks rolled onto the streets of Dhaka. India armed and trained millions of Bengali refugees who joined Indian soldiers to eject the Pakistani army from Bengal. Pakistan bombed Indian airports and India bombed West Pakistan, but the fight was over within days. "Supported by a delirious civilian population," Heay says, the Indians accepted Pakistan's surrender on December 15, when Bangladesh gained its independence as the world's 139th state under the leadership of Awami League.

By that time, colonial rule had thoroughly depleted Bangladesh's phenomenal wealth. Since independence, nation building has been continually frustrated by a seesaw between military and civilian rule, Hindu-Muslim violence, and frequent cyclones, tidal waves, floods, famines, and epidemics. In 1970 a cyclone and tidal wave claimed half a million lives. Four years later, half the country was inundated again and a virtual civil war broke out between millions of homeless, starving people and the police. In 1988 and 1998 record-breaking floods again covered two thirds of the country. Violent floods are expected to worsen in the future. "The fact that flooding continues," Mason says, "is a reproach to the world"; it could be controlled by reforestation and by dams and hydroelectric projects that would save millions of lives, end regular cycles of devastation, and provide electricity to the entire subcontinent, innovations never realized by Bangladesh's strife-torn government. In 1965 Hindus were identified as enemies of the state and their was property seized. Their mass migration has triggered insurgency in the neighboring Indian state of Tripura, whose natives were overwhelmed and marginalized by the Bangladeshi Hindu asylum-seekers. In the Chittagong Hill Tracts, neither the Indian nor Bangladeshi governments have made much effort to halt genocidal violence between migrants and tribal groups.

Bangladesh is the eighth most populous country in the world and the most crowded country in South Asia. The population of 130 million will double by 2035, even if replacement fertility is reached by 2005. Three-quarters of its population are peasants who have been economically disenfranchised by perpetuation of colonial agricultural policies. Plantations growing jute, sugar, and tea for export occupy much of the land, commanding the poorly paid labor of adults and children above the age of six. The average Bangladeshi's income is one of the lowest in Asia, and 80 percent of the people live harsh lives, struggling to get enough to eat in villages where a dozen people share a single-room mud house. Flooding brings frequent outbreaks of waterborne diseases such as cholera and dysentery. Shortly after independence, 3 million wells were bored with international aid to provide clean drinking water to 97 percent of the population, but by the 1990s they were polluted with arsenic and the water they provided causes skin diseases and cancer. The country's weak primary healthcare system serves less than 40 percent of population. Nine of ten children are malnourished and 70 percent of Bangladesh's women are anemic, but literacy is improving and there have been impressive gains in primary school attendance.

The causes of Bangladesh's HIV/AIDS epidemic—an unscreened blood supply, sex work, and drug use—are deeply rooted in this crushing poverty. Needle-sharing among injecting drug users, many of whom are married and sell their blood to hospitals and clinics, is routine. The country has 35,000 paid blood donors and is only now developing blood screening protocols. In 2003 there were 1.7 million male and female sex workers, including 13,000 children and 30,000 transvestites. Ninety percent of their customers report never using a condom, although 43 percent of female and 18 percent of male sex workers have syphilis and almost half have been forced to have group sex. Eighty-five percent are completely ignorant of HIV/AIDS; only 9 percent think HIV is a problem. Bangladesh's brothels, some of the largest in Asia, are big business, but communities have started forcibly ejecting their sex workers. The trouble started in Tanbazar, Bangladesh's oldest and largest brothel, housing 3,000 sex workers and their children. Local politicians contested control of the brothel, which generates large amounts of income and supports other business investments. Sex workers were under siege; customers could not get in, electricity was cut off for nonpayments, and they began to starve until international protests brought closure. More than half of Bangladesh's young males have pre- and extramarital sex with prostitutes and the epidemic is spreading to married women, only 19 percent of whom have ever heard of AIDS.

Many of the conditions governing HIV/AIDS epidemics on the Indian subcontinent are also found in the countries on the second of Asia's great "peninsulas," mainland Southeast Asia and the island nations off its coast. Most of these conditions originate in colonial domination and postcolonial stress, but some—particularly attitudes toward poor and marginal groups—are deeply rooted in the age-old empires of the region. Mainland Southeast Asia's topography defined its early empires as it does the present-day states of Myanmar, Thailand, Vietnam, Cambodia, and Laos. The other half of Southeast Asia is the island realm of Singapore, Malaysia, Indonesia, Brunei, East Timor, and the Philippines. Early Arab, Indian, and Persians traders called it "the land below the winds" after the seasonal monsoons that blow from the southwest from June to November and in the reverse direction from December to May.

By the fifth century A.D. the foundations of Southeast Asia's empires had been laid. Sea travel had become sophisticated enough to support long-distance trading and the spice trade brought prosperity. The mountains had hardwood forests and mines rich in gold, silver and precious gems; the sea yielded fish and pearls. Surplus rice production fed officials, religious leaders, and traders, encouraging social stratification and central authoritarian control over water systems. Giant bronze drums requiring as much as seven tons of copper ore to produce attest to the power of early stratified communities; Chinese sources speak of powerful "barbarians" controlled by aristocratic elites. Rich volcanic soils coupled with a three-month dry season ideal for "ripening" rice still support some of the highest population densities in the world. Rice was cultivated by war captives and debt slaves, many of whom were in better condition than the peasants, who were taxed and conscripted for public works. The major cultural distinction between Malay and Australoid peoples is defined by "Wallace's Line," separating Singapore, Sumatra, Java, and Borneo from the Philippines, New Guinea, and Australia. Although short, "negroid" Australoid hunters can still be found in remote areas of Malaysia, Thailand, and the Philippines, most were driven to New Guinea and Australia by Malay invaders, themselves driven southward by northern empires before the sea level rose between 10,000 and 500 B.C.

Empires rose and fell in Southeast Asia between A.D. 500 and 1500, including Dai Viet (North Vietnam), Champa (South Vietnam), Angkor (Cambodia), Ayutthaya (Thailand), Srivijaya (Sumatra), Mataram (Java), Majapahit (Java and Bali), and Melaka (Malay Peninsula). These powerful and prosperous cultures amalgamated their earlier religious traditions with Hinduism, Buddhism, and Islam, each of which "possessed an efficient, if Machiavellian, statecraft," says Mason. Borrowed religions provided "ambitious rajahs with a blueprint for a society in which elites could control and use the ordinary people." Abundant natural resources drew armies from the east and the north, but they were rarely able to gain a permanent foothold. Kings in Vietnam, Burma, Java, and the Philippines frustrated Mongol China's attempts at invasion, and the sole Indian military victory in the region was not followed by colonization. Between 1500 and 1800 when the mainland kingdoms coalesced, Vietnam and Thailand came to dominate the lesser kingdoms of Cambodia and Laos.

By the eleventh century, "all world trade was more or less governed by the ebb and flow of spices in and out of South East Asia,"[19] says historian Kenneth Hall. Marco Polo's tales of adventure and wealth titillated European fantasies about the "Indies," whose empires were rich in gold and precious jewels that rivaled the wealth of Kublai Khan's China and Mogul India.[20] The ten Spice Islands (Indonesia's Moluccas) were famous in the medieval Europe because they were the world's only source of cloves and nutmeg, held in high esteem for preserving meats and warding off the plague. Until the fifteenth century, spices came to Europe through Italian merchants, who monopolized trade with the Arabs. To break the Islamic-Italian stranglehold on overland trade, Portugal sent Vasco da Gama around the coast of Africa, and when he entered the Indian Ocean in 1498, "he broke into a fabulously lucrative trading monopoly that had eluded the Europeans for centuries."[21]

Portugal took control of the Indian trading network from the Arabs, established a power base at Goa on India's west coast, and from there conquered Malaka in 1511 and took control of the Moluccas in 1512, scattering their Arab traders to other Malay ports. Portuguese merchants hurried to secure Timor (1522) and northern Java (1532), establishing a monopoly over the region's spice trade and control over Southeast Asia's busy sea traffic for almost eighty years. Sultans and rajahs found the opening of the European market highly profitable and the Portuguese crown was realizing one-third of its revenues from the spice trade by 1518. Although the Portuguese employed local administrators and married "Asian wives [who] provided important sources of trade contacts and information on local politics,"[22] as Catholics their zealous hatred of the conquered Muslims meant that the colonies needed constant supplies of ships, men, and guns. These demands, together with greed, corruption, and mismanagement, rendered Portugal unable to meet the costs of its forts and trading posts. In 1578 mainland Portugal suffered a crushing defeat at the hands of the Arab Moors, and fell under Spanish rule.

Spain, in the meantime, had opened an alternative route to the Spice Islands through the Philippines. Thanks to the Pope's intervention, a 1494 treaty with Portugal had forced Ferdinand Magellan to head eastward around the tip of South America in 1519, from which he reached the Philippines in 1521. Magellan died there, but his crew succeeded in returning to Spain in the first circumnavigation of the globe. However, by the time Spain conquered Portugal and was ready to exploit the eastern trade, a new contender had emerged. In 1581 the Protestant Dutch provinces became independent as the Republic of the United Netherlands, and in 1602 the Dutch East India Company was founded to capture Portuguese outposts and trade in Asia. By 1619 it had a trading base in Java called Batavia (present-day Jakarta). In 1641 the Dutch claimed Malaka and the straits, which became the western outpost of their wider Indonesian empire. The "huge intraregional trade network . . . linking all the major ports of South East Asia" was "blown apart," says historian Tim Harper, as one local princeling after another gave way to Dutch guns and their larger, faster ships that made indigenous merchant vessels obsolete.

England and France, latecomers to Asian colonization, ended up as the dominant powers thereafter. During the early years of Portuguese and Spanish exploration in Asia, both had been preoccupied by the Hundred Years' War, which lasted until 1453. They immediately became involved in their own civil wars—the War of the Roses in England and contests between Paris and Burgundy in France. At the end of its civil war, England was finally able to build a navy, but gave precedence to exploration of the Americas. When Charles VIII unified France, he promptly attacked Italy, ruling out foreign exploration until the mid-1500s, when France also turned toward the Americas. Official neglect, however, did not rule out private adventurers. In 1580 Sir Francis Drake returned to England with a small package of cloves from Ternate in the Spice Islands, raising commercial interest in the possibilities of trade. In 1600 the newly-founded British East India Company secured a royal monopoly over trade in the East. The Dutch prevented the English from gaining a permanent foothold in the Spice Islands, so the British East India Company established outposts in India, Thailand, and Burma. Dutch supremacy lasted until the outbreak of the Napoleonic wars in Europe, when all their possessions in Asia passed nominally into British hands, but British control over Malaya was not formally recognized until 1824, when the Anglo-Dutch Treaty was signed.

The fabulous possibilities of trade led early European economic theorists to speculate that a country's wealth depended on hoarding as much gold and silver bullion as it possibly could. Colonies could be virtual gold mines for their parent countries, and since the white race was superior—a "fact" established by the Swedish botanist Carolus Linnaeus in the eighteenth century—seizing the lands and wealth of other races and exploiting their labor was permissible. English, French, and Dutch companies, with the backing of their governments, competed with "manic energy and sheer bloody-mindedness for the rich possessions of Southeast Asia."[23] Asia was not the only target for predatory European colonialists. From 1876 to 1915, a fourth of world's territory "was distributed and redistributed" by European states, and Japan conquered portions of China, Korea, and Russia. Hiram Maxim's invention of the fully automatic machine gun in 1884 was decisive. "Whatever happens, we have got/ The Maxim Gun, and they have not," joked Poet Hilaire Belloc. Henry Labouchere, an anti-imperialist member of the British Parliament, parodied Rudyard Kipling's poem, "White Man's Burden," when he quipped, "Pile on the Brown Man's burden, and if ye rouse his hate, meet his old-fashioned reason with Maxims—up to date."

———◆———

In the race for empire, the Dutch ended up with only Indonesia, but what a prize it was! During 300 years of Dutch rule, the Indonesian archipelago became one of the world's richest colonial possessions. By 1860 a third of the Dutch state's annual revenue came from its East Indies colony, allowing the government to reduce domestic taxation and build the entire Dutch railway network. The Javanese, for their part, were reduced to rural bondage; on the east coast of Sumatra, "plantation laborers were regarded as 'coolie beasts' who needed to be 'tamed' through frequent beatings, whippings, and exorbitant cash fines," say Barwise and White. Tan Malaka, a teacher on Dutch estates in the early 1920s, said the colonies were "A land of gold, a haven for the capitalist class, but also a land of sweat, tears, and death, a hell for the proletariat."[24] The abuse prompted reprisals; several hundred Dutch were murdered by coolies every year. Islam was a source of resistance to European subjugation and the potent basis of an emerging independence movement in the early 1900s, when a "scramble for souls" ensued between Christian and Islamic missionaries. While many Islamic leaders were imprisoned, the Muslim movement grew in strength between the world wars and succeeded in liberating the islands three days after the Japanese surrendered.

The Dutch resisted for four years, but finally relinquished sovereignty to a federal Indonesian government in 1949. During the first nationwide elections in 1955, the Muslim community's insistence that Indonesia become an Islamic state was divisive. Radical Muslim groups are still pushing for Islamic law, but so far moderate Muslim opposition—only one-third of the country's Muslims actually practice their religion—has prevailed. Indonesia measures 3,200 miles from end to end, and has 6,000 habitable islands, and 225 million people. There are at least 300 ethnic groups and as many distinct languages. When Suharto's twenty-two-year-old rule was brought to an end, making way for the first democratically elected regime in more than forty years, the "steely controls he used to cap social unrest" were also gone, says social observer Tracy Dahlby.[25] Java has two-thirds of Indonesia's population and Jakarta's role as the center of politics, finance, and communications fuels the resentment of outlying provinces, such as oil-rich Riau in east-central Sumatra and Irian Jaya, which have much of Indonesia's wealth. The government has brutally executed thousands of tribal minorities, seized their lands, and displaced them through resettlement schemes that upset traditional subsistence patterns. Pledged reforms to contain the legal system's notorious corruption, clean up the banking system, beset by scandals, and distribute the country's wealth more equitably are slow in coming. Since the Asian economic collapse of 1997, Indonesia's infant mortality rate has doubled and a third of children under five are malnourished.

Separatist movements and religious conflicts boil in many parts of the island nation, including Aceh, on the northern tip of Sumatra; Ambon City in
the Moluccas; Ternate; Sulawesi; and Bali, where Muslim extremist bombings
in 2002 are blamed on the Al Qaeda-linked Jemaah Islamiah network. East
Timor claimed its independence on May 20, 2002, after decades of struggle,
but now the 800,000-person nation is fighting with Australia over control of
the oil and gas revenues of the East Timor Sea. Activists claim that East Timor
already paid back the aid it has received ten times over since 1999, when a UN
multilateral force kicked Indonesia off the island. Indonesia had ceded oil
rights to Australia in exchange for Australia's recognition of its sovereignty in
East Timor, the only government to do so. Outside firms prefer to play ball
with Australia, which demands only 30 percent of oil revenues compared to
the 40 percent asked by East Timor, the poorest country in East Asia. Forty
percent of its inhabitants live under the poverty line and half are unemployed.
Indonesia's "scorched earth" withdrawal destroyed the country's infrastructure
and "reduced the country to a smoking rubble," according to a World Bank
advisor. Australia's Green Party senator Bob Brown told the press, "The Australian government is saying on the one hand that East Timor has to stop its
dependency on aid and get on its own two feet, but on the other hand, we are
going to take the resource that [provides] the revenues to build schools, to
build hospitals, to pave roads, to have security." Indonesia gained control of
Irian Jaya (western New Guinea), with the world's largest copper and gold
mines, in 1963. Since 1998 the region has made its desire for independence
from Indonesia explicit.

In 2001 Anthony Lake, one-time head of President Bill Clinton's foreign
policy team, identified Indonesia as one of the world's top five "hot spots" with
problems that could lead to large-scale global disruption.[26] Indonesia is critical
to the global future because it is the world's fourth most populous country
(219 million people) and the largest Muslim nation. Indonesia "sits astride
crucial sea lanes in Southeast Asia," through which half of the world's maritime shipping passes, Lake says, and controls huge investments from American and other foreign oil companies. Some suspect that Suharto's old cronies
are fueling the flames of Christian-Muslim resentment to discredit the government and regain control over the country's enormous resources. Indonesia's internal crises are limiting the Association of Southeast Asian Nation's
ability to deal with regional crises, drawing the UN and the United States into
the vacuum. If it collapses, millions of marginalized minorities will become
desperate refugees. In the meantime, they are losing their jobs as foreign investment and employers pull out to avoid fall-out from the backlash.

HIV/AIDS promises to worsen Indonesia's governance crisis. According to AIDS activist Elizabeth Pisani, Indonesia "has one of the fastest growing epidemics in the world," with rapidly escalating infection rates among prostitutes and injecting drug users. Indonesia has all the ingredients that sparked AIDS growth in Thailand in the 1980s, including a booming sex industry, high STD rates, large numbers of migrants, and low condom use. The country's minister of religion has called for Indonesia's two major Islamic organizations to initiate dialogue about promoting condom use and clean needles, saying that AIDS was an "emergency" and "under Islamic law if there is an emergency, you can change the rules."[27]

Indonesia's Irian Jaya state borders independent Papua New Guinea, which occupies the island's other half. Formerly under British control from 1884 until 1906, when Britain handed over responsibility to newly independent Australia. Papua New Guinea became independent in 1975 and immediately geared up to defend itself from Indonesian takeover. The government was also embroiled in quelling an insurrection on Bougainville Island, where embittered locals vowed to secede because they received no share of the revenues from the Australian-owned Panguna copper mine that was destroying their island. Conflict ended in 1998 but was followed by drought and a series of tsunamis on the Papua New Guinea's north coast. The country's severe terrain challenges political unity, economic development, and the provision of services to its 4.8 million people. Its economy is growing rapidly, but so is the population, most of whom subsist as illiterate, nonmonetarized tribal hunter-gatherers. In 1987 HIV hit Papua New Guinea's capital of Port Moresby and took off rapidly in a population that already had an extremely high STD rates and tuberculosis. There are 8,000 known HIV cases, but the actual number is estimated to be 50,000 to 100,000. HIV is also increasing rapidly on the Pacific islands, historically vulnerable to "virgin soil" epidemics, including waves of sexually transmitted diseases throughout the eighteenth and nineteenth centuries brought by their first European contacts.[28] Most gained independence in the 1970s, although the French still hang on to several island groups.

—◦—

Besides grabbing the Indian subcontinent, Britain took control of Ceylon (present-day Sri Lanka), Burma (present-day Myanmar), Malaysia, parts of Brunei, and a few Pacific islands; held a six-year suzerainty over Tibet; and concluded an alliance with Nepal. Britain's divide-and-conquer strategy had much the same effect on the rest of its colonies as it had in India, creating or reinforcing permanent animosities that made subsequent nation building difficult or impossible. Sri Lanka is still plagued by internal civil war between the Buddhist Sinhalese who first settled the island in 500 B.C. and Hindu Tamils, brought to the island between 1870 and 1930 when the Sinhalese refused to be indentured laborers on British tea plantations. Ethnic strife has strained the economy since independence in 1948, when the first prime minister's Sinhala-only campaign brought power to lower-class Sinhalese, left out by the British, but excluded Tamils. Open hostilities broke out between the island's 13.5 million Sinhalese and its 3 million Tamils, and claiming more than 100,000 lives since 1993. Years of fighting have threatened social sector improvements that gave Sri Lanka one of the best education and healthcare records in South Asia, along with the island's aspirations to become South Asia's financial center. High literacy and the status of women, however, have kept AIDS relatively low.

In Myanmar, however, the epidemic is full blown, fueled by conflicts with ethnic minorities and governance crises originating in colonial times. Although smaller than India, Burma was a much harder conquest for the British. It took them sixty-one years and two wars to pull the country into Raj, and they never succeeded in conquering the Hill Tribes (Shan, Kachin, Karen, Chin, Mon, and Rakine), allied as the autonomous Frontier States of "Outer Burma." At the time of conquest in 1885, Burma was fabulously wealthy—there was said to be more gold on the central stupa of Yangoon's Shwedagon Pagoda than in the Bank of England; the golden orb at its peak is studded with more than 4,000 diamonds topped by a 76 carat stone—and it was a highly cultivated society that thoroughly resented Britain's exploitation. At the outbreak of World War II, the Burmese allied themselves with Japan against their former colonial masters but later switched sides to help the British eject the Japanese, who had proven even more burdensome. Burma gained its independence in 1948, but continuous rebellion by the Hill Tribes led to takeover by a hard-line military regime in 1962. Chaos has reigned ever since, and much of the violence centers on control of the drug trade built by the British. In 1987 and 1988 massive demonstrations against twenty-five years of hardship and repression were brutally quashed by the regime, which gunned down thousands of students, declared martial law, suspended the constitution, and unilaterally changed Burma's name to the Union of Myanmar. When the opposition National League for Democracy (NLD), led by Nobel Prize winner Aung San Suu Kyi, won the 1989 election, the military refused to give up power and NLD leaders have been repeatedly jailed or put under house arrest.

Serious human rights abuses prevail, including murder and rape. Many people have died in service to the army as conscripted porters, and hundreds of thousands, perhaps millions, of ordinary Myanmar citizens are forced to "contribute" their labor to construction projects in the country. One of these is the reconstruction of the ancient capital city of Pagan, one of the most dazzling cities Marco Polo described in his travels. Thousands of villagers have been forcibly evicted to make room for hotels built with the cooperation of western investors. The junta is rapidly rebuilding old temples from the ground up in bright red brick, along with a 200-foot observation tower that dwarfs all but one temple, resulting in what one archaeologist calls the Disneyfication of the ancient city. When the UN's cultural organization, UNESCO, withdrew Pagan's designation of as a World Heritage Site because of these activities, millions of dollars of support and expertise were lost. An agreement with the UN's International Labor Organization (ILO) to end forced labor was suspended in May 2003 after government-backed groups attacked an NLD convoy, and citizens cooperating with the ILO were sentenced to death for high treason according to Amnesty International.

The ILO reports that forced labor is common in ethnic minority settlements on Myanmar's borders with Thailand and Bangladesh. Many minorities have fled to Thailand, where they have settled permanently in refugee camps. The Rohingyas, a Muslim ethnic minority living in the Rakhine state on the Bangladesh border, have repeatedly sought asylum from summary executions, rape, torture, and harsh forced labor. The Bangladesh government claims they are "economic migrants," while Myanmar's government claims the Rohingyas are illegal Bangladeshi migrants. Although they are not recognized as an official ethnic group under Myanmar's 1982 constitution, Rohingyas voted and ran for office in the 1990 elections. In 1995, the UN High Commission on Refugees persuaded Myanmar to issue temporary registration cards to the Rohingyas, but they cannot travel outside their villages even for emergency medical care or work. They pay to register births and pregnant women must have their photos taken. As one Rohingya said, "We Muslims now live inside a cage."[29] The army has settled on confiscated land and conscripts villagers to build them houses, provide food, tend their livestock, and bring firewood and water. Rohingya land has been taken for fish and shrimp farms and commercial rice fields and plantations, and to resettle retired civil servants and ethnic minorities from other areas. Taxes are routinely collected from Rohingyas but not from Buddhist Rakhines.

With hard shoves from China and Thailand, annoyed with border problems and the disruption created by Burma's drug mafia, Myanmar's new prime minister promised a constitutional convention in August 2004. The military regime faces other intractable problems. The economy is in shambles, except for the drug trade, and most foreign assistance has dried up. According to Johns Hopkins epidemiologist Chris Beyrer, the HIV/AIDS epidemic is the worst in Asia and Myanmar "is perhaps the most likely to become like an African country in terms of the spread of the virus," citing government denial, the collapsing health sector, an unclean blood supply, injecting drug use, a growing sex industry, the underpaid and undereducated army, and internal refugees as contributing factors.[30] Ninety percent of Burmese drug users are HIV-infected, the highest rate ever reported anywhere.

One former British colony, Malaysia, has so far managed to escape the crushing burden of HIV/AIDS, largely because it took a hard line on drug trafficking in the 1970s. Britain grabbed control of peninsula of East Malaya from the Dutch in 1795; island Malaya came into British hands through the exploits of Sir James Brooke. The colony was famous for its tin mines and plantations, and also controlled shipping and trade through the Malaka Straits. Although Britain regained control after World War II, communist guerillas who had resisted Japanese occupation ousted the British and gained independence in 1957. In 1963 Singapore, primarily Chinese, joined East and West Malaya to form the Malaysian Federation but withdrew two years later because of growing ethnic tension. In 1969 riots between the Malays (60 percent of the population, primarily Muslim) and Chinese (25 percent, Buddhist) led to a twenty-two-month suspension of Malaysia's parliament, but the country's relative prosperity, high education levels, and a thousand-year-old history of positive ethnic interaction helped sooth ethnic differences. Islam is the national religion but the federal constitutional monarchy did not adopt Islamic law.

Malaysia's prosperity—it is one of the fastest-growing Asian markets for BMWs and other luxury automobiles—is based on an expanding industrial sector, concentrated in West Malaysia, which gave the country an 8 to 9 percent annual growth rate from 1987 to 1997. Migrants from all over Asia are attracted to its job market, but in 2002 more than 400,000 Indonesians and Filipinos working in mines, factories, and domestic service were expelled from the country. Some 100,000 Indonesian women still work as maids in Malaysian households, where incidents of "maid abuse" are so frequent they prompted riots in 2001. The abuse has become so severe—in May 2004 *Asia Pacific News* reported a Kuala Lumpur woman arrested for beating, burning, and pouring boiling water on a teenager who found shelter in the Indonesian embassy after displaying scars from five years of bondage—the government of Malaysia has signed a Memorandum of Understanding with Indonesia to oversee the training, recruitment, and employment of domestic maids by the end of 2004. Malaysia's HIV/AIDS epidemic has been contained to injecting drug users and sex workers by good health care, high education levels, strong employment, and the relatively high status of women.

The Sultanate of Brunei, wealthy from 1,000-year trade contacts with the Chinese, successfully fended off would-be colonialists until it lost half of its lands to James Brooke and to the British North Borneo Company, which annexed the island of Labuan as a coaling station on the India-China route in 1846. Happy as a British protectorate, the UN forced independence on Brunei in 1984, but a defense agreement with Britain has allowed the sultan to retain a battalion of Nepali Gurhkas and his sovereignty. When oil was discovered in 1929 at Seria, the sultan became the world's richest man. In May 1985 the Brunei National Democratic Party was allowed to register, "but oil-induced wealth has proved a formidable anesthetic to democracy."[31] Brunei's 250,000 people were "soothed by affluence." The island state of Singapore, whose population of four million is primarily Chinese, like Malaysia has controlled its drug trade and the incidence of HIV/AIDS.

———◆◆◆———

The French, relative latecomers to the race for Asia, made up for lost time by grabbing control of Vietnam, Cambodia, and Laos in the mid-1800s. Its colonies in Indochina were so fabulously lucrative that the French refused to let go until they were forced to do so by an international conference in 1954. By then France had convinced the United States, ridden with Cold War anti-Soviet paranoia, to bankroll its war for colonial restoration in North Vietnam by describing it as an anticommunist struggle. In the decade-long Vietnam War that began in 1965, the United States dropped five times the tonnage of bombs on Vietnam, Laos, and Cambodia than were dropped in all of World War II. In 2001 the United States was still spending more than $20 million a year on recovery operations in the three states.

French involvement in Indochina began when Louis XVI, at the request of Vietnam's nobility, sent 1,650 soldiers to reestablish royal rule in 1787. Between 1858 and 1885 the French conquered Vietnam and divided it into three parts, Cochinchina (the south), Tonkin (the north), and Annam (the center). Having already established a protectorate over Cambodia, the French brought Laos into the Union Indo-Chinoise as a safety net against British expansion from Burma, and the three territories were united as French Indochina in the 1890s. Opium, rubber, and rice plantations made the French rich while most of their subjects lived very marginal lives. After World War I, Ho Chi Minh, under the tutelage of China's Mao Zedong, began organizing the impover-

ished peasants. The Japanese withdrawal after World War II left a power vacuum and the communists seized control in the north in 1945. They battled
with the French and gained control of the North when the country was divided at the 17th parallel by the international conference. In the South, the
French transferred power to the United States instead of a Vietnamese successor state. In Laos the French passed power to the conservative elite who were
immediately challenged by communist insurgents. French control had already
passed back to Cambodia's monarch in 1953, who played off American and Soviet interests to keep Thais and Vietnamese at bay until the war in Vietnam
spilled over to Cambodian soil in the 1970s.

At the close of their war with the Americans in 1975, Vietnam was a politically united state but it had been shattered in every other respect. Following the example and advice of their northern big brother, the Soviet
Union—history dictated Vietnam's resistance to an alliance with communist
China—centralized socialist planners bogged Vietnam down for the next ten
years. In 1986, Vietnam's communist party made the fortunate decision to
begin living in the present and liberalized Vietnam's economy, opening the
country up to foreign trade and investment. Not only has the country's economy zoomed, but social development has not been neglected and enormous
gains have been realized in literacy, health services, nutrition, and poverty al-
leviation. Vietnam did not abandon the positive legacies of socialism,
women's rights and children's entitlements, so all citizens enjoy the bounties
of the Party's mandate from heaven.

Unfortunately, the Vietnamese chose to deal with their terrible post-war
legacy of injecting drug use by adopting communism's "social evils" approach
to containing HIV/AIDS, and imprisoning drug users and sex workers in rehabilitation centers. As in China, confinement was no solution, and Vietnam's
epidemic is now increasing at the rate of 7 percent per year.[32] HIV has spread
into rural areas from the country's major cities and along its borders with
Cambodia and China. Half of all new cases are among 20- to 29-year-olds, and
more than three-quarters of all new infections are heterosexual, as more
women are infected by their husbands. In a 2002 survey, 66 percent of the
pregnant women interviewed who were afraid of becoming HIV-infected were
afraid of infection by their husbands.[33] One-third of all men who have sex with
men in Vietnam are bisexual or heterosexual, and 55 percent said they had either paid someone or had been paid for sex. As in other countries of the region, widespread temporary or seasonal migration is also a critical factor in
epidemic's spread. The Ministry of Health says there are 130,000 Vietnamese
currently infected and that the number could rise to 1 million by 2010. In

2004 the United States and Vietnamese militaries announced that they were strengthening cooperation for HIV prevention, and the country was also chosen as the last of fifteen in the U.S. president's special $15 billion global AIDS initiative, the only country selected in Asia.

The devastation of Cambodia began at the end of the Vietnam War, when Pol Pot's communist Khmer Rouge killed at least 1.7 million people in three years. Southeast Asia's former colonial powers made no effort to stop the bloodbath, but in 1979 a Vietnamese invasion forced Pol Pot's revolutionaries into the countryside. They ended the killing, but touched off another twenty years of fighting. UN-sponsored elections in 1993 led to the formation of a coalition government, and in 1998 after a second national election and the surrender of the remaining Khmer Rouge forces, political stability returned. Cambodia is now a multiparty democracy under a constitutional monarchy, but its post-conflict legacy is nightmarish. Under Pol Pot, the educated urban middle class had been systematically tortured and executed and the health, transportation, and educational infrastructure was destroyed. Cambodia's economy registered slight growth in 1999, the first full year of peace in thirty years, and the country has achieved between 5 and 6 percent growth each year since then. Foreign investors are still cautious, however, because of governmental corruption and the potential for renewed instability. Cambodia's history of civil violence had one positive outcome, however. The country is one of the few Southeast Asian states where injecting drug use has not yet played a major role in the epidemic. Also—perhaps because of their extreme fragility— Cambodia is one of the few countries in Souteast Asia where the government has had the commitment to make HIV/AIDS prevention work. In the mid-1990s, when the government learned that three-quarters of the police and military and two-fifths of male students reported using sex workers, it instituted a "100 percent condom use" policy among brothel-based sex workers that stopped the spread of the epidemic into the general population.

By contrast, leaders in Cambodia's northern neighbor, Laos, seemed to have their head buried in the sand. After winning independence from the French, the country was plunged into twenty years of civil war between royalists and communists backed respectively by the United States and Vietnam. It bore the brunt of U.S. bombing raids during the Vietnamese War, and when the Lao People's Democratic Republic was proclaimed by the communists in 1975, some 350,000 refugees, most of them Hmong who had served as U.S.-funded irregulars, fled. Communist leadership slowed the country's development until 1986, when Laos followed Vietnam's lead and began encouraging private enterprise and economic decentralization. Growth has averaged 7 percent per year since that time, but the base was so low that most of the population still lives in poverty with marginal health and education services. Life expectancy is 54 years, more than half the population is illiterate, and 80 percent of the country's six million people still earn their living from agriculture.

More than 30 percent of Lao citizens are classified as "ethnic minorities," including many hill tribes. The majority (68 percent) are Buddhist Lao Loum—Lao of the Valleys. The Lao Theung—Lao of the Mountainsides— (upland areas, 22 percent) and the Lao Soung—Lao of the Mountaintops— (highland areas, 9 percent) were once contemptuously called *ka*, or slaves. Through the 1990s, government relocation killed up to 30 percent of some re-settled groups, and their children are still being sent to "ethnic minority boarding schools" to speed cultural assimilation. Over the past few years, relo-cated tribal people have been allowed to return home and the government is building infrastructure to service the remote areas of the country.

Unfortunately, this policy reversal has opened remote parts of the country to the spread of HIV/AIDS. Udomxai in northern Laos, for example, finds it-self at the intersection of super north-south and east-west highways being constructed with the Asian Development Bank funding to connect southern Chinese cities to the Southeast Asian capitals. It is rapidly being transformed from a sleepy market town into a frontier "hot spot," where truckers and con-struction workers meet pretty, young, impoverished, and uneducated girls from surrounding Hill Tribes who come to town to sell sex. The government has no money for HIV/AIDS prevention campaigns or testing. David Fein-gold, an anthropologist and Hill Tribe expert, says "there is the potential for some of these groups to be both physically and culturally wiped out." When a condom education campaign was conducted in Udomxai, truckers began to stop at small restaurants outside the city, looking for "clean" girls who did not ask them to use condoms. Drivers might have more than one "minor wife" along their route, creating liaisons with families who accept regular stipends for their daughters' services. Highway construction also promises to spread the disease through northern Thailand from the Chinese border along High-way 3, which will replace a dirt track hacked through precipitous jungle moun-tainsides and lined with untouched Hill Tribe villages for most of its length. It has been designated as a major China-Thailand corridor, and small armies of construction workers are arriving to begin work.

In other parts of the country, seasonal migration is spreading HIV/AIDS. Rice farmers surrounding Luang Prabang, the former northern capital turned tourist city, make extra money selling sex to tourists in the dry season. A boom-ing sex industry in Vientiane involves girls and boys as young as 10. Rice farmers from around Savanahket in central Laos were the first to realize the benefits of migration across the Mekong to Thailand, and the area now has the country's largest number of HIV-infected people. Stark differences in standards of living between rich Thailand and poor Laos draw at least 100,000 Laos to work in Thailand each year, and migrant workers account for 35 percent of total HIV cases, the highest of all occupational categories. Migration, however, is still officially banned by the Lao government, so the young people get no AIDS education before they leave and no help when they return infected. Laos also sells timber and 80 percent of its hydroelectric power, worth over $30 million each year, to Thailand, although most Lao homes still lack electricity.

Vietnam built roads from Savannakhet to Da Nang on the South China Sea in the late 1980s to bring in gasoline from the Soviet Union, and in exchange took Lao teak and rosewood. Standing outside a small lunch spot on the highway toward Vietnam, my vision is blurred by the log truck after log truck hauling valuable tropical hardwoods to Vietnam. They are paying Laos' unfinished debt with the relentless outflow of its ancient rain forests, contributing to massive deforestation, soil erosion, and the loss of life and livelihood for upland Laos and other minority groups. In 2001 the Australian mining company Oxiana Ltd. received generous tax concessions from the Lao government to develop gold and copper mines in exchange for 2.5 percent of the mines' earnings. Laos's inexperience with these types of ventures meant that investigation into their environmental and social impact was minimal. AIDWatch, an international watchdog organization, says that "mines characteristically leave a massive legacy both environmentally and socially," and that "no mine has ever avoided leaking cyanide-laced water and waste into the ecosystem."[34] Cyanide is used to extract gold from its ore. Waste earth is being dumped on villagers' land, threatening endangered species in a nearby river, and the water table is dropping. Oxiana made no agreement to recruit locally or to control the influx of outside labor, and two villages have already been moved although no compensation was provided to the farmers, says AIDWatch.

———◦◆◦———

Thailand, one of the world's few HIV/AIDS success stories, is also one of a handful of developing countries that have never been colonized. While close to 1 million Thais have been infected (in a population of 58 million) and 300,000 have died, a vigorous "100 percent condom" campaign enforced in the nation's licensed brothels turned a skyrocketing epidemic on its ear. Thanks to the campaign, the proportion of Thai men visiting sex workers dropped from 25 to 10 percent in under a decade. Although the epidemic slowed, Thailand still has 695,000 HIV-positive people, about 2 percent of its men and 1 percent of its women, and 30,000 new infections occur annually. About 50,000 Thais die from AIDS each year, a number expected to remain constant through 2006. Thailand's excellent public health system provides voluntary counseling and testing and public education to its highly literate population. The government was one of the first to institute prevention of mother-to-child transmission countrywide through its clinics and hospitals that put a stop to virtually all vertical transmission. It has implemented antiretroviral treatment nationwide and manufactures its own generic anti-AIDS drugs. However, prevention among intravenous drug users has not been totally successful, and the proportion becoming HIV positive has increased. Infection rates are highest in the north and in Bangkok, and there are undocumented sex workers, many from the Hill Tribes. More recently, the "100 percent condom use" requirement of Thai law for brothel-based sex workers has driven casual sex into the workplace and school. Although these contacts occur with lower frequency than commercial contacts, they are largely unprotected.[35]

When the Chakri dynasty, which rules Thailand to this day, moved the government to Bangkok in 1782, a succession of King Ramas succeeded in evading the control of all would-be European invaders while carrying out a series of social reforms, including the abolition of slavery. They also modernized the government and transportation system. Forced by France to relinquish control over Cambodia and Laos, Siam allied itself with Britain in World War I. At the beginning of World War II, Thailand allowed the Japanese to advance on the British-controlled Malay Peninsula, Singapore, and Burma, and in 1942 it declared war on Britain and the United States. At the war's end, Thailand was forced to return territory seized from Cambodia, Laos, and Malaya. Thailand's military controlled the country from 1932 until 1992, when a civilian government rode in on the back of massive public demonstrations. The monarchy continues, but rule is in the hands of a prime minister at the head of a majority coalition. Thailand enjoyed the world's highest growth rate from 1985 to 1995 and growth rebounded after the Asian financial crisis. Low unemployment draws many illegal migrants from surrounding countries and makes Thailand's economy critical to Southeast Asia as a whole. With a population of close to 65 million people, its sophisticated cosmopolitan society has achieved below replacement-level fertility and a life expectancy of 71 years. Thailand has high levels of school attendance and literacy, but for some Thai minorities, access to social benefits and services is restricted.

A crackdown on drugs in February 2003 resulted in the deaths of 2,000 suspects by the end of April. The deaths were blamed on criminal gangs, but human rights groups say they were encouraged by government authorities.[36] Extrajudicial killings and the blacklisting of offenders accused of being "security threats" sent injecting drug users into hiding and increased syringe sharing because of the shortages. The "war on drugs" became an attack on small-time users rather than a consistent effort to eliminate major dealers and thugs. Thailand is a relatively minor producer of opium, heroin, and marijuana, but it is an international transit point for heroin from Myanmar and Laos and a major center for drug money laundering. Southern Thailand is emerging as an operational and logistic beachhead for violent transnational Islamic movements. Its porous maritime border "makes it a logical staging point for external jihadists seeking alternative operational hubs in South East Asia," says expert Andrew Holt.[37] Black market activities, central to the economy of these provinces, include gambling, gun running, human trafficking, prostitution, and drug smuggling by criminal gangs.

◆•◆•◆

Colonial powers turned their "white man's burdens" into profitable enterprises that carried their own economies to much high standards of living while Asian economies stagnated. The deliberate economic, social, and economic distortions that were the hallmark of the colonial period created entrenched and widespread poverty, massive illiteracy, and almost continual violence that has ended only recently if at all. The last of Asia's great "nomadic invasions"— the incursions of European colonial powers—was a time of brutality, peasant rebellions, and unendurable poverty from which states in South and Southeast Asia are just now raising their heads. The vision of enlightened leadership has lifted many from poverty, but in many states an age-old Asian leadership pattern re-emerged. The "avaricious elite" reaps the benefits of colonial disorder, while the benefits of new economic growth bypasses the lower classes, leaving income distribution badly skewed and many groups totally disenfranchised.

The breakdown of traditional communities leaves many people vulnerable, especially minority ethnic groups, women, and young people, whose status declined under colonial rule. In most states these groups have been the last to benefit from postcolonial growth. As a result they have been driven into sex work and the drug industry, increasing their vulnerability to HIV/AIDS. The position of women has risen in some states along with rising economies, but in many, women's position is as poor as ever, with women placed in a perpetual bondage of human degradation, a subject treated more fully in chapter 6. Young people have suffered from lack of education and employment, and are especially vulnerable to HIV/AIDS infection, a topic taken up in chapter 7. But the colonial powers broke the backs of all their Asian subject states in a way that was much more harmful and has an even more direct link to the epidemic and to the spread of HIV/AIDS around the world, a subject taken up in the next chapter.

Historian Tim Harper says that one of Southeast Asians' most powerful personality traits, "present-mindedness" or "a willingness to embrace and act upon new things," stems from their historical middleman position in the East. Southeast Asians have been able to interact with the modern world economy more easily than some of their larger and more culture-bound neighbors. Throughout history Southeast Asian tenacity and resourcefulness has helped small countries deal with, tolerate, and even defeat much larger countries. Thailand and Cambodia have demonstrated this resourcefulness against the largest enemy they have ever faced—HIV/AIDS—and Vietnam looks as if it may follow suit. If so, they will be three of only five developing countries—along with Senegal and Uganda in Africa—that have vanquished HIV/AIDS as well as their colonial past.

FIVE

ASIA AND THE WORLD DRUG INDUSTRY

BINH LIFTED HIS HEAD AND LOOKED AT RAGEENA with his one good eye. "I wasn't trafficked," he said, "but I began selling myself to other men when my habit got bad. I was weak and couldn't drive my *tuk-tuk*"—he looked at the puzzled faces and laughed—"you know, my taxi—anymore. After I started using heroin, I never felt much like working at anything."

Molly looked at the handsome boy—well, half of his face was handsome—and wondered what had happened. The right side of his face looked as if it had been burned. Maybe they used kerosene for cooking in Vietnam, too, she thought. She'd seen some pretty nasty burns from cooking fires in Africa. "Drug use isn't common in Africa—at least not injecting heroin," she said. "People use *bangi*—that's marijuana—and young guys use *khat*, the stuff that looks like sticks but keeps you up all night if you chew on it. Why do so many young people in Asia use heroin?"

"Heroin is so cheap, a lot cheaper than alcohol, and there are a lot of dealers pushing it, even offering it free the first time to get you hooked. I was an addict by the time I turned 14," Binh said. "I started using in 2001. I'd come to Ho Chi Minh City from my parents' farm, more than 300 miles away. I stayed on the street for a while, looking for work, but I was getting discouraged. A man approached me one evening and said he could offer me a place to sleep at his house. He said that his wife wouldn't mind. It didn't take me long to realize he didn't have a wife—at least not a female one—and I didn't have a job, so he started paying me for sex. One time he shared his heroin with me. After a while I found a street gang and stayed with them instead, so we didn't see each other very often, but I think I got my habit and my HIV from that man. I began roaming the streets with my gang. We took odd jobs and sometimes helped ourselves to people's money.

"We defended ourselves against the older kids and the local communist party. They tried to round us up and put us in rehabilitation centers," he said, "if you can call them that. Nobody gets rehabilitated from anything in those places—not the addicts, not the sex workers. The detention center I went to near Ho Chi Minh City housed about 1,200 boys and men in a space built for 750. We were locked in the health unit until we detoxed, and then they put us to work. We had to grow our own food and work on the roads. The old guys hit on us for sex, and there were plenty of drugs to be had in the place if you didn't mind sharing needles. What addict ever minds that if that's the only way he can get high? I got drugs, but I hated the place. I can remember just counting the days, hours, and minutes until I got out, and the minute I did, I found some friends of mine that were on the street and got a hit from them within an hour."

Vladimir looked up. "I did the same thing. I was on the street, then in prison, then on the street, then back in prison. You know how it goes." He laughed. "But in Russia, prison was much, much worse. We couldn't grow our own food—too cold for that. I lost ten kilos in the first month. By the time I came out, I was being treated for tuberculosis, but the drugs didn't work, so they put me in a hospital and finally found some drugs that worked. Prison was rough. I was raped by the older guys—they didn't know I was HIV positive, and I wasn't going to tell them. They were gangsters, and you should have heard their stories about running women, drugs, and guns. Even big weapons." He looked at Binh, "By the way," he asked, "what happened to your face? Did somebody throw acid on it or something? That's what the big dealers used to do to us if we didn't pay them."

Binh touched his face and shook his head sadly. "Our dealers never wasted any acid on us. They just put us to work as prostitutes so we could keep paying them. No. I caught herpes and it spread to my face. I didn't have any money to pay for drugs—to fix it, I mean—and by the time I could pay for a doctor, it took my eye."

Molly winced. "Wasn't there anyone there to help you?"

"My parents and family all rejected me when they learned I was HIV positive," Binh told her. "And the government was more interested in rounding us up. They called us social evils because we took drugs and most of us were sex workers, too. I had women customers," he smiled, "but mostly men. At least I used to. When I lost half my face, they weren't so interested any more. That's when I went to the Friends Helping Friends center. They were mostly old guys who had become addicted during the Vietnam War, but they let me come to their meetings and one of them let me sleep in the center. They're all still addicts, but their children have to help them, so they're okay."

———•◆•———

Each time he visited, Wallace was stunned by the beauty of the Banda Islands, which were dominated by the regal profile of an active 1,800-foot volcano thrusting up from the bottom of the turquoise Banda Sea. At its peak were silver and white clouds created by disturbance of the wind flow that made him feel that it was about to erupt. "Almost every year there is an earthquake here," reported Wallace, "and at intervals of a few years very severe ones, which throw down houses and carry ships out of the harbor bodily into the streets." The Bandas, he knew, had earned their nickname, the "Jewels of the Moluccas," for a different reason than their sheer beauty. They had been the source of the Indies' wealth, nutmeg, and mace, over which the Dutch established control in the seventeenth century. By the time Wallace visited 120 years later, traveling on the regular Dutch steamers he used to tour much of colonial Indonesia, Banda was a highly cultivated nutmeg "garden." It had been snatched by the Dutch from the control of the *orang kaya*, or "rich men," who had controlled the southern Spice Islands trading fraternity because they alone had vessels large enough to sail to the Asian mainland. Rather than trade with them, the Dutch provoked the *orang kaya* into armed resistance, and then systematically eliminated them. A few escaped but the majority were hung or decapitated by Japanese mercenaries. Fewer than 600 native Bandanese survived from a population of 15,000.

By the time Wallace arrived, there were not many wild specimens for him to collect and the only new bird he found was a pigeon that lived off a peach-sized fruit. When Wallace cracked it open, he saw that the shiny, dark brown seed (nutmeg) was encircled in a lacy net of bright crimson (mace). The pigeons dispersed the nutmeg seeds by swallowing the fruit whole so the seed passed undamaged through their gut. Thriving only on the Bandas, the nutmeg trees yielded two crops a year. The Dutch, who traded New York's Manhattan Island to the English for control of the tiny Bandas, harvested a billion guilders' worth of nutmeg and mace during two centuries of colonial rule. Wallace was silent about the slavery that still existed on the islands when he visited, voicing his approval of the Dutch state monopoly which allowed them to fund education and bring a "civilizing influence" to the unruly natives. He argued that monopoly of nutmeg production, not essential to native survival, kept it out of the hands of rapacious and exploitative business interests. The Dutch monopoly had been undercut by corruption in Banda and Amsterdam, and they handed the plantations back to their native owners less than a decade after his visit. By then, the French, who had smuggled nutmeg seeds to its Mauritius plantations, dominated the trade and the Bandanese farmers were unable to compete. Twenty years after Wallace's visits, a new generation of *orang kaya* had emerged who earned their living in the same way Wallace had, by collecting wild specimens. Unlike Wallace, however, these new entrepreneurs harvested the birds of the islands to near-extinction to meet the demand of European milliners for 50,000 skins from Birds of Paradise and other exotic species each year.

Wallace collected only one or two examples of each species he encountered in the Malay Archipelago. In six years, he logged 14,000 miles on sixty to seventy separate journeys through the islands, covering an area equivalent to the continental United States and collecting 125,660 specimens, all of which were meticulously prepared and cataloged, then shipped to European scientific institutions.[1] While Darwin studied, theorized, and experimented in relative luxury, supported by inherited wealth, Wallace had to work. He was a mere "fly catcher" who filled the time between collecting expeditions philosophizing about changes in species. Fourteen years Darwin's junior, the upstart collector was inspired by Darwin's *Voyage of the Beagle* and William Edward's *A Voyage Up the River Amazon* to begin his career in natural history as a commercial venture in 1848 at the age of 25. Wallace came from a working-class background, and when his father died he and his older brothers supported their mother and younger siblings by teaching, surveying, and construction. Largely self-educated, Wallace and his brother John had developed an early passion for insect collecting. When their livelihoods from the English building trades lagged in 1847, they resolved "to go abroad into more or less wild countries," leaving the competitive and crowded business of British surveying to seek their fortunes on other continents. Three years later, Alfred was in the Amazon and John was in the California goldfields.

Although Wallace lost much of his South American specimens in a freak fire that destroyed the vessel he'd chosen for his return to England, he made enough to consider another collecting expedition in Asia. He was inspired by a growing scientific curiosity as well as the need to make a living. Wallace had read Thomas Malthus's *Essay on the Principles of Population*, "the first work I had yet read treating of any of the problems of philosophical biology." In the work, Malthus described "checks on the increase of the savage races" (disease, accidents, war, famine), an idea that both Wallace and Darwin later applied to animal populations when they sought to explain how new species came into being and old ones declined. In Asia, Wallace knew he would find more evidence of the gradual change in plant and animal species he had witnessed first hand on his Amazonian expeditions.

His reputation in scientific biology had grown sufficiently to earn him a first-class complementary ticket from the Peninsular and Oriental Steam Navigation Company at the behest of the British Admiralty. He left Southampton in March 1854 on the P&O steamer *Euxine*, which took him via Gibraltar and Malta to Alexandria. In the days before the Suez Canal, passengers sailed from Alexandria to Cairo, then proceeded in a horse-drawn carriage across the desert to the north end of the Red Sea, changing horses every five miles. At Suez, Wallace boarded the steamer *Bengal*, which was faster and more comfortable than the *Euxine*. After a stop at Aden, the *Bengal* put in at Galle, an old Dutch port city south of Ceylon, and at Penang island in the straits of Malaka. Wallace arrived in Singapore on April 20, 1854, met James Brooke, and began collecting specimens in Sarawak. By 1855 he had written the first version of his law on species change and the 1858 paper he sent Darwin solidified his early ideas into a theory of evolutionary change. Wallace had initiated correspondence with Darwin in October 1856, and in his second letter told Darwin that he anticipated preparing a much fuller presentation of his theories when he returned to England and could access libraries and collections.

When Darwin received the package containing Wallace's complete 1858 essay, he kept it for some time before he sent it to Lyell on June 18, when he wrote that "all my originality [is] smashed. I never saw a more striking coincidence. If Wallace had my MS. Sketch written out in 1842, he could not have made a better short abstract! Even his terms now stand as heads of my chapters." In fact, Lyell told Wallace some years later that he preferred to use *On the Tendency of Varieties* over Darwin's *Origin of the Species* "because there are some points laid down more clearly than I can find in the work of Darwin itself." Darwin, desperate to preserve his "priority," wrote Lyell again a week later, offering to write a précis of his 1844 sketch, but confessed that "I cannot persuade myself that I can do so honorably. I cannot tell whether to publish now would not be base and paltry." Lyell contacted Hooker and together they devised the scheme of presenting both scientists' papers to the Linnean Society. "Both authors having now unreservedly placed their papers in our hands," their fate was laid before the "jury." Darwin's material, though incomplete, was presented first.

Fortunately, Wallace's paper was read in its entirety and transcribed into the proceedings, because the original disappeared from Lyell's correspondence.

The envelope in which Wallace had sent his paper from Ternate and eight letters he sent Darwin between 1856 and 1858 laying out other aspects of his theory also disappeared from Darwin's scientific correspondence. Darwin's son explained that he periodically destroyed old letters to create space for new ones. Darwin retained letters from other scientific contemporaries; was the gap part of a conspiracy by the scientific aristocracy of the day to protect Darwin's interests in this "delicate situation," as he characterized it to Hooker? After the Linnean Society meeting, Darwin wrote Hooker: "You must let me once again tell you how deeply I feel your generous kindness and Lyell's on this occasion; but in truth it shames me." Wallace preserved all of Darwin's replies to his letters, pleased to have corresponded with a man so esteemed by British science. Later in his life, he said that his greatest achievement had been to prompt Darwin to publish his own theory.

———◆•◆•◆———

Nutmeg and mace may have driven the first phase of European colonization in Asia, but it was a different "spice" entirely that drove the second phase of colonial exploitation in the nineteenth and twentieth centuries. This spice—traded by early Asian merchants as a medicine—was opium. Its cultivation and sale was at the heart of the European contest for control in Asia, and its commercialization and marketing as heroin around the world "is the culmination of four hundred years of Western intervention" in that region, according to international drug trafficking expert Alfred McCoy.[2]

By the fifteenth century, opium—cultivated in Persia, Egypt, the Middle East, and India where it is called *Mash allah*, "the work of god"—had become an established, widely used drug and an important trade item. Cultivation of opium poppies spread across Asia from the eastern Mediterranean and reached China via the Silk Road. It was an important source of revenue for India's Mogul empire, which encouraged extensive cultivation in Bengal and Maratha. Observing its widespread use by Indian laborers, Portuguese explorer Alfonso de Albuquerque wrote his king from India in 1513 advocating its cultivation in Portugal to keep the poor compliant. A century later the Dutch were making spectacular profits exporting 50 to 60 tons of Indian opium to Javanese villagers. It was the British and French, however, who "transformed opium from luxury good to bulk commodity" by introducing it to the Southeast Asian mainland where "state-licensed opium dens became a unique Southeast Asian institution, spreading and maintaining addiction," says McCoy. "In no other region of the world did so many governments promote mass drug abuse with such unanimity of means and moral certitude." British and French colonial administrators relied on the opium trade to finance their operations. In French Indochina, there were 125,200 addicts and more opium dens per capita than doctors. Even independent Siam earned 14 percent of its annual revenues from its 164,000 addicts, the largest group in the region by 1900. Most were immigrant Chinese, who consumed 84 tons of opium every year.

The commercial opium trade began with the Portuguese, who by the early seventeenth century were selling opium grown in India's western coastal province of Goa to the Chinese, displacing Muslim traders. Recreational use of the drug, mixed with tobacco and smoked in primitive "dens," was known in Dutch trading settlements in Java by 1610. The Dutch brought the practice to Taiwan in the middle of the 1600s, and when the Fukien Chinese took over the island, they brought the habit back to coastal China. By 1700, the Dutch were carrying Portuguese shipments of Indian opium through Macao into China so regularly that millions of Chinese had become addicted. Beijing issued its first edict banning the drug in 1729, flogging dealers and intermediaries and then executing them by strangulation. Unable to curb the trade, Peking imposed an import duty in 1753.

When the British East India Company took control of Calcutta and Bengal, Robert Clive excluded native, Dutch, and French merchants from the opium trade and industrialized it as a commercial venture by 1773. The Company contracted with the Bengal government to pay advances to cultivators, refined the raw opium to standard quality, and pressed it into uniform bricks stamped with the East India Company's mark. It also prohibited opium use in Bengal because it lowered productivity among the growers. The Company got around the British government's ban against the trade by selling opium to private exporters at auction in Calcutta. It now had a commodity the Chinese wanted to trade for tea and silk, already in high demand in Europe, and soon the Company's directors were realizing £500,000 annually from the trade. Profit margins were high. In 1800 when impoverished Bengali farmers threatened to quit growing poppies because their share was too low, Company agents forced them to continue. Britain's prime minister, concerned about depletion of British bullion for Chinese tea, overruled the British governor general's proposal to end the monopoly to improve the conditions of the growers. By this time, the Company had competition from the Portuguese in Goa and American commercial ships had begun trading Turkish opium in the Canton market. In 1819 the Company bought out the Portuguese, introduced poppy cultivation into fifteen new districts of India, and began collecting an export tax from other shippers. They were so efficient in expanding production that prices fell as output rose in the 1830s.

Opium was also very popular in other parts of the world. Throughout the 1700s, European and American physicians experimented so widely with the drug that by the end of the century it was being used to treat everything from the cough of a cold to the "vapors." By 1800 "a powerful international supply network was well established," says historian Richard Davenport-Hines, and throughout the 1800s opium became increasingly popular for recreational use in Europe and the United States.[3] The English poet Samuel Taylor Coleridge installed himself in the Highgate home of his physician in 1816 so his opium consumption could be regulated. Antislavery advocate William Wilberforce attributed the success of his public speaking to small doses of opium, Robert Clive used it to alleviate severe gallstones and chronic malaria, England's George IV became an addict while he was still Prince of Wales, and Frederick the Great of Prussia carried his opium pills in a small oval box around his neck. Physicians gave young women opium for menstrual cramps and prescribed it for morning sickness and "nerves" during pregnancy. It was used liberally in patent medicines, was prescribed to keep restless children quiet and induce sleep, and was even a popular way to commit suicide or murder. Drug use had long been associated with sexuality in romantic works like *The Count of Monte Cristo* and *L'education sentimentale*, and opiates were commonly prescribed to cure sexual problems, including excessive desire, masturbation, "hysteria" among young girls, and syphilis.

During the California gold rush of 1848, Chinese laborers, subject to harsh conditions as indentured mine workers, became regular opium smokers. Between 15 and 20 percent became so addicted they had no money for their return passage. The habit spread to their American bosses and to gamblers and prostitutes who patronized smoking "shops" in towns around the gold mines. From there it spread to the middle class, and the consumption of drugs quickly become a youthful rite of passage in the United States. During the late 1870s and early 1880s, middle-class teenagers rebelled against their parents by frequenting opium shops and disrupting their communities. Over the next thirty years, eleven states passed laws against opium smoking, forcing the habit underground. Other drugs gained popularity in its stead. While youthful opium addicts were being treated in the Philadelphia General Hospital in 1916, marijuana was being smoked by New Orleans and Chicago schoolchildren. Recreational use of drugs was not limited to the United States. In 1911 an English geography teacher, noticing that most of his elementary school class was dozing or asleep, learned that they had passed around a bottle of laudanum (liquid opium). Moscow opened a clinic for homeless young cocaine addicts in 1926, and when French writer Andre Gide visited Zurich in 1927, he remarked on the number of opium smokers and cocaine addicts he saw in the streets.

Hashish was introduced to Europe in 1801 by Napoleon's returning troops, who had picked up the practice from Egyptian laborers who were then consuming twenty to twenty-five tons of hashish each year. Marijuana, used in traditional healing and by laborers in many parts of the world to alleviate the strains of work, was also put to use to cure conditions as varied as sciatica, tetanus, asthma, bronchitis, flatulence, diabetes, rheumatism, and gout. Physicians revived exhausted soldiers with opium and cayenne in European and American conflicts. Opium poppies were cultivated by both sides during the American Civil War to treat dysentery, malaria, and diarrhea among the troops. Cocaine, popularized by black stevedores in New Orleans who sniffed it for energy while they worked, was distributed by employers to plantation workers in the American south, construction workers on public projects, and miners in Colorado, who became addicted and dependent on their work as a source for their habits. In the United States, cocaine was popularized through medical and military use; the dying president Ulysses S. Grant was treated with a mixture of brandy, morphine, and cocaine. The Coca-Cola Company had to remove it from their drink in 1901 when many states began prohibiting the drug, driving the cocaine trade underground.

In the late 1800s, other mind-altering substances developed by enterprising chemists emerged from the lab into popular use. Amyl nitrate was administered to women during pregnancy and childbirth, and the rush of blood it caused when inhaled popularized its use as a sexual stimulant. Homosexuals found it relaxed the anal sphincter, improving the experience of sodomy. The fact that many children were given the drug for asthma may have contributed to the epidemic of masturbation that so frightened late Victorians. Arsenic was also used for mood alteration and by women to clear their complexions. Popular stories about the virile and amorous arsenic eaters of southern Austria and northern Slovenia turned arsenic pills into the Viagra of the late 1800s. Peyote came into experimental use in the 1890s. Hypodermic syringes were perfected in the 1850s, raising levels of addiction. Morphine, the principal alkaloid of opium, was refined in quantity for use as a pain killer in the middle of the century. It was prescribed to help patients overcome their addictions to opium. Its popularity as a recreational drug was unwittingly abetted by physicians (many of whom were addicted themselves). Heroin was first concocted by an English chemist in 1874 by cooking morphine with acetic anhydride. When tests showed it was eight times more powerful than morphine as an analgesic, the medical establishment was more careful about its introduction. By the first decade of the 1900s, doctors had quickly become more conservative in their prescriptions and hospitals began restricting narcotics use.

By the late 1800s, opium use had been demonized as a feminizing, effete vice that reduced productivity and civic responsibility, but criminal prosecution occurred in only a few U.S. cities that banned its use. In Europe, as addiction to Indian opium grew, social reformers began raising public sentiment against Britain's colonial trafficking. Sir Stamford Raffles, Java's lieutenant governor, first protested the trade in 1817, saying that it had "struck deep into the habits and extended its malign influence to the morals of the people." He predicted that it "is likely to perpetuate its power in degrading their character and enervating their energies as long as the European governments, overlooking every consideration of policy and humanity, should allow a paltry addition to their finances to outweigh all regard to the ultimate happiness and prosperity of the country." Ironically, after the British colony of Singapore was established by Raffles in 1819, it earned half its revenues from its opium franchise.

In the 1830s a Swedish diplomat publicly denounced the British raj for enriching itself from the trade, which "poisoned" the Chinese and denigrated the Indians. Britain imported large quantities of Indian opium into Burma after it occupied the southern half of the country in 1852. The Shan state in northern Burma grew its own poppies, but the British bought out the warlords to reduce their production. The British administrator of India's Assam Province on the Burmese border lamented that migrant laborers brought from other parts of India to establish tea cultivation were being infected with "opium-mania—that dreadful plague which has depopulated this beautiful country, turned it into a land of wild beasts [and] has degenerated the Assamese from a fine race of people to the most abject, servile, crafty, and demoralized race in India." Opium had so "kept down the population" by addicting youths, who died or became crazed thief and murderers, that he despaired of having enough labor to grow tea. Administrators in Malaka reported that "excessive duties have increased the thirst for opium; and quadrupled the number of murders and other crimes committed in order to obtain the means of procuring the drug."

By the late 1700s, China had 300 million addicts. Fashionable among the rich and with mandarins, opium smoking was believed to deter homosexuality in young people. The trade quickly spread northward and westward from southern coastal provinces. In 1799 the Chinese government once again forbade the import or use of opium and the cultivation of poppies, but use had already spread to the poor. China was importing more than 2,000 tons of

Indian-grown British opium annually despite the ban and the number of habitual users had grown to ten million, many of them soldiers and government officials. In 1839 the emperor ordered his commissioner, Lin Zexu, to seize 1,500 tons of opium from British ships in the Pearl River Delta and destroy it in lime pits just north of Hong Kong.

Lin petitioned the English Queen to stop the trade, but Parliament voted for a punitive expedition to China despite William Gladstone's protest against "a war more unjust in its origin, a war more calculated in its progress to cover this country with permanent disgrace . . . Our flag is become a pirate flag to protect an infamous traffic." Gladstone, later Britain's prime minister, denounced Britain's Opium War with China as "unjust," saying that he stood "in dread of the judgements of God upon England for our national iniquity towards China." Gladstone may have been under the influence when he delivered his address, for he often took laudanum with his coffee to relax before he addressed the House of Commons. Britain and other Western powers forcibly occupied mainland concessions and Hong Kong was ceded to Britain in 1842. The opium trade flourished and imports doubled between 1830 and 1850. The government could not control imports or deter farmers from growing poppies in China. By 1870 Chinese opium growers were producing a drug so potent it could be smoked seven or eight times, compared to three times for the imported strains. Opium poppies were cultivated in all but two provinces by the mid-1880s; Szechuan and Yunnan were the two top producers. In 1890 the government decided to completely flout importers by making opium production legal in China.

In 1893, badgered by the Quaker businessman Sir Joseph Pease and his Society for the Suppression of the Opium Trade, Gladstone appointed a Royal Commission to investigate Britain's opium traffic. Testimony at the commission's London hearings in 1893 were overwhelmingly negative, so in India in the following year the commission stacked their public hearings with Indians willing to testify that suppression of the opium trade would cause another Sepoy Rebellion. They held no hearings in China or Malaysia at all. According to a contemporary journalist, the commission's report concluded that "everything is for the best in the best of all possible worlds . . . It is impossible to prohibit the use of opium in India, even if it was desirable, and it is not desirable." Britain's economy was as dependent on the opium trade as individual users were on the drug itself. The commission reported that "Oriental people" used opium judiciously for nervousness and fatigue and that "in many Oriental countries [opium is used] not as an idle or vicious indulgence, but as a reasonable aid in the work of life."

In 1881 French administrators in Saigon established Opium Regié, a state marketing monopoly, and the approach was adopted by all Southeast Asian states by 1900 except the Philippines, where Chinese opium "farms" thrived. To increase revenues, colonial governments forcibly spread sales to areas that resisted opium use, while businessmen paid their wages with it in plantations and mines. Unlicensed Chinese traffickers across Southeast Asia encouraged addiction with free samples. "The opium trade created a nexus of corruption that spanned the whole of Indies colonial society," says McCoy. "Opium dens were the centerpiece of [a] floating world of vice where gamblers, prostitutes, outlaws, and opium police congregated." By 1905, opium growth and sales were a significant proportion of colonial revenues in British Malaysia (53 percent), French Indochina (16 percent), and Dutch Indonesia (16 percent).

Siam's monarchy had legalized opium in 1851 and franchised opium distribution, lotteries, gambling, and alcohol to four Chinese concerns. With a ready market among Chinese immigrants in Bangkok, opium became a mainstay of royal finances. Siam had been importing Chinese laborers to construct canals across its central plains from the early 1700s, and by 1880 half of Bangkok's 1 million residents were Chinese immigrants. In 1908 King Chulalongkorn proclaimed that he would eliminate the trade, remarking that it "casts degradation upon every country where the inhabitants are largely addicted," but he worried over "the considerable shrinkage in the State revenues to be faced." By 1920 tax on opium sales constituted 20 percent of royal revenues. In 1928 the king established a royal monopoly that doubled imports to 180 tons to sustain Southeast Asia's largest population of addicts. In 1932 when the king again threatened to ban opium, Colonel Phibun Songkhram seized power and expanded opium production in northern Siam and Burma. In 1938 he became prime minister, changed Siam's name to Thailand, and began openly promoting poppy cultivation among the Hill Tribes to cut imports and control smuggling. Hill tribe farmers from Laos and Burma migrated to Thailand, but expanded poppy crops were insufficient and Siam still had to import most of its opium from India and Iran. When World War II cut these sources, Phibun agreed to support Japan in exchange for control of the Shan states in northeastern Burma. When Japan's fortunes declined, he allied with the Nationalist Chinese army in nearby Yunnan. Defeated by China's communist forces, they retreated into Burma and worked with the Thais to develop opium production, processing, and export. Their efforts bore fruit domestically and internationally. The number of Thailand's addicts increased from 110,000 in 1940 to 250,000 in 1970.

The opium trade had long flourished in neighboring Yunnan Province under control of Muslim merchants, known as Panthays, who marketed drugs, gold, gems, and tea over the caravan routes to India, Siam, and Laos. In 1856 they allied with the Hmong and Yao Hill Tribes and established an independent kingdom in Tali, a city 100 miles from Burma in Yunnan's western mountains. After fifteen years of fighting, the Chinese blasted through the Muslim fortress with modern guns and slaughtered Panthay, Hmong, and Yao defenders. Survivors fled into Burma but in the 1870s the Chinese attacked again, sending waves of opium farmers into Vietnam and Laos. When hostilities died down, the Muslim traders integrated the refugees into an overland trading network that stimulated opium production in the Golden Triangle (northern Thailand, Myanmar, Laos, northeast India, and parts of southern China). A British explorer crossing northeastern Burma in the 1890s saw "miles of slope covered with poppy . . . fields climb up steep ravines and follow the sheltered side of ridges." By 1935, Hill Tribe networks offered illicit opium at one-third of official rates, forcing Bangkok to cut its prices. To control prices on the official market, French Indochinese officials forced the Hmong to cut production and the British reduced production quotas from their licensed opium growers in Burma's Shan state. When Hill Tribe production was cut, opium growing surged in China and India.

Although the Vietnamese had outlawed opium in 1820, the French immediately established a state opium franchise when they took control of North Vietnam in 1858. Sales of Indian opium "put the new colony on a paying basis only six months after they annexed Saigon in 1862," McCoy says. In 1899 a new refinery in Saigon processed Indian opium into a special mixture that burned fast, forcing addicts to buy more, and the French imported cheap, low-grade opium from Yunnan to expand sales to the poor. Opium accounted for one-third of all France's colonial revenues, making them immune to international moralizing during the 1920s and 1930s, and by 1938 French opium revenues were the highest in Southeast Asia. By World War II, there were 100,000 addicts in Indo-China and the French were importing 60 tons of opium annually from Iran and Turkey to meet demand. "Plantation workers, miners, and urban laborers spent their entire salaries in the opium dens," says McCoy, and "many died of starvation." A Vietnamese novelist describing the typical village official of the period said, "if he were white, he would have been a European; if yellow, he would have been an Asian; if red, an American; if brown, an Australian; and if black, an African. But he was a kind of green, which is indisputably the complexion of a race of drug addicts."

When the United States annexed the Philippines in 1898, the new governor learned that he had inherited a Chinese opium monopoly retailing 130 tons each year. He banned opium farms, sales, and smoking, driving the trade underground. Opium use spread rapidly among poorer Filipinos, who had been unable to afford the Chinese monopoly's prices. Desperate to stop continued imports, the governor pushed the U.S. government to strengthen the international movement prohibiting nations to grow and market opium. "Faced with the threat of diplomatic censure," McCoy says, "the major trafficking nations were forced to restrict their trade, resulting in an eighty-two percent decline in the world supply of opium, from 42,000 tons in 1906 to 8,000 tons in 1934." Britain's Parliament had ended India's trade in 1906 and developed a deal with Manchu China to phase out Indian imports and Chinese production. Opium production was revived when the Manchus lost power, but it came to an official end in 1919. By then, Chinese growers were already producing enough to satisfy the country's internal demand. Southeast Asian opium monopolies reduced their sales by 65 percent in response to international pressure, but found that the cultural and economic roots of mass opium addiction nurtured during the colonial period were too deep to cut. Soldiers sent to end the trade quickly began to collect unofficial "levies" instead of official taxes.

Inspired with messianic fervor by the "clean up" of the Philippines, the United States passed the Food and Drug Act in 1906 to regulate patent medicines at home. But cold powders containing cocaine, illicitly sniffed by children as well as adults, were still available, and U.S. coca leaf imports increased drastically. Morphine had already supplanted opium among the country's recreational users by 1900, and after 1910, where opium and morphine were banned, cheap heroin supplanted both. Gangs of urban youth used heroin and marijuana openly, and both became even more popular when alcohol was prohibited the 1920s. A 1937 ban on marijuana remained in place even after a 1942 medical study reported that its use resulted in "no permanent deleterious effects." Despite the ban, it was widely used by African American migrants from the rural South to northern U.S. cities in the 1950s. Influenced by U.S. propaganda against marijuana, in 1955 the World Health Organization claimed that it increased the risk of committing unpremeditated murder, and British experts declared that it led to insanity. The uproar only made marijuana use more fashionable.

In 1909 U.S. President Theodore Roosevelt spearheaded the formation of the international Opium Commission, which passed an International Opium Convention in 1912. All developed countries signed the Convention banning opium and cocaine except Germany, which was a major manufacturer of cocaine. Overnight, the Convention transformed habitués around the world into criminals. Harsh punishments against users became the rage, forcing most of the international drug trade underground. Prohibition was a windfall for criminals, who responded to the challenge by creating new international trafficking networks and clandestine drug laboratories. Drugs were associated with foreign subversion as more traffickers began selling arms, and also with sexual unconventionality, homosexuality, and perversion. Prostitutes, who often earned extra money by selling drugs to their clients, were targeted by police. Despite the international ban and official efforts to discourage drug use, it escalated during World War I.

In the unstable post-war period, the Dutch established the world's largest cocaine manufacturing plant in Amsterdam to process coca leaves from colonial Java. They dominated the market, although Latin American countries beefed up production as a way of stimulating economic growth. Persia took over sales to the Far East from Britain, trafficking opium and heroin through Russian royalist refugees in the central Manchurian city of Harbin and Ukrainians in Vienna. Banned throughout the British Empire for supplying opiates to the Far East in 1925, Swiss drug manufacturer Hoffmann-La Roche and many German pharmaceutical manufacturers that got their start by producing illicit drugs, began shipping drugs to New York under false labels.[4] French investors built three huge factories in Istanbul that exported more than two tons of morphine and four tons of heroin in the first six months of 1930. In Serbia, Turkey, and Bulgaria, peasants raised poppies in addition to subsistence crops. With one-third higher morphine content than Asian varieties of poppies, their opium was in high demand. The Turkish Chamber of Commerce pronounced itself happy with the opportunity prohibition of the trade in India had presented.

By the early 1920s, heroin had become the drug of choice for millions of Chinese opium smokers. A cartel in Shanghai—then known as the "World's Whore"—was marketing the millions of "anti-opium pills" it produced as "the best medicine in the world," and imported 10 tons of heroin in 1923 alone because it could not keep up with consumer demand in China. When a new international agreement added heroin to the existing bans on opium and cocaine in 1928, the city's drug lords stepped up production and by 1934 more heroin was being smoked in Shanghai than opium. Shanghai laboratories also supplied American syndicates after European heroin dried up. In 1936 jails in Hong Kong, which had 24,000 heroin users and 40,000 opium smokers in its population of a million, were overflowing. The cartel became so powerful it helped Chinese nationalists bust communist labor unions and allied with the Japanese in northern China and Manchuria to expanding opium growing. Japanese heroin production was "the largest and best organized in China.

While Japanese navy gunboats regularly carried opium down the Yangtze River, twenty-four known laboratories in northern China manufactured heroin 'under the protection of Japanese authorities,'" says McCoy. When the Japanese invaded China's coastal provinces, opium sales were negotiated across the battle lines from the Nationalist stronghold in Szechwan.

With the outbreak of World War II, Middle Eastern opium shipments skipped Russia and went directly to Japan, where they were converted to heroin. Small farmers in Japan and Taiwan also grew poppies and both countries became major exporters of manufactured drugs. When the war cut supply lines from the Middle East, the French encouraged the Hmong in Laos and northwest Tonkin to expand production. It jumped from 7.4 tons in 1940 to 60.6 tons in 1944. By doubling local taxes and allowing the Hmong to pay in raw opium, the French motivated farmers to shift from subsistence to cash-crop farming. In this period, Southeast Asia became self-sufficient although production was considerably short of modern levels. Laos, for example, was producing 30 tons a year compared to 150 tons in 1968. The Golden Triangle produced less than 80 tons in total, compared to 1,000 tons in 1970.

The United States entered World War II's Pacific theater with the explicit goal of ending opium traffic so its troops would not become addicted, forcing the Dutch, British, French, and Portuguese to abolish opium smoking in their territories in return for U.S. help with the war. At war's end, only Thailand allowed opium smoking, but bowed to international pressure and prohibited it in 1959. However, while international drug agreements closed the door on official production and trade in the region, military and intelligence forces filled the vacuum and began funding their operations with clandestine drug sales. Production reached modern levels in just ten years. Although several governments in the region (Singapore, the Philippines, and Malaysia) eliminated drug abuse, in most countries the expanded trade fed growing populations of addicts and a burgeoning epidemic of corruption.

In 1949 the Chinese People's Liberation Army won Yunnan, closing the border to nationalist counterattacks and opium shipments. Yunnan's poppy fields were reclaimed for food production, and China's new communist government instituted a massive detoxification campaign, sending the world's largest population of addicts, some 40 million, to local drug clinics and labor camps. But Cold War paranoia made this clean-up effort shortlived. The U.S. Central Intelligence Agency (CIA) supported Chinese nationalists exiled in Burma, encouraging the drug trade to fund campaigns against the communists in Yunnan. Remnants of the old Chinese nationalist army and newly recruited hill tribesmen from Burma's Shan province were shipped to

Taiwan to harass China from that front. The U.S. government denied allegations of involvement but the U.S. ambassador to Rangoon resigned after complaining in an official cable that CIA operations had "brought chaos to the eastern Shan states and have been conducted in flagrant disregard [for] Burmese sovereignty."

When Burma's General Ne Win seized power in 1962, his "Burmese Way of Socialism" crippled the country's legitimate economy. Opium exports helped balance trade deficits, so the government entered the drug business, buying raw opium from the Shan rebels—who they were fighting—and processing it into high-grade heroin. The drug deals transformed Khun Sa, leader of the Shan's freedom fighters, into an opium warlord who traded drugs for guns on Bangkok's black market. Shan rebels increased their own heroin production from 550 to 2,500 tons during the 1980s, half the world's supply, and the Golden Triangle was producing 3,050 tons of raw opium, almost three-quarters of the world's supply, by 1989. Burma's military regime—still producing narcotics itself—allied with the United States and Thailand, receiving U.S. helicopters for a promise to suppress narcotics.

When the Chinese communists won in 1949, the nationalist-allied Shanghai cartel migrated to Hong Kong and the crime scene there mushroomed. The cartel's chemists manufactured heroin and took control of Thai morphine and opium exports. By 1970 Hong Kong had the highest proportion of drug users anywhere in the world—150,000 in a population of 4 million. Most addicts had been driven to heroin by government suppression of opium use, 85 percent of the colony's prison population was addicted, and teenage addiction was rising sharply. In 1969 the Hong Kong cartel sent master chemists to the Golden Triangle to expand heroin laboratories under the control of warlords in Burma, Laos, and Thailand. By 1971 the largest of the region's seven heroin factories could process 100 kilograms of raw opium per day to make 3.6 tons of heroin a year. To fund anticommunist activities during the Vietnam War, says Davenport-Hines, the CIA helped Laos' Hmong tribesmen increase poppy cultivation, transport the crops to laboratories in the Golden Triangle, and ship their high-grade heroin to South Vietnam. According to Davenport-Hines, "Many senior military officers and politicians in producing countries such as Thailand and consuming countries such as Vietnam participated in the traffic." Blaming the Vietnamese Communists, the CIA "protected the heroin business of its warlord allies while its operatives distributed heroin in Vietnam,"[5] addicting American troops. It was the same model used by the French in Indochina in the 1930s and 1940s, when the "French Connection"[6] significantly expanded the drug trade from Southeast Asia to the United States.

During the Vietnam War, the Thai, Lao, Vietnamese, and American governments "made critical decisions that would expand Southeast Asia's opium production and transform the Golden Triangle into the largest single opium-producing area in the world," says McCoy. In 1947 a coup in Thailand brought the military to power and Thai politics were dominated for the next ten years by a rivalry between two powerful cliques that vied for control of the lucrative opium trade from Burma. By becoming vehemently anticommunist in the 1960s, the dominant clique gained Washington's support and staged frequent "seizures" and "arrests" in which it confiscated and redistributed opium and heroin from the Shan states. During the war "Thailand had changed from an opium-consuming nation to the world's most important opium distribution center," according to McCoy, and the "national police force had become the largest opium-trafficking syndicate in Thailand."

In 1997 the U.S. secretary of state described the government of Burma—by then renamed Myanmar—as "drug traffickers and thugs," spearheading growing domestic and international criticism of Southeast Asia's drug trade. Under international pressure, Myanmar's generals gave Shan drug lords until 2002 to phase out production and negotiated unsuccessfully with Washington for foreign aid in exchange for Shan drug lord Khun Sa. When the Thais ended their support for the Shan separatists in exchange for timber and water concessions from Myanmar, Khun Sa surrendered and retired to a luxurious villa in the hills of Myanmar, beyond Washington's reach. Before his retirement, he introduced the manufacture of low-cost methamphetamine tablets in the Golden Triangle, "unleashing an epidemic of cheap stimulants that soon swept Southeast Asia," says McCoy.

Abuse of legally manufactured stimulants and depressants had become widespread by the 1930s, and during World War II the troops' use of analgesics, amphetamines, and barbiturates popularized them with the general public. Although the U.S. Federal Bureau of Narcotics declared them dangerous in 1957, by 1958, 8 billion pills were manufactured in the United States alone. In 1965 the United States restricted their use to medical purposes but production increased to 12 billion pills by 1971. When these substances were finally restricted in the United States and Europe in the late 1960s, pharmaceutical companies began marketing them in Latin America, Asia, and Africa. The companies also turned the growing reaction to manufactured psychotropic drugs to their advantage. Since few countries had the resources to regulate new substances, companies advocated a global regulatory treaty but proposed very low standards and hijacked the 1971 international regulatory conference. As a result, the new treaty put hallucinogens under much stricter control than stimulants and depressants. As late as 1989, the U.S. Drug Control National Strategy did not mention barbiturates, amphetamines, and comparable substances, and they were not included in the National Drug Policy's claim that "drugs represent the gravest present threat to our national well-being."

In this unrestricted environment for stimulants, Khun Sa's retirement legacy quickly became a bonanza. In 1998 Myanmar's new drug warlords, the Wa, learned through an informal market study that overproduction in Afghanistan and the increasing costs of bribes and indictments had made the opium and heroin markets unattractive. The government had stepped up seizures, so Myanmar's opium growers cooperated with the UN crop replacement program while the Wa shifted into amphetamine production, investing the profits in Yangoon airline, banks, and telecommunications businesses. By 1999, 257,000 Thais were regular amphetamine users, surpassing the country's 214,000 heroin addicts. By mid-2000 the Wa were exporting 600 million methamphetamine tablets worth $2.8 billion to Thailand each year, growing to 800 million by 2002. As methamphetamines supplanted heroin, three-quarters of Thailand's 2 to 3 million users found a new addiction. New methamphetamine users in the Philippines were supplied by manufacturers in Hong Kong and the Netherlands until the late 1980s, when they began domestic manufacture and started marketing the drug in Indonesia.

The few Southeast Asian countries that were successful in controlling addiction were never used by their colonizers for opium production or trade, and have relatively high standards of living and equitable distribution of income. Singapore reduced its addict population from 25,000 in 1947 to 8,000 in 1970 by attacking syndicate leaders instead of cracking down on small-time users. The Philippines executed a Chinese heroin manufacturer by firing squad in 1973 and now has the smallest addict population in Southeast Asia. Malaysia went after drug traffickers and users in the 1970s, instituting the death penalty for possession of more than 15 grams of heroin, although it has been unable to completely control through-shipping and local production of heroin because of its proximity to Thailand. Driven from Singapore, the Philippines, and Malaysia, drug cartels sought refuge in Thailand in the 1970s and 1980s. Transit traffic was protected by the police "because it met the strategic and financial needs of the nation's military," McCoy says, but in 1990, after Thai politics were freed from military control, Bangkok "cut its ties to the opium armies." A UN crop-substitution program in northern Thailand has helped sharply reduce supply in Thailand, but Myanmar's harvest doubled in the same period to compensate. Although opium and heroin use has declined, some 300,000 Hill Tribe farmers in Myanmar still produce opium and half a million

Burmese are still addicted to heroin and 63 percent of them are HIV positive. In 1999 Laos announced a program to eliminate opium production by 2006.

———————

CIA covert action solidified trafficking patterns and infrastructure in Southeast Asia just as it had in the Mediterranean in the late 1940s when the Agency was "combating" drug smuggling from Turkey by the Italian Mafia. After the United States withdrew from Vietnam in 1973, the Golden Triangle continued to supply one-third of the heroin brought to the United States and Europe. Having not learned their lesson in the Golden Triangle, the CIA supported the start-up of drug warlords in Afghanistan and Pakistan (Osama bin Laden was one) who pledged to combat terrorism in the 1990s. Covert CIA operations in Afghanistan "transformed Central Asia from a self-contained opium zone into a major supplier of heroin for world markets," says McCoy. As late as 1975, Central Asia's historic patterns of opium production dating from the sixteenth century had remained unchanged. Iran absorbed all the opium the region could produce. Its huge population of addicts was second only to China's, but drug use in Pakistan and Afghanistan was uncommon. Eleven percent of Iran's population, or 1.3 million people, smoked in their homes and in opium dens where child prostitution was common. Iran had been a major producer until 1955 when the Shah, concerned about the health of military recruits, responded to international pressure and abolished opium growing, stimulating expanded production in Afghanistan, Turkey, and Southeast Asia's Golden Triangle.

When the Communist People's Democratic Party of Afghanistan came to power through a military coup in 1978, it tried to radically transform Afghani society through violence and coercion. "Along with their attempt to implement various policies like land reform, literacy programs, and so on, the Communists had a massive campaign of terror to eliminate groups that they thought were rivals, which included first of all other factions of the educated elite," says foreign policy expert Barnet Rubin. Rivals were swept away easily "because Afghanistan did not have political parties and an autonomous political structure through which it could mobilized people." The communists killed 12,000 urban dissidents in the central prison of Kabul alone, and they eliminated between 50,000 and 100,000 local Islamic and tribal leaders and *zamindars* in the countryside. Their brutality incited rebellion, and in March 1979, even the military began to revolt. When Russian officials were executed, the Soviet Union invaded in December 1979.

U.S. military aid, CIA-donated eastern bloc infantry weapons, and shipments of arms from China and Saudi Arabia flowed in for the northern warlords. The Soviet-sponsored faction quickly lost legitimacy, "large portions of the rest of the army defected, and the state structure began to melt away," Rubin says. Student rebels and any of the educated elite who had not fled were executed. By the mid-1980s, one-third of Afghanistan's population of 10 million were in exile and by 1989, when the Soviets withdrew, 1.5 million Afghans had died. During the 1980s, 50,000 had been killed in Kabul by the indiscriminate shelling by the U.S. government, and another several thousand lost their lives when the United States drove the Taliban out of power in 2001. The United States also sent $3 billion in military aid to Pakistan, where a massive drug operation under CIA cover was shipping Afghanistani opium processed in Pakistani heroin laboratories into international markets. Pakistan's harvest rebounded to 800 tons, while Afghanistan doubled its harvest to 575 tons.

The war destroyed "everything in Afghanistan that supported governance and development [including] formal government [and] social structures that enabled people to run things by themselves." Rubin says that the Pakistanis even tried to persuade the Afghani *mujahedeen* "to blow up a huge dam near Kandahar and flood the city but the *mujahedeen* refused and sent guards to save the dam from Pakistani agents." McCoy says that "after spending $2 billion to expel the Soviets from Afghanistan," the United States "found itself responsible for a nation with a ruined central government and ruthless warlords running the provinces." President Hamid Karzai and his internationally backed government rule in Kabul only, while the bulk of rural Afghans are the subjects of self-appointed warlords. Pakistan extremists, backed by Saudi Arabia and Iran, have infiltrated rural areas, and violence is increasing. When Karzai threatened to resign unless warlords submitted to government authority and paid part of the customs they gather as privateers to the central treasury, he was ignored. Clerics who support the Karzai government and denounce the Taliban's call for jihad were being assassinated.

Of Afghanistan's economy, Rubin says, "if it hasn't disappeared, it is already entirely illegal." Afghani farmers had depended on labor-intensive irrigation works destroyed in the war; even their fruit orchards were cut down, and they cannot bring any produce to market because the roads had been destroyed. Afghan farmers, unable to plant wheat, were driven to sell their livestock. Farmers in the east, south, and north began freely planting opium poppies and opium production doubled to 4,600 tons in 1999. Afghanistan now produces 75 percent of the world's crop. Opium growing accounts for half of all employment—especially for women, who had been banned from education and employment in other sectors—and demands nine times the labor of food production but yields twenty times the profit. Opium uses only half the water of wheat and its cultivation fosters investment, accumulation of capital, and development of credit systems. McCoy says that "opium filled an economic void inside Afghanistan, helping rebuild a shattered society with networks of credit, labor and commerce." Because it was nonperishable and could be stockpiled, it was a source of savings and tided farmers over in lean periods. Merchants are reputable members of their communities, educated influential landholders, and former civil servants and professionals "who sold opium to survive the chaos of civil war."

"I know the poppy is poison for everyone," a young farmer said, "but are you ready to tell me not to cultivate it? We will die from lack of bread and food." Rural areas have no health workers or teachers to speak of—two-thirds of Afghanis have no healthcare and two-thirds of the children are not immunized—and epidemics spread easily. The northern province of Badakhshan has one of the world's highest maternal death rates. Returning refugees, warned of millions of land mines and unexploded bombs, found their villages destitute. Opium production has become the basis for postwar reconstruction, supplying money and employment that enables millions to survive. Commentator Edward Girardet claims that "without the pool of money created by aid, peacekeeping, and illegal traffic in opium and other commodities, reconstruction would grind to a halt," and unless livelihoods are restored, the country will descend into turmoil.[7] By 2000 international aid had plummeted to $13 million even though the country had suffered a devastating drought. Noting that Afghanistan opium was the basis of only 5 percent of America's heroin, President George W. Bush said that Britain and Germany would have to pay the price to curb production.

———◆•◆———

The end result in Pakistan has not been much better. The CIA's covert war in Afghanistan transformed Pakistan into a narco-state where drug money dominates politics, says Pakistan expert John McCarry. The 3.3 million Afghan refugees who poured across the border brought weapons and "a heretofore nonexistent heroin trade." Tribal warlords fended off any attempts at police control with automatic weapons, reducing Presidents Bhutto and Zia to puppets. The Pakistani army controlled the heroin network while the government provided its banking services. When Asia's monsoon rains failed in 1978 and 1979, Afghan-Pakistani heroin laboratories geared up production. By the early

1980s, Pakistan was the world's second largest opium grower and heroin earnings were one-quarter of the entire gross domestic product. "The heroin boom was so large and uncontrolled that drugs swept Pakistan like a plague in the early 1980s," McCoy says, "leaving it with one of the world's largest addict populations"—1.3 million.

At independence, Pakistan had inherited little of British India's industrial infrastructure and had few educated workers, most of whom were Hindu and fled for India. The country had been a breadbasket for the British raj, and agriculture still leads the economy although Lahore and Karachi have some textile manufacture. Eighty percent of Pakistan's fast-growing population are farmers, one-third of whom do not own their own land. Agriculture is not mechanized, but Pakistan has the world's largest contiguous irrigation systems, with 38,000 miles of canals covering more than 39 million acres. Less than half of the population is literate, and primary schooling is available to only half of the country's children. Arid mountains occupy most of its western border with Iran and its northern border with Tajikistan and China. The eastern half of the country is a broad, fertile plain that includes the fertile Punjab area in the north, where the five tributaries of the Indus River join as they descend from the Himalayas, and the Sindh region, which borders the Great Indian plain on the south. The plain ties Pakistan geographically to India, but its cultural ties are with the Middle East. Its official language is Urdu, related to Arabic and Persian; its economic assistance comes from Iran and Saudi Arabia; it is officially an Islamic state, although *sharia*, strict Islamic law, has not been adopted in all parts of the country.

The 1,000-mile Afghanistan-Pakistan border is occupied by the Pashtuns, fierce tribal groups that have kept the region "pure and veiled" since 600 B.C. At independence, when Pakistan was created, the Pashtuns wanted their own state. The plan was supported by Gandhi and Jawaharal Nehru but ignored by the British, despite the warning of Afghanistan's emir that "these frontier tribes will be your worst enemies." The fiercely Islamic territory is administered as a semiautonomous region whose local *maliks*, or bosses, receive government payouts of $80,000 per year. Since the U.S. war with Afghanistan started, the territories have become a hideout for Al Qaeda and Taliban fighters, who are fellow Pashtuns and Sunni Muslims. Area khans are descendants of Persians, Greeks and Mongol invaders, seminomadic fighters who subsisted on nuts, apples, tomatoes, corn, dates, and wild honey before the drug trade opened up. "Now heroin supports most of the tribal economy," says area expert Eliza Griswold,[8] and the tribesmen "are formidable smugglers, trafficking hashish, opium, and heroin around the world."

In 2001 General Pervez Musharraf ousted Pakistan's parliamentary government, suspended the constitution, and named himself president. The constitution was restored in 2002, when Musharraf's presidency was extended for five years by a parliamentary referendum. On May 25, 2004, a pro-Taliban cleric who supports Osama bin Laden became head of the opposition in Pakistan's parliament, strengthening the military-religious alliance. Secular politicians, who hold more seats, say the continuous conflicts in Kashmir and Afghanistan have given military and hard-line religious leaders an excuse to co-opt national politics. Musharraf's UAF party, known as the Military-Mullah Alliance, is pretending to hunt terrorists while providing them sanctuary. Pakistan's economy grew six percent per year in the 1980s and early 1990s but now that one-third of the budget is devoted to the military or to interest payments on national debt, it is deteriorating. The government finances itself with black market arms deals that include nuclear as well as conventional weapons. A 2003 International Atomic Energy Agency probe into nuclear leaks to Iran found that Pakistan's Khan Research Labs was at the hub of a network of suppliers and middlemen in the Middle East and Asia that provide enriched uranium, designs, and equipment for nuclear bombs to Libya, North Korea, Russia, Malaysia, and China, and to private businesses in Germany, Belgium, Britain, and Dubai. Despite the implications of the Agency's findings, Musharraf granted a pardon to KRL head Abdul Qadeer Khan days after he confessed. Pakistan tested a long-range ballistic capable of traveling 1,200 miles in March 2004.

———•◦•◦•———

Post-partition conflicts spread violence in other parts of the region. India's 400,000 troops lob bombs over the cease fire line drawn by UN peacekeepers in Jammu-Kashmir in 1949, ducking bombs aimed at them by 200,000 Pakistani soldiers. Pakistan and India have been fighting over the tiny state since 1947. When the subcontinent of India was partitioned by the British, the state of Jammu and Kashmir (composed of two districts) was the largest of 562 princely states that covered 45 percent of its land mass. These Hindus, Muslim, and Sikh fiefdoms were controlled by feudal potentates called maharajas and nawabs who had acknowledged British power and complied with its rule. Kashmir was a vulnerable anomaly, a primarily Muslim state headed by a Hindu maharaja, Hari Singh, whose ancestor had purchased the state from the British in 1846 for a nominal annual tribute of one horse, twelve perfect shawl goats, and three pairs of Kashmir shawls. At independence, Jawaharlal Nehru wanted to demonstrate that a mixed state with Hindus ruling primarily Muslim populations could work. The arrangement worked in reverse in two other Indian states, but in Jammu and Kashmir, "the distance between the privileged Hindu elite . . . and their Muslim subjects was particularly vast," says London School of Economics political scientist Sumantra Bose.[9] "The poverty of the Muslim masses is appalling," a contemporary journalist reported. "Dressed in rags and barefoot, a Muslim peasant presents the appearance of a starving beggar. Most are landless laborers, working as serfs for absentee [Hindu] landlords." Hari Singh was "self-absorbed and hopelessly incompetent"; his subjects were indentured to the small landed elite and state officials. Muslims could not go to school, had no press, could not be military officers, and few held positions in the civil service.

Pakistan's leader, Mohammed Ali Jinnah, who had already given up more than he wanted in the Partition, squared off against Nehru over Jammu-Kashmir. Muslims had organized a "Quit Kashmir" Movement to oust the maharaja, and over the years, the fighting has escalated. China grabbed an adjacent territory, Aksai Chin, in their 1962 war with India, which intensified India's determination to control Jammu-Kashmir. Pakistan, an agricultural state, wants to protect the headwaters of three of its major rivers—the Indus, the Jhelum, and the Chenab—arguing that Kashmiris had been Muslim since the fourteenth century. The once pristine state has been torn apart by violence, bringing tourism, once its main income-earner, to a halt. In 1987, when Indian officials rigged the elections, Muslim insurgency grew into a full-blown separatist movement fueled by genocidal rage. Only 5,000 of the 150,000 to 300,000 Hindu Pandits, once the most successful and well-educated minority among the country's 8 million inhabitants, remain outside of refugee camps. Muslim rebels have imposed harsh Islamic regulations, burned down government schools, closed down movies and bars, and forced women to veil. In the mid-1990s, Saudi Arabia and Iran funneled money for Pakistan to send Taliban zealots, Afghanis, and soldiers of fortune from Libya and Chechnya into the conflict. Between 1998 and 2002, at least 70,000 Kashmiri civilians and militants, Indian and Pakistani soldiers, and civilians were killed.

Kashmiri Muslims are tiring of the intrusion of outsiders. They have their own interpretation of Islam, evolved over years of isolation, and their economy and culture are collapsing in the turmoil. Their chance for self-determination is diminishing as the struggled becomes international, spanning many states and interest groups. But Bose says that "Kashmir's people have not yet made the transition from being subjects to being citizens," because few see Kashmir as a single, sovereign unit with the right to determine its own future.

The cause of the conflict "comes down to the great truism of real estate: location. Kashmir perches like a raja's jeweled turban in the Himalayas at the very top of the great subcontinental landmass," says Kashmir expert Lewis Simons. "It is a gateway—or barrier—between [India and Pakistan] as well as between them and China and Afghanistan."[10]

———◆◆◆———

The effects of colonialism and subsequent partition on the politics of India, Bangladesh, Afghanistan, Pakistan, and Jammu and Kashmir are paralleled in the central Asian republics of Kazakhstan, Uzbekistan, Turkmenistan, Tajikistan, and Kyrgyzstan, where weakened governments left at sea by the 1991 breakup of the Soviet Union are falling prey to radical Islamic extremists. Marco Polo called this high, arid central plain the "roof of the world." The "vast, empty landscape dotted with oases of vibrant populations and political ferment, sitting on the world's last great untapped natural energy reserves" is as unknown to most westerners today as it was in Polo's time, says journalist Ahmed Rashid, because it was deliberately isolated during Soviet rule.[11] The rising instability created by radical Islamic groups is raising the area's visibility as "the new global battleground," Rashid warns, the result of a "new political phenomenon at work amongst small groups of extremists around the Muslim world." As Russia, the United States, Iran, Turkey, Pakistan, and China compete for the right to the region's reserves of gas and oil, the countries in the region have been caught in the "Great Game" again.

The war in Afghanistan "sent shock waves of instability throughout Central Asia." In the 1990s Afghanistan's production of heroin fueled the growth of a vast illicit international trading network that deals in drugs, arms, women, and money laundering through Central Asia, Russia, and Europe. It also "fueled an eruption of ethnic insurgency across a 3,000-mile swath from Central Asia to the Balkans," financing wars in Chechnya, Georgia, Turkey, Bosnia, and Uzbekistan. In Kyrgyzstan alone, the base for a northern smuggling route controlled by Chechnya, Tajik, and Azeri gangs, 4 million people were employed in drug trafficking by 1998, and the country was exporting more heroin than Myanmar by 2000. By the end of the Tajik civil war (1992 to 1997), one-third of the country's gross domestic profit was generated from drug trafficking. In the first six months of 1999, heroin use jumped 4.5 times 1998 rates, and HIV was erupting along the path of injecting drug use that ran from Central Asia to Eastern Europe. Al Qaeda's militant Islamic network is just one player in the game. McCoy says that "Extraordinary profits from drugs and guns have produced mafia gangs, criminal diasporas, tribal warlords and rebel armies." The warlord Juma Namangani, backed by Osama bin Laden, coordinated a trafficking network across Central Asia that controlled 70 percent of the trade and was extending guerrilla operations into Uzbekistan and Kyrgyzstan before he was murdered.

The contest for Central Asia is an inevitable function of its location between great states. The region has changed hands regularly for over 2,000 years. The present conflicts stem from the chaos accompanying the dissolution of the Soviet Union, the latest of the great empires that occupied the region. After Russia conquered all of Siberia to the Pacific Ocean, Peter the Great conquered Central Asia between 1865 and 1895 when Russia's cotton supplies were cut off by the American Civil War. In the "Great Game," the Russian and British empires struggled for control of Asia and used Central Asia, Afghanistan, Nepal, and Tibet as their pawns. Russia built a railway network through Central Asia to the borders of Afghanistan, Iran, China, and British India to better control the region. When Tsarist armies tried to conscript Central Asians to fight in World War I, a massive revolt broke out. The Russians subdued the rebellion, increased taxes, and expropriated wheat for its armies. Tens of thousands of rebels died, and a Cossack army carried out reprisals against the Kyrgyz, killing a quarter of their population, burning villages, and sending the survivors fleeing to Xinjiang in China.

The region now has 52 million people in more than 100 ethnic groups, dominated by the Uzbeks, with 22 million people in Uzbekistan and substantial minorities in the other republics. The 10 million Russians forcibly moved there to weaken indigenous ethnic groups before the Soviet breakup constitute one-fifth of the population. In 1929 Joseph Stalin divided the region into five socialist republics along their present-day boundaries and set about systematically exploiting all of them. Cotton was irrigated by massive networks that have drained the region's water supplies, causing pollution and permanent environmental damage. When forced to collectivize their farms, many Central Asians killed their herds rather than deliver them to the communists. Teachers and holy men were sent to the gulag or the firing squad. As many as 3 million people died, mostly from famine. "For many people of the Soviet Union," says area expert Mike Edwards, "Kazakhstan became, like Siberia to the north, a great corral into which suspected enemies of the state were driven."[12] In the 1980s thousands of Central Asians were drafted to fight the Afghani *mujahedeen,* and the economies boomed because the region was the supply depot for the war. When the Soviets abruptly withdrew in 1988, Central Asian leaders faced not only the loss of income but the threat of militant Islamic takeover of their own countries.

The Soviet Union exploded its first atom bomb on August 29, 1949, from its Kurchatov facility in northeastern Kazakhstan where almost 500 nuclear devices were detonated over the next forty years. The Soviets used nuclear bombs to build reservoirs, mine for diamonds, and staunch oil well fires. "People were rabbits for experiments," said a Kazakh ecologist; it was "a crime . . . fascism." The government periodically tested radiation levels in Kazakhstan, but the people were never given results or treatment. Thousands of children suffered birth defects and disfigurement, and the Soviet government made no attempt to help the victims because, in the words of one government official, "Kazakhstan was just a Soviet colony." Zinc and lead smelters and a small uranium processing plant polluted eastern Kazakh cities, and the Aral Sea was poisoned by the runoff of fertilizers and starved by irrigation projects. The residue of pesticides and fertilizers on the shrinking seabed are deposited on villages by wind, causing immune disorders, cancer, hepatitis, and respiratory diseases. The Kurchatov nuclear facility came under Kazakh control after the breakup of the Soviet Union, but the staff was left to develop its own new business applications by the bankrupt Kazakh government.

From 1923 until 1991, Central Asia was deliberately isolated by the Soviet Union, its borders with Iran, Turkey, Afghanistan, and China closed. It had no contact with the outside world, no autonomy, and its political development was quashed. When independence finally came with the breakup of the Soviet Union in 1991, "Central Asians, ideologically speaking, were still back in the 1920s." The crisis in Central Asia today is "directly related to this stunted political and ideological growth," says Rashid. Central Asia's republics begged for admission to the new Commonwealth of Independent States (CIS). The republics' economies, oil pipelines, roads, electricity, industry, and agriculture—even all the international telephone lines—were all tied to Russia. They had no armed forces, and Tajikistan survived on Soviet subsidies. Their leaders were unaccustomed to taking autonomous actions. Economic deprivation, ethnic rivalries over scarce housing and other shortages, and growing anti-Russian feelings led to violence, especially among unemployed young people. "Living standards plummeted, inflation galloped upwards, unemployment grew, and critical raw materials for industry and agriculture became unattainable," Rashid says. According to the World Bank, since 1991 the volume of irrigation water across Central Asia fell by half with a loss of 20 to 30 percent of the region's agricultural output. Increases in rural birth rates show no signs of abating, encouraged by radical Muslim extremists who are trying to build a population base. Ethnic conflicts and border disputes are common, and leaders responded with more repression.

When freedom was theirs, the people of Central Asia, forced to renounce Islam for seventy-four years, "at last saw an opportunity to reconnect spiritually and culturally with their Islamic past," Rashid says. Military service in Afghanistan had helped them reconnect with their Muslim neighbors, and Islamic missionaries from Pakistan, Saudi Arabia, and Turkey helped build mosques and translate the Koran into Russian and local languages. Central Asian Muslims learned about Iran's 1979 Islamic revolution, Palestinian resistance to Israel, and wars of resistance in Kashmir, Algeria, Egypt, the Philippines, and Indonesia. "The speed of Islamic resurgence caught the elite by surprise." By October 1991 there were 1,000 new mosques in each republic, with more opening each day. An indigenous Islamic revival blossomed, but it was "quickly radicalized by outsiders."

With the exception of Kyrgyzstan's President Askar Akayev, Central Asian leaders failed to recognize the stirring nationalism and "lumbered along the well-trodden path they knew best—the suppression of dissent, democracy, popular culture, and eventually the Islamic revival, jailing and torturing many of its new leaders." The newly awakened Muslims had a convenient place to turn: Afghanistan. Central Asia's first war broke out in 1992. Islamic rebels and democrats fought against the Tajik regime until 1997, a civil war that killed at least 50,000 people. Now, only Tajikistan, which created a coalition government through fair elections that includes Islamicists, neo-Communists, and clan leaders, has succeeded in stilling the chaos. In 2000, however, it experienced its worst drought in seventy-four years, leaving one fifth of the population destitute. "People have sold the doors and windows of their houses to buy food," said a Red Cross official. "We have seen children digging among rat holes in wheat fields, searching for grain hoarded by the rodents for the winter." At least 65,000 children could not attend school because they had no shoes or clothes. Uzbek Islamic extremists entered Tajikistan, threatening the fragile coalition government.

In the early 1990s, the Islamic Movement in Uzbekistan "had come out of hiding," says area expert Rashid,[13] challenging Uzbek strongman Islam Karimov from bases in Tajikistan and Afghanistan. The United States, Russia, and China gave Karimov military aid to defeat the rebels, and since then, Rashid says, Karimov has increased human rights abuses, secure in his position as a U.S. ally. He and other Central Asian bureaucrats have not, however, tried to improve what Rashid calls the "horrific" economic, political, and social conditions, so the radicals have little trouble getting money from Saudi Arabia or

Afghani drug and gun trafficking or garnering new recruits to join the Chechen, Caucasian Dagestani, and Xinjiang Uighur rebels at their core. On their side, Central Asian regimes use the involvement of outside militants as an excuse to brutally suppress dissent, playing the United States, China, and Russia against one another for more foreign aid.

The region's Hizb ut-Tahrir al-Islami (HT, the Party of Islamic Liberation) has also declared jihad in Central Asia, but wants to unite the republics under a seventh-century style caliphate. It too lacks any program of social, economic, or political reform, but its utopian vision is popular with college students, who are being jailed by the region's hard-line regimes. Rashid says that "every act of state repression has pushed these movements into taking more extreme positions, distorting their original message." The ultimate irony, he says, is that neither movement is based on the region's two indigenous forms of Islam: Sufism, a tolerant form of Islamic mysticism that advocates direct communication with God, and Jaddidism, a modernist reinterpretation of Islam. The Taliban guerrillas' "knapsacks full of dollar bills" are rapidly converting the new generation. Sixty percent of the population is under age 25 and most are unemployed, poorly educated, and hungry.

In Central Asia, Rashid concludes, "the Great Game has changed. In the nineteenth century, Russia and Great Britain used the Central Asian states as pawns; today the superpowers are finding themselves at the mercy of forces they helped unleash but that are now beyond their control." Extremist groups and organized criminals seek to weaken national borders and foster a contraband war economy "based on looting, smuggling, or trafficking in drugs, arms, or even human beings," says political expert Barnett Rubin. The "truck and transport smuggling mafia" and drug traffickers benefit from weakened state authority, which allows "their business interests and Islamic agendas to flourish," explains Rashid. Pakistan wants Central Asia's regimes replaced by radical Islamic leaders who will look to it rather than to Russia or China for alliances. There has been an "explosion of self-interest groups in Pakistan, both Islamic and non-Islamic, who have benefited from the Afghan civil war and Islamic insurgency in Central Asia," Rashid says, and they "see no need for peace." U.S. energy companies, Rashid argues, are themselves using the conflicts "as a lever to extract maximum benefits" from their client states instead of using their power to encourage strategies to ensure long-term stability.

Central Asian states, like their parent state Russia and its cousins, the East European states that were formerly part of the Soviet Union, is courting chaos. Poverty, organized crime, and drugs "are creating previously unforeseen problems," says Rashid, the worst of which is a burgeoning AIDS epidemic. The five Central Asian republics have more than 300,000 HIV-positive people. In Kazakhstan, corruption is rampant, particularly in the burgeoning oil and gas industries and human rights abuses are fueling the epidemic. Drug users and sex workers are subject to routine and violent harassment, says Human Rights Watch, driving them away from needle exchange facilities and preventing condom use.[14] In Uzbekistan and neighboring areas of Tajikistan, HIV/AIDS is also increasingly fueled by injecting drug use and illicit drug trafficking. In Kyrgyzstan, prison populations are going up rapidly, and 80 percent of the prisoners are drug users, with very high rates of HIV, tuberculosis, hepatitis, and other sexually transmitted disesaes. Prisons are crowded, food is short, and medicine is lacking. The Fergana Valley has been named one of the world's three "hottest danger zones" for global security by the European-based International Crisis Group, which says that the dire poverty prevailing in Central Asia, along with despair and outrage over corruption and repression, could ignite a regional conflict.

As in Pakistan, Afghanistan, and Kashmir, Central Asia's Islamic extremists "have no economic manifesto, no plan for better governance and the building of political institutions, and no blueprint for fostering democratic participation in the decision-making process." The fact that they distort the historical reality of Islam is of little concern to the leaders of the Taliban, al Qaeda, or the Islamic Movement of Uzbekistan because they reject historical experience, scientific evidence, and the other forms of knowledge in favor of the personal vision of a single leader that Muslims have historically revered. The chosen one's "character, piety and purity rather than his political abilities, education, or experience will enable him to lead the new society," says Rashid. In the hands of these leaders, *sharia*, or Islamic law, is not a way to create the just society envisioned by Muhammad, Rashid claims, but a way to regulate behavior, suppress women, and create a climate of fear. In destroying Bamian, Afghanistan's 1,500-year-old statues of Buddha, the Taliban was rewriting history, expunging any memory of the long reign of Buddhism in northern Afghanistan. In pursuing the lesser jihad—rebellion against injustice, struggle for social and political change—Rashid says, they ignore the greater jihad, the inner-seeking struggle for personal goodness, which Muhammad put first.

———— •◦• ————

Its annexation of Siberia, Central Asia, and the Caucasus made the Russian Empire second in size only to Britain in the nineteenth and twentieth centuries, and with the inclusion of its Eastern European satellites, the Soviet

Union became the largest empire since Dar al-Islam and the Mongols. For four centuries Russia has been "a country of daunting proportions," the largest state in the world. In the sixteenth century, Europeans believed that Russia was larger than the surface of the moon. Russian poet Alexander Pushkin said that Russia's "vast plains absorbed the force of the Mongols and halted their advance at the very edge of Europe." The Cold War was inevitable because Russia "could scarcely be ignored," say policy analysts Fiona Hill and Clifford Gaddy of the Brookings Institution, a U.S.-based economic thinktank.[15] Covering a sixth of the world's surface from the Baltic to the Pacific, when Russia was formed it was larger than the two of its three competing empires (Austria-Hungary and the Ottoman). In the nineteenth century, Britain, with its colonial possessions, was larger, a fact that led to the face-off in Central Asia's Great Game. Siberia alone occupies a twelfth of the world's landmass. "You could take the whole of the United States of America," wrote a nineteenth-century explorer, "and set it down in the middle of Siberia, without anywhere touching the boundaries of the latter territory. You can then take Alaska and all the States of Europe, with the single exception of Russia, and fit them into the remaining margin like the pieces of a dissected map."

The Russian conquest of Siberia "was the largest and most enduring land grab ever made by Europeans, and yet—curiously enough—it was scarcely noticed in the annals of discovery,"[16] says historian Tim Severin. The invasion of Siberia, launched by Tsar Ivan IV in 1577 ("the Formidable" to Russians, "the Terrible" to English speakers), was carried out by a small band of brigands. Severin says that "the ageing half-mad Tsar Ivan, worn out by nearly half a century of despotism," was "like Kublai Khan three hundred years earlier." Kublai's descendent, Kucham Khan, "the blind ruler of Siberia, had also come to his throne in a welter of dynastic murder." Heir to the Mongol Empire, he believed the Russians should pay him tribute. "A steppe warlord in the old Mongol tradition," he ruled the last surviving khanate of the Horde. Two others, Kazan on the Volga and Astrakhan on the Caspian, had fallen to Ivan in the 1550s.

Yermak, the man who would connect the emperors and determine their destinies, "sprang from the soil like the crop of dragon's teeth, ready armed with a host of warriors at his back." Yermak, "part mystic, part robber-baron," was the grandson of a coachman who ran away to soldier with the Cossacks, mercenaries who hired themselves out to state armies. Their name is derived from the Russian *kasak*, a word of Turco-Tartar origin, meaning "freebooter." An *ataman*, he led his own band of escaped convicts and ruffians, collecting protection money in the "twilight zone between nation, culture and frontier,"

Severin says. In the summer of 1577, Ivan had sent his own soldiers against the Cossacks, who had become too bold and robbed a Russian embassy on its way to Persia, scattering them before the wind.

Yermak's band ended up in the eastern frontier province of the Stroganoffs, a powerful merchant family who knew "that to attempt to settle a Cossack Host was to try to pen the wolf." The Stroganoffs, granted a royal charter to mine the Urals for iron and salt in 1517, had amassed an enormous fortune from their land holdings and trading rights. Their charter required them to build and garrison new forts, so they offered to supply and equip Yermak and his men if they would march east across the Urals to attack the Siberian khan and claim new territory. He set off with 540 of his own men, 300 Stroganoff soldiers, and various monks and scribes in July 1579. Until that time, only a few fur traders had penetrated the land beyond the Urals, returning with tales of Samoyeds, or "self-eaters." Also charged with converting the Siberian pagans and Muslim Tartars, Yermak and his band were sent away carrying icons on their shoulders, their banners embroidered with the images of saints, preceded by trumpeters and endowed with supernatural weapons. In Russian legend, Yermak is remembered as a Cossack outlaw who became "an apostle of Christianity." Tartar spies warned Kucham that "when [the Cossacks] shoot from their bows, there is a flash of fire and great smoke issues, and a loud report like thunder in the sky."

Yermak passed along Siberia's rivers like "a new virus . . . injected into north Asia's circulatory system . . . a deadly contagion, reaching into every corner of north Asia," Severin says. He tricked the Tartars into firing on vessels manned by stuffed dummies and lured them into ambushes. Ten thousand Tartar cavalry were helpless against Cossack guns. Kucham ordered his mullahs "to shout their prayers . . . because their gods were asleep," but to no avail. Yermak claimed Siberia for the tsar in 1582. He sent the Tsar 2,300 sable pelts, 20 black fox skins, 50 beaver pelts, and a note asking for reinforcements because less than 400 of his men had survived. Through trickery, he managed to fend the khan's counterattacks until Russian soldiers arrived at the beginning of winter in 1584. Finding the Cossacks short of food, they survived until summer by eating the bodies of their dead. Yermak drowned the following summer trying to escape an ambush; Kucham Khan survived until 1599, when he was hunted down with his family and exterminated by Tartar rivals. When his successor Seydak was called to parlay, he and his men were served drugged wine and massacred. "Henceforth," wrote a chronicler, "there was great fear among all the infidels of the Siberian land, and all the Tartars, both near and far, did not dare to go to war against the sovereign's cities." With the khanate gone, there was no one left to halt Russians armed with muskets who built a chain of fortresses and trading posts, opening Siberia up across its entire width only eighty years after Yernak's arrival.

Russia stretches through eleven time zones. It has 40 percent of the world's natural gas reserves; 25 percent of its coal, diamonds, gold, and nickel; 30 percent of its aluminum and timber; and 6 percent of known oil reserves. Unfortunately, most of these reserves are in remote and unreachable areas, making them expensive or impossible to tap with existing technology. Many are in Siberia, so cold that winter temperatures average minus 30 to 40 degrees centigrade. "In such conditions," says historian Anna Reid, "mercury turns to lead, brandy to syrup. Living trees explode with a sound like gunfire, chopped logs strike blue sparks, and exhaled breath falls to the ground in a shower of crystals, with a rustling sound called the 'whispering of the stars.'"[17] The Russian Federation, the remains of the Soviet Union, is rapidly running out of time, defeated by the very characteristic that gave its ancestors enormous power: its forbidding size.

Although it is still the world's biggest country, its economic potential is poor. Although Russia occupies 11.5 percent of the global landmass, it has only 150 million people, or 2.32 percent of the world's population, and they control only 1.79 percent of its purchasing power. In a December 2002 presentation on the country's persistent economic problems, Andrey Illarionov, President Vladimir Putin's economic advisor, said that "the unavoidable conclusion here is a cruel one. Human history has no precedent of a gap this wide between 'territorial power' and economic 'insignificance' holding for any extended length of time." Problems of maldistribution created by Soviet planners cannot be solved by improving transportation or communication networks because while new infrastructure will make inhospitable places more livable, from an economic perspective, few people should be there in the first place. Hill and Gaddy say Russia has to "shrink" by helping people move from cold and distant cities to locations that are more productive from an individual and state perspective.

Even during tsarist times, Russia's size was a burden. In the nineteenth century, it maintained the largest standing army in Europe, a force of 1 million men stationed at its borders or in potential trouble spots such as Poland. During wartime, the army consumed three-quarters of Russia's revenues although the country spent less per soldier than Germany or France. This left no money for transport, so Russia's soldiers went everywhere on foot. During its 1875 conquest of Central Asia, after the Russian commander's request for additional troops was approved, the troops had to walk from Europe to Asia and did not arrive for a year. In 1904 it took Russia's Baltic fleet nine months to sail to Japan, "only to be blasted from the water by the Japanese navy at the Battle of Tsushima Strait." After the 9,000-mile trans-Siberian railway was completed, getting to Manchuria still took several weeks. Russia's weakness, one contemporary observer wrote, was its "unwieldiness"; troop movements consumed vast outlays of capital, so that in the end, Russia "was not a Great Power, but a country teetering on the edge of domestic disaster." The cost of the army's repeated losses in World War I led to widespread rioting in the major cities of the Russian empire and to the 1917 overthrow of the 300-year-old Romanov dynasty. By 1993, two years after the breakup of the Soviet Union, Russia still had 1.2 million men in uniform.

Post-Soviet planners unable to rectify the economic distortions created by the Bolshviks simply by imposing a market economy still want to develop and repopulate Siberia. "Russia's size and ideas of battling the elements continue to define the modern state," say Hill and Gaddy. After the breakup of the Soviet Union, Russia has tried to engineer a market economy on a "nonmarket distribution of labor and capital across its territory. People and factories languish in places communist planners put them—not where market forces have attracted them." The expense of developing production and transportation capabilities in Siberia prohibits development of its natural resources—no matter how rich—at prices competitive in the world marketplace. If the country's regions interact solely with one another, Russia can operate at only a marginal profit. Although Australia, Canada, and the United States are also vast, they are much more productive than Russia because their populations cluster in more temperate areas, close to shipping and transportation networks.

Russian economist Andrey Parshev says that economists must adopt "isothermal fatalism" if Russia's development is to move forward. "The fact that our production is noncompetitive is no secret. The secret is that the factors causing it to be noncompetitive cannot be removed."[18] Distance and temperature make the cost of mining Russia's gold deposits, for example, higher than the value of the reserves. The cost of Russian labor must include subsidies for living in the cold, which make wages "high by world standards. The proof of that statement is the fact that they are alive. Simply surviving under our conditions is expensive," says Parshev. The cost of construction, raw materials, and other physical inputs, transportation, energy, labor, and taxes send potential investors running elsewhere. The World Bank estimates that Russia spends between 2 to 3 percent of its gross domestic product every year supporting its northern population. The cost of poor Soviet centralized planning can be measured by other effects as well. Air, water, and land pollution went unchecked. Russia's first president, Boris Yeltsin, declared, "We've inherited an ecological disaster." Every major river in Russia is polluted, one-quarter of the drinking water is unsafe, and 35 million people live in cities where the air is dangerous to breathe.

During the 1991 transition, three-quarters of state enterprises were fully or partly privatized. Much of the money went into the pockets of Yeltsin's buddies, and crony capitalism enabled "a small number of oligarchs to become fabulously wealthy," says Fen Montaigne.[19] The collapse of the ruble in 1998 made importing impossible and boosted domestic production, so the economy grew 5 percent in 1999 and 8 percent in 2000. But it was not enough. In 2001 20 million of Russia's 145 million people (14 percent) were living below the official poverty line of $31 a month. High tax rates caused rampant evasion, sending the economy underground, and "every year a tiny layer of super-rich Russians—fearful of general instability and a shaky banking system—ships an estimated 20 to 25 billion dollars out of the country to foreign banks, much of it from the sale of Russia's abundant natural resources," says Montaigne. In the transition, two Russias emerged, one composed of "well-educated, hardworking people slowly building a humane society" and the other "a land where a worn-out populace endures corruption and a lack of decent civil institutions." Montaigne said that in 2001 "There is virtually no mortgage banking system, less than 2 percent of the population use credit cards, and only 7 percent have checking accounts."

Yeltsin resigned on December 31, 1999, and acting president Vladimir Putin was elected president in March 2000. Putin, also surrounded by get-rich-quick cronies, is popular although he has "little commitment to democracy or a free press and little stomach for tackling critical problems like endemic corruption and the creation of a viable legal system," says Montaigne. Putin also continued the war against Chechnyan separatists, "draining the country's treasury and spilling the blood of its citizens." Human Rights Watch and Amnesty International say the wider international community is "glad to be deceived" about the impact of war in Chechnya, now in its fourth year, which they call "one of the greatest threats to stability and rule of law in Russia."[20] The war has taken thousands of lives, and numerous acts of terror, torture, illegal arrest, and mass murder have displaced 300,000 Chechnyans into neighboring areas of Russia. After the terrorist attacks of September 11, 2001, Putin characterized the war, with roots in a ten-year-old separatist movement, as a containment action against international terrorists. However, the news blackout was not complete and Russians saw thousands of Chechnyas slaughtered; television recorded "Russia's brutality to a people it still claims as its own." Service says that the severity of the attacks were a "plague upon the

Russia state and society" that have "infected every aspect of political, administrative, military, economic and social affairs." Yeltsin and Putin lost the moral high ground; their retaliation against the Chechnyans looked like genocide even to the Russian public.

According to demographer Nicholas Eberstadt, "In barely a decade, Moscow has plummeted from the status of imperial superpower to a condition of astonishing geopolitical weakness."[21] The economy has shrunk to the size of Sweden's, and export revenues are lower than Singapore or Belgium. Military strength has evaporated, and dire economic problems have caused Russia leaders to sell off military hardware to China and Iran. Russia is "an unintentional menace, a burden" to the international community. Since the breakup of the Soviet Union, peoples' health has worsened, and death rates are rising across the board. Only one-quarter of Russia's children enjoy good health, and life expectancy has declined to 67 years of age, where it was four decades earlier. Russia also experienced a thirty-three-fold jump in sexually transmitted disease rates in the 1990s and almost quadrupled its rate of tuberculosis, including drug-resistant forms. One observer says that deregulation of the economy has led to "rampant crime and prostitution, relentless drug trafficking, mile-long queues for nonexistent food and a general end-of-the-world aura."

At the end of 2002, Russia was spending only $6 million of its own budget on HIV/AIDS, less than a third of what Moscow had pledged to UNAIDS that year. The government has access to individual HIV test results, which discourages voluntary testing, and waited until May 12, 2004, to reform its narcotics law, ending criminal penalties for small-time users. The reform will alleviate some of the crowding in jails, but authorities must now see that users have clean needles. Prior to the May reform, police systematically disrupted needle exchange programs and undermined access to health services for injecting drug users.[22] "Moscow seems to have settled on a posture of malign neglect toward the gathering problem," Eberstadt says, and the results will have dire economic consequences for a country that is already on a downward trend. Russia's growing social crisis has left 700,000 children on the streets, compared to 600,000 after World War II, and the number is rising by 20,000 per year. There are already 200,000 children in orphanages, "and statistics show that 30 percent of them will end up in criminal gangs and in jail."[23]

The three Baltic republics—Estonia, Latvia, and Lithuania—had begun to break away from the Soviet Union before August 1991. Of the eleven old republics left, nine merged into the Commonwealth of Independent States (CIS), while Ukraine and Belarus declared their independence. AIDS is spreading rapidly in many of these countries for the same reasons it is in Russia. Declining economies and increasing lawlessness have encouraged crime, prostitution, and drug use. The CIS countries are transit centers for illicit drugs, weapons manufacture and trafficking, and production of synthetic drugs for export to the West. "Ukraine is the epicenter for global badness," says reporter Peter Landesman. "It's worse than Pakistan. It's a one-stop shopping infrastructure for anyone who wants to buy anything."[24] In 2002 Ukraine's president was caught personally directing illicit weapons sales.

According to an April 2004 UN Development Program (UNDP) report on the HIV/AIDS situation in the CIS, the region has some of the fastest-growing epidemics in the world. Only Poland, the Czech Republic, and Slovakia were cited for building their "vibrant democracies into effective responses to HIV/AIDS." Estonia and Ukraine have the fastest growth. Social conditions feed the epidemic. The report called the regions' prisons and jails HIV "incubators," which interact with injecting drug use and prostitution to amplify epidemic growth. And government responses border on negligence. Prevention programs are small or nonexistent, voluntary counseling and testing is not widespread, and of the estimated 80,000 who need AIDS treatment, only 7,000 now receive it. In the UNDP's judgment, "It is already too late to speak of avoiding a crisis" in Eastern Europe and the CIS. "Of all the social and political challenges to an expanded European Union," said UNAIDS Director Peter Piot, "AIDS is one of the greatest, requiring determination and sustained action now."

<hr />

The UN Office for Drug Control (UNDOC) says that of the 200 million people in the world consuming illicit drugs, the number abusing heroin and opium stabilized at about 15 million between 1999 and 2002.[25] Some 163 million use marijuana, 34 million are addicted to amphetamines, 15 million use cocaine, and 8 million use ecstasy. Opium production remained level at about 4.5 million tons, although the amount of land devoted to poppy cultivation actually declined by 25 percent. Seventy-six percent of the world's supply of opium now comes from one country, Afghanistan, where irrigation fields increase the yield four times over the Golden Triangle's rain-fed crops. As a result, production in the Golden Triangle has declined by 40 percent, while production in Southwest Asia increased by 16 percent. This shift is reshaping global patterns of heroin abuse, fostering increased consumption in South West and Central Asia, the Russian Federation, and Eastern Europe. Lower prices mean that individual transactions are less profitable than in Western Europe, so dealers are widening their consumer base.

"The global drug trade . . . [links] First World and Third in a complex commerce that interpenetrates every aspect of contemporary society," says McCoy. The contemporary drug industry is fed by a commodities market created by European colonial powers that could "promote cultivation where needed (India) and suppress it where not (Southeast Asia)," while integrating the whole into the global economy. Global prohibition beginning in the 1920s added another layer: "criminal syndicates emerged to link highland growers and urban addicts in a global illicit market." Each subsequent effort to suppress production and use has had a chain of unintended consequences that has bolstered the drug trade and increased markets. Nearly eighty years of failed eradication efforts show that "the illicit drug market is a complex global system, both sensitive and resilient, that quickly transforms suppression into stimulus," says McCoy.

Suppression unleashes "unpredictable market forces that might ramify invisibly through the global system for years to come, contributing to a spread of narcotics production, drug consumption, and HIV infection." The price of failed eradication "has been extraordinarily high: extensive defoliation, forced migration, and military conflict in drug-source nations; mass incarceration, rising HIV infection, spreading drug use, and social polarization in the consuming countries." Since the end of the Cold War, nations have opened their boundaries, making containment even more difficult.

In 1986, while the CIA was helping to build drug infrastructure in Asia's Golden Triangle, the United States began certifying countries around the world as "partners" in the war on drugs and penalizing noncompliant countries with loss of foreign aid and trade sanctions. In 1989 the U.S. Department of Defense took the lead in administering this law and now "U.S. counter-narcotic training is barely distinguishable from counter-insurgency training to . . . military units notorious for human rights abuses." Through enforcement efforts, the United States has created "an unequal partnership in which the USA judges, certifies, impoverishes and degrades human rights in the subordinate combatant nations," says Davenport-Hines. "Washington continues to blame foreigners for nearly a century of failed US drug prohibition."

Drug suppression policies were being formed in an atmosphere that was extremely hypocritical in another respect: it favored addictive but licensed pharmaceutical company products for adults over the illegal substances preferred by young people. In the 1960s, the growing popularity of LSD and mescaline, used by younger "deviants," provoked extreme opposition from

U.S. and European authorities—unlike the stimulants and depressants used by older consumers. Drug use became increasingly associated with the radical youth culture, which was also sexualized by anti-drug proponents to make its behavior appear more deviant. In 1969, U.S. President Richard Nixon—who was addicted to anti-depressants, alcohol, and sleeping pills–announced that "to erase the grim legacy of Woodstock, we need a total war against drugs." Nixon was also worried because many U.S. soldiers in Vietnam used marijuana and 10 percent were regular heroin users.

Funding for the U.S. Drug Enforcement Agency, originally created as part of the war on drugs to suppress imports and domestic drug use, grew from a $3 billion in 1986 to $15 billion in 1997 as the Agency assumed an ever-larger international role. Domestically, drug suppression has not been successful. By 1985 one-third of 18- to 25-year-olds reported cocaine use in the past year. In 1997, 60 percent of 18- to 25-year-olds confessed to having tried marijuana at least once, and 44 percent in New York City said they sold it at least once. Severe criminal drug penalties increased the U.S. prison population threefold between 1980 and 1994, so the country had the highest per capita rate of incarceration in the world. One-third of all African Americans were either in jail or on probation in 1995. On average, first-time crack offenders were getting longer prison sentences than rapists, and many untreated addicts with repeat offences were jailed for life. With domestic conditions like these, it is difficult for the United States to be taken seriously when it recommends more enlightened policies to HIV/AIDS-threatened Asian governments trying to contain injecting drug use problems.

McCoy says that many drug enforcement officials are idealists, but they are co-opted by politicians with "other, less lofty agendas—racial repression, colonial dominion, partisan politics, covert operations, or, most recently, mass incarceration of unemployed minority males." Conservative administrations have housed the most militant antidrug advocates while their covert operations expanded drug production and supply. The CIA's covert wars "transformed tribal warlords into major drug lords and protect [them] from criminal investigation," says McCoy. In Southeast Asia, the CIA was seminal in developing the Golden Triangle and supporting the military regime in Thailand, where drug trafficking problems still linger. It played a major role in promoting opium growing among the Hmong in Laos and supported heroin production and sales that addicted thousands of U.S. soldiers in Vietnam. It stimulated a still-growing network that has caused massive addiction and criminality in Central Asia, Russia, and Eastern Europe, and operations in Central America have had a similar effect on the drug trade there. In each case, the CIA stayed long enough to achieve economic take off and sustained development for its partner warlords. And in each case, opium growth and heroin production have been the only means for post-war economic reconstruction in the absence of international aid. "Over time, narcotics production not only sustains a traumatized society during its postwar recovery, but it also reinforces its isolation from the legitimate economic resources of the international community," transforming recovering societies into "significant sources of international instability," concludes McCoy.

The opening of borders over the past twenty years has drawn new countries in Asia into globalized drug trafficking networks. India is still the world's largest producer of legal opium, but most of it is not sold to pharmaceutical companies. The country is a transit point for narcotics produced by neighboring Myanmar and Pakistan, an illicit methamphetamine producer, and a money-laundering hub. Mass unemployment and social insecurity, coupled with the erosion of rigid social control, has created a perfect setting for the rapid growth of the drug trade, which underpins the economies of many Asian states. Efforts to control drug trafficking, largely focused on the user rather than the gangsters who are profiting, have succeeded in contributing to the spread of HIV/AIDS. UNAIDS Director Peter Piot told the 2004 meeting of the international commission on narcotics that "from the Baltic to Central Asia, around the Mediterranean and Middle East, in South East and East Asia, injecting drug use is responsible for between 30 and 90 percent of the HIV epidemics." Changes in social norms associated with globalization and economic liberalization have set many people adrift without jobs or safety nets. Young people who feel hopeless and alone are drawn into experimentation with drugs. Young people in many Asian countries are also endangered because their countries are not supporting their needs for schooling, vocational training, and employment. Frustrated by their unrealized needs, pessimistic for their futures, sex and drugs gives them the perfect way to rebel.

SIX

GENDER, RELIGION, AND ECONOMICS IN THE EAST

"IN RUSSIA, THE POLICE HARASSED US AND HARASSED the people who gave us clean needles," Vladimir said. "We mostly lived on the street, and stole what we could. But there wasn't much to be had. Everyone was as poor as we were." He grimaced as the group laughed. Then he reached across and toyed with the end of Rageena's green scarf. "But I think it's time for the women to talk. I want to hear the end of your story."

Rageena pulled the scarf away from his hand and shrugged. "I think you probably already guessed the plot," she said. "But maybe you are too thick-headed, like most men, so I'll tell you the rest of the story." She winked at Molly and laughed. "Remember how my husband sold me to the carpet man after he brought me to Kathmandu?" The group nodded. "Mr. Sharma's fac-tory was not far from our house. When we got there, Sharma sent me off with an older woman, Jyoti, who helped me get undressed and bathed. She washed my hair, all the time crooning to me and comforting me like a child. The next day she helped me become accustomed to the factory. She was one of the few kind people I met, and I shall never forget her.

"Sharma, it turns out, owned several carpet factories in Kathmandu, and many of the girls who worked there came to him through trickery and deceit. Some of the rug makers refused to employ children, but others are not ashamed to do it. It goes against Nepali law, but in a country where so many parents are very poor, it is unavoidable. I learned this later, from Jyoti and the other girls. All of us worked twelve hours a day or more at our looms and so we had plenty of time to talk.

"I did not dare to leave. I believe I had shamed my parents and they would never take me back. I believed that Sharma owned me. At that time—I was only twelve—I had no idea of Nepali law on this matter. Besides, I had no idea how to get home. The other girls were friendly, and the work was no harder than at home. Sometimes the older women in the factory joked with us, saying that we had been ensnared in the threads of our carpets like birds in a net and that we should never escape because we were *randi* and could not be trusted. But they were kind to us, took care of us when we were ill, and tried to protect us from Mr. Sharma's sexual attentions.

"It wasn't too long before he came to stand at the side of my loom, watching me intently as I worked. I had just started a new carpet and was studying the pattern that lay on the ground beside me, so I didn't even hear his footsteps. 'Little girl,' he finally said, grinning wide, 'how are you enjoying your new work?' I stood quickly to greet him, dusting off my skirt. I told him that I was well and thanked him for his help. He only laughed at me, shook his head and walked away. 'No good deed goes unrewarded,' he tossed the words back over his shoulders. 'I am glad you like it here. Because it would be a hard thing for you to leave.' I shivered. The girls had told me how he liked to take his time with you, playing with you like a cat with a mouse.

"It wasn't too long before my day came," Rageena said. "Mr. Sharma was waiting for me when I finished. I tried to avoid his eyes and didn't greet him, but he put his big bulk right in my path. 'You are doing such a good job, Rageena. I have noticed your work. The women tell me you are polite and clean, and never complain about the work. Are you glad your husband sold you to me?' He laughed and tried to grab my wrist, but I pulled it back from his grasp and tucked it quickly behind my back.

"I stared at the ground and said nothing, hoping he would let me go. Shoba, one of the older women, came to stand beside me and put her arm around my shoulders. 'We need this one, Sharma,' she said, 'to meet your lousy production quotas. Let me take her to help us with dinner.' Sharma darkened and stamped his foot like a small boy. 'Don't tell me what to do, Shoba. It could cost you your job.' Her arm fell from my shoulders and she scurried away with the rest of the women.

"He turned back to me. 'Now, Rageena.' He stamped his foot again, angry at Shoba's intervention. 'Let me take you to my office. I have some new ideas for carpet designs that I would like you to see.' From that day on, I did nothing but look at his new 'carpet designs' until I could stand it no longer and tried to run away. He beat me severely, then sold me to a trafficker from India after my bruises healed. The trafficker sold me to a large brothel with almost 2,000 sex workers in it. It was like my parents' barn. Each of us had a little stall and were raped more than twenty times a day. When I got sick, I still owed the gangsters that owned it money, but they paid my bus fare home anyway because I looked so terrible no one would pay to be near me. That, my friends, is how I came to catch HIV in a Mumbai brothel. We even called it 'the Mumbai disease,' because there were so many like me. By the time I got HIV, 'respectable' Nepali women were becoming infected just like me because their husbands played around. Marriage is no insurance against this terrible disease."

"Damn Mr. Darwin!" Christabel exclaimed, slamming her fist hard on the table. Her mother looked up. "Oh!" Emmeline said, "you've got new gloves. How pretty. Wherever did you get them and how did you manage the money . . ." Her voice trailed off. Christabel was glaring at her. "Mother! I'm trying to have an intelligent conversation here!" she cried. "Yes, dear, I am too," Emmeline replied. "But having the proper clothing is so important for women who do what we do. I do like the white dresses with purple and green sashes, don't you? I think it's a very strong symbol . . . Christabel, really. You shouldn't make faces. Listen please, dear. I do want your opinion on this. You are always so good at gauging public opinion. And if we don't wear the right clothing, the public just won't sympathize with us."

Christabel frowned. "I'm not sure the public will sympathize with us no matter what we wear! I was talking with a group of women the other day—women, mind you. Women, mother!—who said we shouldn't be given the right to vote because we aren't capable of independent thought. In fact, they told me that, according to Mr. Darwin and others of his ilk, we are not very far from children when it comes to ratiocination." Emmeline's pretty eyebrows knit. "Ratiocination," Christabel continued. "You know, mother! Thinking!" "Yes, of course, dear," Emmeline said, laughing. "How Richard loved that word. You are so like your father, dear! As to women thinking, why I understand when Mr. Darwin was a young man, he decided to take a wife because she would be a slightly better companion than a dog, and much more fun to play with! Now as to those dresses . . ."[1] But Christabel frowned again.

"You know I've tried to read Mr. Darwin's *Origin of the Species* and his far more interesting *Descent of Man*, where he expounded on the relative positions of the races and of the female sex," Emmeline said, "but I am far too busy with our own revolution to keep my mind focused on such dry stuff. I know it is important, because Mr. Darwin and his band openly scorned the female sex as lower on the evolutionary scale than the male, and his thinking is still so influential. But I vastly prefer Mr. Wallace. Do you know, Christabel, that he once told a reporter from the *Humanitarian* that 'it is to the women of the future that I look for the needed reformation'? Look," she continued, "I saved the article because it was so important. He said, 'educate and train women so that they are rendered independent of marriage as a means of gaining a home and a living, and you will bring about natural selection in marriage, which will operate most beneficially upon humanity.'"

Christabel smiled at her broadly, thinking of how extraordinary she was. Emmeline continued reading. "'I want to see women the selective agents in marriage,' Mr. Wallace said, 'as things are, they have practically little choice. The only basis for marriage should be a disinterested love.'" She cleared her throat, thinking as she often did of her dear Richard. "Here, Christabel, is the part I like the best. He concluded the interview by saying, 'I believe that the unfit will be gradually eliminated from the race, and human progress secured, by giving to the pure instincts of women the selective power in marriage. You can never have progress so long as women are driven to marry for a livelihood.'"

"Here! Here!" Christabel said, laughing. "I stand corrected. Some evolutionists are positively human." Her mother smiled, too. "Not only that, my dear, but Mr. Wallace just sent a wonderful letter to *The Times* saying that 'All human inhabitants of any one country should have equal rights and liberties before the law; women are human beings,' he says, 'therefore they should have votes as well as men. The term 'Liberal' does not apply to those who refuse this natural and indefensible right.' The next time you lecture, you can tell those women that natural selection is as female as it is male. Now, about those dresses . . ."

Emmeline was too busy for evolutionary theory, and she was also too poor—and too determined—to succumb to the fashion of drug use so popular among many Victorian women. But she knew the same thing had not been true of Herbert Gladstone's aunt Helen, for all their brother's hammering on the evils of the Britain's opium trade in India. Helen had been a hopeless laudanum addict. Emmeline knew that William was often "not himself" either, but no one talked about his habit because he was a man and a very powerful one at that. It was alright to lay into women for being indolent opium delinquents, but men could use the stuff to prepare for their speeches to parliament. She'd been infinitely amused by Randolph Churchill's comment that listening to Gladstone's oratory was like taking morphia. "The sensations are transcendent," he'd said, "but the recovery is bitter." She and Richard had approved of Gladstone's stand against Britain's pretensions to empire, however. Richard had said that empire building was totally inappropriate when so many people were starving right at home in Britain. In fact, he'd often said that he thought the reason why so many politicians avoided giving the franchise to women was because they knew that women would be more interested in home issues than in building military might.

It was fortunate, Emmeline thought, that Helen had traveled with her personal physician frequently because she was so disruptive and embarrassing to her family. Gladstone once confessed after traveling to Baden-Baden to coax her of her habit that "she was in danger of death! She is poisoned much in body and, more, in mind, by the use of that horrible drug." He tried to repair her moral disorganization by reading to her, but after a particularly stirring rendition from a book of Protestant divines, he found the volume in the family water closet where it was being used as toilet paper. When the family stopped persecuting Helen for her conversion to Roman Catholicism, she was able to give up the drug for long periods at a time.

Emmeline had seen many poor women spend their savings on quacks' nostrums and tried to dissuade them from wasting their money, but to no avail. She had become very angry with physicians, whose attitudes toward women were truly shameful. If they had not made the women so stupid with laudanum in the first place, they might find them a little more intelligent than they gave them credit for. She remembered her shock on hearing a leading physician hold forth on women as "hypersensitive, unreasonable, and having no sense of proportion." Opium had been liberally deployed, she knew, to control women's feelings and contain their behavior in ways that men preferred. One of her friends had been given so much opium during the early stages of her pregnancy for what Emmeline felt was very natural symptoms—having carried five children herself—that she fell into despondency. Physicians believed that opium relieved nausea, which might be true, but most women she knew could stand a little discomfort and would prefer it to debasing addiction.

Many ideas inherited from Darwin's day have come up for closer scrutiny. With the advance of molecular genetics, we've learned that all the flap about races and their relative endowments and intelligence is ridiculous because there is more genetic difference within human "races" than between. Unfortunately, we've also learned that aversion based on sex and age is stronger than aversion based on race.[2] These ideas are being challenged, but still have incredible power in our day-to-day lives. Take this story from Laos, for example, as a start . . .

———•◦•———

"See that hotel with the green sign?" My colleague, a Lao HIV/AIDS and migration expert, gestured across the river. If the Mekong had dried up that instant, the Thai hotel with its huge bank of beckoning neon would have been an easy walk from the café where we sat. "Chinese businessmen on sex junkets use their cell phones to call across the river and in two hours pimps on this side deliver a fresh bunch of Lao schoolgirls to their hotel room doors. In their uniforms. And they have to be virgins or the Chinese won't pay." The flirtatious schoolgirl, winking through her oversized hornrimmed glasses while she tugs at a short plaid skirt that barely conceals her buttocks is an old cliché of American pornography. The literature of women and AIDS is rife with stories of molested innocents who were introduced to the school of hard knocks at the same time as they were learning their ABCs. Adopting the schoolgirl sexpot as an icon of the predicament of women in the world of AIDS might not be a bad idea, expressing as it does the deep sense of gender conflict—the outright misogyny—underlying the rapid spread of HIV in all corners of the world.

The Global Coalition on Women was launched in February 2004, some thirty years after the epidemic started, and—many would argue—thirty years too late. It has been twenty years since women's biological and social disempowerment has been recognized as key to epidemic spread, yet little has changed in any real way except in the negative direction. After a visit to several African countries in January 2003, the UN Special Envoy for AIDS Stephen Lewis said "Women are at the center of the pandemic, as they are acutely vulnerable to infection on the one hand, doing all the care-giving for the sick and the orphans on the other. [But I] saw precious little evidence of efforts at women's empowerment, sexual autonomy or gender equality. And there was certainly no effort whatsoever to relieve their unfair share of the burden. In fact, male hegemony was ubiquitous."

Two-thirds of the world's illiterate adults are women. More than half a million women die in pregnancy or childbirth each year. Women are four times more vulnerable to HIV/AIDS. Almost one-third of all women in the world are victims of domestic violence, and 130 million suffer genital mutilation. More than 100 million women are "missing" from the world today, according to Nobel Prize-winning economist Amartya Sen.[3] They have been eliminated because they are unwanted, eliminated because they have no power to fight back and preserve their own right to life. They are eliminated before they are born or shortly afterward, aborted or victims of infanticide. They are strangled, smothered, burned, and mutilated. Every year worldwide there are 80 million unwanted pregnancies and 20 million unsafe abortions. The only reason women are not at the absolute bottom of the global feeding chain is because children are weaker.

Or are they? The Convention on the Rights of the Child (CRC), passed by the UN in 1990, gets much more respect than CEDAW, the Convention to Eliminate All Forms of Discrimination Against Women. Countries that ratify CEDAW agree to take active steps to eliminate discrimination against women in all spheres and to modify social and cultural patterns of conduct to eliminate prejudices and customs based on the idea of inferiority or superiority of either sex. CEDAW has been around for ten years longer than the CRC and has accomplished less. Nepal ratified CEDAW in 1991; Article 11 of the Nepali Constitution guarantees equal right to women. Like India, it is a state where women still commit *purdah*—suicide upon their husband's death—(little wonder since their lives as widows is so full!), and girls service men eager to improve their spirituality in temple precincts. "When my father died, my mother became a nonperson," my young Nepali friend said bitterly. "She knew the family would probably marry me off, even though I was much too young, so she sent me to join my sister at her American school. She took the brunt of their hatred. She could never wear red again. It was her favorite color. Jewelry was out of the question. She could never wear the tika spot on her forehead or participate in religious events. She sat in the house and withered. When she wasn't physically beaten, the family crushed her mind and spirit. They called her 'husband killer' even though my father had clearly died of a heart attack. Finally,"—her green eyes drilled into me—"she killed herself. Rat poison. My mother! And what crime had she ever committed, except the one of being a woman?"

Laos ratified CEDAW in 1981, but fresh schoolgirls are still shuttled regularly across the Mekong. The United States has signed the convention but never ratified it because it affirms the reproductive rights of women, rights consistently challenged by religious fundamentalists. By December 10, 2003, 174 other countries, more than 90 percent of all UN member states, had become parties to the convention and committed themselves to end all forms of discrimination against women, including legal protection and access to opportunities in education, health, and employment. But it looks like it will take a third wave of international feminism, much like a second wave was needed in industrialized countries in the 1960s and 1970s, before the scorecard evens out. And by then it will be too late for many women in Asia and Africa.

At the opening of *Children of AIDS: Africa's Orphan Crisis*, author Emma Guest says, "A 13-year-old Kenyan AIDS orphan gave away her virginity in exchange for an apple. Asked why, she replied, 'No one's ever given me anything before.'"[4] All around the world, poverty and lack of opportunity reduce women to the state where their only currency, to borrow Helen Epstein's phrase, is sex.[5] Almost 70 percent of the 1.2 billion of the world's extremely poor people are women. High-fertility and hypersexuality are the only ways women can demonstrate their value, reinforcing existing cycles of poverty and degradation. As R. Barri Flowers argues, recent increases in the worldwide sexual exploitation of women and girls "is largely attributable to a booming sex tourism industry in Asia, Europe, and South America, to Third World poverty, to the economic depression of the former Eastern bloc, and to weak or inconsistent laws that effectively encourage prostitution in many countries by minimizing penalties against pimps, purveyors, panderers, sex tour promoters, brother owners, customers of prostitutes, and other sexual exploiters of women and girls."[6] In *Sex Slaves*, author Louise Brown connects sexual exploitation to disenfranchisement and labor exploitation in the global economy. Politicians and economists collaborate by failing to include women's work, largely unpaid, in national economic accounts.[7]

A 2002 UNAIDS survey in three dozen countries found that even where infection rates were high, 66 percent of women said they were either at no risk or low risk for AIDS. In countries where 20 to 30 percent of the population is HIV positive, this belief is at best naively optimistic. Half the respondents to 2000 and 2002 surveys in twenty-eight countries say they are unconcerned about getting sexually transmitted diseases (STDs), and 38 percent take no measures to protect themselves.[8] In Southeast Asia, only 13 percent of young women could correctly identify two ways to protect themselves from getting HIV. Half of young Vietnamese women think they can get HIV from a mosquito bite, and 30 percent of young Cambodian women think they will get it if they are cursed. In Central Asia and Eastern Europe, almost half of all young women believed a healthy person could not be carrying HIV or have AIDS. While 72 percent of Chinese women have heard of HIV/AIDS, half who were illiterate had not. Over three-quarters of the women, of all ages and from all backgrounds, said it was "impossible" for them to get HIV.

Even if women are aware, their right to refuse sex is limited. In Asia as in Africa, men who have sex outside of marriage experience no stigma, but if their wives demand condom use, they risk partner violence. As health expert

Chris Breyer pointed out in 2001, in Asia, "the single most important risk factor for HIV infection among women is marriage."[9] Women who seek voluntary counseling and testing for HIV or ask their partners to use condoms often face violence from their partners, so much so that major international effort is being put into developing "couples counseling" programs that will counsel husband and wife together. Preaching abstinence, partner reduction, or condom use is cynical "for the majority of women and girls in many cultures and situations," says Noerine Kaleeba, founder of The AIDS Support Organization in Uganda, one of the first home care programs on the continent.

According to Human Rights Watch, widespread rape and brutal attacks on women by their husbands are contributing to a resurgence of HIV/AIDS in Uganda, a country that succeeded in stopping the spread of HIV in the mid-1990s.[10] Almost half of all women in Ethiopia, Uganda, and Kenya, a third in Canada, and a fifth in the United States have been beaten by their husbands, the most common form of violence against women in every country. The Centers for Disease Control (CDC) estimates that the health-related costs of rape, physical assault, stalking, and homicide by intimate partners exceeds $5.8 billion each year in the United States alone. The ultimate costs are even higher because many women and children do not seek medical assistance. According to U.S. Health and Human Services secretary Tommy Thompson, "Violence against women harms more than its direct victim. It also harms the children, the abuser and the entire health of all our families and communities." In Asia many women believe they deserve a beating (as long as it does not leave visible marks) if dinner is not ready on time or if they go out without their husband's permission, and men agree. Women with HIV are much more likely to have a physically violent partner, and almost half said they could not deny their husbands sex after a beating or if they feared HIV infection. "Women especially at risk are those in a heterosexual marriage or long term union in a society where men commonly engage in sex outside the union and women confront abuse if they demand condom use," says Human Rights Watch.[11]

In 1997 women accounted for 41 percent of the world's HIV/AIDS cases; that proportion is now 48 percent.[12] In sub-Saharan Africa, with the oldest epidemics, women comprise 57 percent of all HIV/AIDS cases, and while the proportion is lower in Asia, it is rising fast. Globally, women comprise 62 percent of new infections, meaning their overall share will continue to increase. Among infected South and Southeast Asians, 25 percent are female and 28 percent of the new infections are among women. In Eastern Europe and Central Asia, 33 percent are women and the proportion is rising fast. Experts predict that as the epidemic spreads more widely in the general population, the proportion of women infected in Asia will exceed men just as it has in Africa. On International Women's Day, UN Secretary General Kofi Annan asked, "Why are women—usually not the ones with the most sexual partners outside marriage, or more likely than men to be injecting drug users—more vulnerable to infection? Usually because society's inequalities put them at risk." Why are HIV/AIDS cases increasing faster among women than among men around the world? Why does gender discrimination persist although it results in ill health, violence, death, and lost productivity? The reasons are many.

First, women are more biologically vulnerable. Physiological differences in the genital tract mean that women run a higher risk of HIV infection than men with each sexual encounter. Many STDs that increase the risk of HIV infection are asymptomatic in women, and women often face shame, discrimination, and partner violence when they seek treatment.[13] Women have more illnesses than men but are less likely to receive medical treatment for any condition. Women are more likely to need blood transfusions after childbirth, especially if they are anemic and malnourished, exposing them to infected blood supplies and their government's irresponsibility. No woman-controlled form of HIV prevention has yet been developed and widely distributed.

The female condom, developed in the early 1990s, was judged to be too expensive for developing countries. Although acceptability surveys find that up to 95 percent of men and women who have used the female condom find it "user friendly," only 64 million have been distributed in 100 countries, and only Brazil makes it a central component of its prevention efforts. When used correctly and consistently, they are more effective than male condoms (97 percent compared to 90 percent). A new, less expensive version is expected in 2005. Microbicides—gels, creams, films, sponges, or suppositories inserted in the vagina or rectum before sex, which can be used without the partner's knowledge—prevent sexual transmission by killing or inactivating the virus. After almost two decades, their use is still being worked out. Human trials are underway in Brazil, India, and Zimbabwe, but of the $775 million needed to bring a product to market by 2007, only $230 million has been committed so far. Even male condoms are not widely available. Less than half of all people at risk of HIV infection can get them, and availability is especially low in poorer parts of the world.

The second reason is economics. Women have not been empowered because their unpaid labor in food production and domestic work is too valuable. In developing countries, where household and agricultural chores are labor intensive, women provide no-cost labor for farms and homes so men can work for very low wages. Women who are marginalized in this way can easily be exploited for sex work, which, as we will see below, is big business. In poor countries, where unemployment is high, keeping women in the home or in the brothel has the distinct advantage of sopping up a lot of otherwise unemployed and potentially restive people. Women provide unpaid labor to care for sick family members and girls, not boys, are taken out of school to replace lost labor from AIDS deaths. In many Asian countries, like India, Afghanistan, and Pakistan, women cannot own or inherit property, which helps concentrate the distribution of wealth in the society. Ironically, while inequality for women has many economic benefits for the elite, the economic loss to the society as a whole is substantial. A World Bank study in sub-Saharan Africa showed that gender discrimination has reduced per capita economic growth in the region by at least 0.8 percent each year since 1960, roughly the same annual loss experts attribute to AIDS.

Third, economic vulnerabilities are controlled by social systems, which set the rules that perpetuate gender inequities. Without education, women's ability to get information of any kind—but especially about sex and STDs—is vastly reduced. There are no social safety nets, unemployment insurance, or social security systems in most Asian countries because governments work with employers to hold cost down and maximize profits. Brown says that "families provide protection but they can also be a prison in which the worst abuses take place . . . . The girl is easy prey when families fail." But there is no other protector of women's virtue, no economic or social status for females, and no other social support systems. "When they do not belong to one man," Brown says, "they belong, by default, to all. Women like these constitute a large proportion of the prostitutes of Asia." Asian women marginalized by their national education and labor systems who feel obliged to support their parents in addition to their children can find ready employment, usually more lucrative than comparable jobs, in the sex sector.

Fourth, economic and social systems are solidly reinforced by cultural beliefs. Gender norms limit what "good" women are supposed to know about sex and sexuality, so their ability to accurately determine their level of risk and learn how to protect themselves from infection is reduced. Women must rely on their husbands to know about these things, but many of them are just as ignorant as their wives or more so. Women also rely on their husbands to be honest about sexual relations outside the union. Gender myths about sexuality encourage the promiscuity of men and lack of marital fidelity and sustain the sex sector. These are linked to wider myths about normality and productive functioning. For example, many Indian truck drivers believe their safety as drivers depends on having regular sex, which helps release the body "heat" that builds up while they are driving. In many cultures, male identity is tied to having many sexual partners, whether the man is married or not.

Social systems also control women's ability to speak out, either within their family or in a public setting, and determine whether women can own property and build up economic security on their own without relying on a man. They determine where females live when they are children or as single or married women, and how much say they have in their own lives relative to their families of birth or marriage. Organized religions, the primary source of beliefs about women's essential nature and the essential nature of the universe in which they reside, have over time become increasingly aligned with the prevailing power structures of their day and reinforce damaging cultural stereotypes and social structures.

"Children and women are considered to be the possessions of the traditional Asian family," says Brown. "Women and girls are treated as property . . . and marriage for most women in Asia is the principal means to a livelihood and social status." In the face of enduring tradition, women's gains can easily be lost. In 1949 Chinese communists moved quickly to eliminate systematic discrimination against women, but with liberalization in 1978, the changes evaporated. "China buys and sells its women and girls today in much the same way as it did a century ago. Only now it does so in the name of the free market," Brown says. In Thailand, "daughters are cast in the role of caretakers of the family. As in the rest of South-East Asia girls are expected to pay back their 'breast milk money,'" Brown says. In the Philippines, girls must pay their *utang na loob*, "debt of gratitude," to their parents, and Chinese children are eternally in their parents' debt for giving them life. Male children are less obliged to support their parents because they will be responsible for supporting their own wives and children in these predominantly patriarchal societies.

Fifth, communities and families help children learn cultural stereotypes, teaching women to be their own best enemies. A gender system—cultural ideas of what women can and cannot do—is a form of control that helps keep about half of the population in line with tradition and uncomplaining, even when it means death. Geeta Sodhi, director of an Indian organization devoted to women called Swaasthya, says that cultural ideals promote sexual coercion. "The woman [accepts] sexual assault without ever raising a voice, because that's what's expected of a good woman, a good wife, a good daughter-in-law. She's caught in the trap of a social-cultural context which promotes and propagates sexual coercion, which actually contributes to her vulnerability to HIV/AIDS and other negative outcomes of sexual intimacy, like unwanted pregnancy."[14] As anthropologist Margery Wolf learned from her extensive work in Chinese villages, "cultural conceptions of gender are systematically linked to the organization of social inequality."[15] Power "crosses conventionally established boundaries between politics and everyday life, between the state and the family," and concepts of gender and sex are one of the pathways it follows. Wolf says, "many women in Taiwan villages were quite good farmers, and they were competent to make decisions, but they needed a male voice to announce them in the public part of the house. That . . . is why women are called 'pillow ghosts.'"

When a woman becomes infected with HIV, gender myths lead to stigmatization by the community. Women are perceived as the "bearers" of HIV. HIV-positive women whose status is known are more likely to be abused, abandoned, or even killed. Even if they caught HIV from their husbands it is assumed that they are "bad" women who sought sex outside of marriage. The statistics on "bad girls" are mind-numbing. At least 4 million are sold into sexual slavery every year. Women and men are socialized to behave according to community expectations. Men generally use alcohol and drugs, which increase the likelihood of risky behavior, where "good" women do not. "Bad" women, on the other hand, exchange sex for money. In Brazil, says anthropologist Linda Rebhun, "locals use sexual behavior as a . . . symbol of moral status in women, and . . . spoiled sexual reputation interacts with other stigmatized statuses."[16] The real story is different. First sexual intercourse for about one-third of all women in the world is forced, and sexual coercion continues to threaten women throughout their lifetimes. In Papua New Guinea, a ritual of group sex of one woman and many men called *lainap* may be contributing to transmission of HIV both to the women involved and among the men who participate. In this ritual of male bonding, "an urge to assert male superiority over women, the intent to punish, and an ethos of sexual opportunism and violence are all stressed."[17] One-third to one-half of all women in New York City are likely to be raped or brutalized at least once in their lives.

While communities can be the source of harsh rules, they can also be a vital source of protection. The breakdown of traditional communities leaves many people vulnerable, especially minority ethnic groups, women, and young people, whose status declined under colonial rule. In colonial times, community breakdown was encouraged in a number of ways, and community social and cultural norms deliberately violated by colonial authorities aimed at control or modernization. Molestation of female workers by their colonial overlords was common. In Sri Lanka, Tamil laborers struck in 1914, demanding an end to the attacks. In many modern Asian countries, poor communities and ethnic minority communities are now brutalized by their own governments.

Women are especially vulnerable to abuse and exploitation. The March 2004 Banguio Declaration of the Second Asian Indigenous Women's Conference lists their top problems, including theft of their lands, water, and other resources, which leaves them poor and in ill-health; militarization and violence against their villages by governments and the "private armies of private companies, especially in communities targeted for development;" individual physical and sexual violence against themselves and their children; violation of their right to citizenship, especially in Thailand, which cuts access to education, public services, property rights, and social mobility for them and their children; and the weakening of women's roles. Aruti Chakma, a Bangladeshi delegate, told the conference that militarization is the government's main tool of subjugation, and ethnic minority women are raped "to maintain discipline. The government is also spoiling our young generation by supplying them with drugs." A Nepali delegate said that violence by and against communist insurgents has made them poorer, promoting the trafficking of women.

Sixth, for the sex sector to thrive, the political system it calls home must support it, either explicitly or tacitly. A government accomplishes that by ignoring its commitments to CEDAW and making no positive changes in law and policy. As sex work becomes an increasingly profitable sector, there is less incentive to push legislative reforms for women's rights, and more opportunities for corrupt officials to evade them. Few countries have behaved like Vietnam, where the rights of women were enshrined in a Marxist slogan: "Knowing that they must work to eat, women no longer simply *follow* their fathers and mothers, *follow* their husbands and sons, as though they were in a state of perpetual bondage." Most governments in Asia and the world are controlled by men, who ensure that women's access to power is low. Only 15 percent of the seats in Asian parliaments are held by women, 14 percent in the Pacific, and less than 4 percent in Muslim countries. Only in Nordic countries do women approach fair representation, averaging 40 percent of the total seats, and it is in those countries that women's social safety nets are strongest. Most industrialized countries average only 15 percent. American women are sixteen years away from celebrating the 100th anniversary of obtaining the vote, yet only eight women currently serve as governors and women hold only 14 of 100 U.S. Senate seats and 48 of 435 seats in the House of Representatives. Only 29 women have ever held cabinet positions in the country's history.

HIV/AIDS epidemics in sub-Saharan Africa show that the disease can reinforce women's political vulnerability. In South Africa, second only to India in HIV infections, and in Zambia and Zimbabwe, more women than men are infected and 75 percent of infections among young people are in women. Political observers are speculating that this will cause a major loss of franchise for women, who will be outnumbered politically, underrepresented in government, and have a smaller share of all voting ages except the very oldest. South Africa's Governance and AIDS Programme's April 2004 report said that "women in particular risk disenfranchisement, as they were most often affected by the epidemic." Malawi is also reporting similar problems, because women taking care of the sick are too busy to vote, as are people sick with AIDS themselves.[18]

The final reason women are so disempowered is because international collusion supports perpetuation of national systems of gender inequality and the disinclination to change them. For more than twenty years, the United States has failed to ratify CEDAW, which elsewhere has helped reduce sexual slavery, increase women's education, and improve education. UN Secretary Genderal Kofi Annan says, "This 'Women's Bill of Rights' stands as a milestone. It reflects the principle of universal and indivisible rights sacred to all nations, foreign to no culture and common to both genders." As of January 2004, 175 countries had ratified or acceded to the treaty, including every other industrialized country, but the United States has elected to join Afghanistan, Iran, Syria, and Somalia in rejecting it. The United States also supports a foreign policy that interferes with condom use, electing to advocate abstinence for the prevention of HIV/AIDS instead.[19] In 2003 the first "Global Women's Scorecard" gave the Bush administration a high mark for rhetoric on global AIDS policies, but failing grades on policies to protect the rights of women and vulnerable groups from infection, and for restricting family planning services worldwide by cutting back on condom distribution. Although the administration promotes itself as compassionate, its actions have been exceptionally damaging to human rights and the effort to prevent the spread of HIV/AIDS around the world, the group said.[20] Abstinence-only education is being promoted at home, too, although the United States has the highest rates of STDs and teen pregnancy in the developed world. Research demonstrates that abstinence-only education does not work because most women are subject to the sexual coercion of men.

———◦•◦——

The age of the brothel "madam"—the *mamasans* of Malaysia and the *gharwalis* and *didis* of western India and Nepal—is over, says the Bangkok-based Global Alliance against Traffic in Women (GAATW), because "control is shifting from the hands of women into that of men. The sex trade in Asia is rapidly acquiring the characteristics of an industry, including high levels of organization, wages for work, a factory-like atmosphere, anonymity, and a complete alienation at the workplace. "The courtesans and geishas peppering literature and folklore have become dehumanized and objectified into anonymous bodies on a dance floor," says Zi Teng, a Hong Kong-based sex workers' association. "With well-organized, male-dominated thugs moving in to control prostitution," says a representative of an Indian sex workers' collective, sex has been reduced to "purely a commercial transaction."

According to a 1998 International Labor Office (ILO) study in Indonesia, Malaysia, the Philippines, and Thailand prostitution in Southeast Asia has grown so rapidly in recent decades that the sex business has assumed the dimensions of a commercial sector, one that contributes substantially to employment and national income. "The stark reality," said the study's coordinator, economist Lin Lim, "is that the sex sector is a big business that is well entrenched in the national economies and the international economy. . . . Prostitution is deeply rooted in a double standard of morality for men and women, as well as in a sense of gratitude or obligation that children feel they owe their parents." Asia's economic crisis may have fueled its growth by throwing millions of women into unemployment. Lim said, "If the evidence from the recession of the mid-1980s is any indication, then it is very likely that women who lose their jobs in manufacturing and other service sectors and whose families rely on their remittances may be driven to enter the sex sector." Demand never slowed down as men lost their jobs. "Poverty has never prevented men from frequenting prostitutes, whose fees are geared to the purchasing power of their customers," observed the ILO report. Now that sex work is internationalized, recessions make sex work cheaper for tourists.

The four governments earn between 2 and 14 percent of their gross domestic product directly from the sector. In Indonesia, the sex sector earns between $1.2 and $3.3 billion a year, or 0.8 to 2.4 percent of the annual gross domestic product. The ILO study estimates between 0.25 and 1.5 percent of all females in the four countries are sex workers. Indonesia has at least 230,000 sex workers; Malaysia, about 140,000; Thailand, about 300,000; and the Philippines, about 500,000. Authorities collect licensing fees and taxes on the many legitimate businesses, hotels, bars, restaurants, game rooms, tourist agencies, escort services, spas, and special clubs that flourish around the sex sector. In countries where prostitution is illegal, bribes are collected from businesses the sex industry uses as fronts, including nightclubs, cocktail lounges, karaoke bars, discotheques, saunas, and massage parlors. The income it generates is crucial to the livelihoods of millions of workers in peripheral businesses, supporting tens of thousands of cleaners, waitresses, cooks, parking lot attendants, and security guards. In Malaysia, physicians are employed for regular checkups, food vendors near sex establishments have more customers, and property owners earn good rent. In Laos, locals carefully directed me to one of the few spas in Vientiane where services did not automatically include sex. In the border area of Vietnam, my local field trip included a karaoke lunch at a "motel" whose elegant equipment included a bevy of comely and very demure young serving girls.

In Thailand, close to $300 million is transferred annually by urban-based sex workers to rural families, more money than any rural development program provides. A minimum of $90 million is sent home every year by Jakarta's sex workers, and sex workers make similar transfers in other Asian countries where the amounts have not been quantified. Rural remittances, as they are called, constitute a "poverty relief" program that allows the poor in subsistence agriculture to survive in the absence of government concern and programming. It "is often the only viable alternative for women in communities coping with poverty, unemployment, failed marriages and family obligations in the nearly complete absence of social welfare programs," says the report. Seventy percent of Philippine sex workers said they are supporting poor parents, their own children, or their spouses and boyfriends, the same incentive most commonly mentioned by Thai sex workers. Half had previously worked on their family's farm, in rural cottage industries, or in domestic labor until they became sex workers.

Society fixes the bargain to compensate for the risk. In exchange for the distastefulness and danger of their labor, sex workers earn much more. Sex work provides significantly higher earnings for young, often uneducated women than other forms of skilled labor. High-end sex workers in Indonesia's big cities can earn as much as $2,500 a month, more than mid-level civil servants, although at the bottom of the pile, sex can cost as little as $1 and incur substantially more risk of HIV infection. Despite the financial incentives, the study says that "in the experience of most of the women surveyed, prostitution is one of the most alienating forms of labor." Half the Philippine sex workers interviewed, most of whom are Catholics, said they carry out their work "with a heavy heart," conscious that what they do as a living is a sin. Half said they felt nothing for their clients, and the other half said the work saddened them. Few women work where they were born or grow up. Most go to cities or across borders, and there has been a rise in "ruthlessly efficient" networks of traffickers who recruit, transport, and sell women and children. Eighty percent of Asian women legally entering Japan in the 1990s said they were "entertainers," a common euphemism for prostitutes. Most were from the Philippines or Thailand. The ILO study says that "flows of prostitutes throughout south and southeast Asia are described as almost 'commuter-like' in their regularity and complexity."

Other Asian countries also have large populations of sex workers. Bangladesh is estimated to have 1.7 million, and India's 1,000 "red-light districts" employ 2.3 million women, one-fourth of them minors. Their conditions vary greatly, from highly remunerative, freely chosen sex work to virtual slavery. Most child prostitutes fall into the latter category, where they are "helpless against the established structures and vested interests of the sex sector," says Lim. They are more susceptible to getting HIV and other diseases, "to debt bondage, trafficking and physical violence and torture, and lifelong physical and psychological trauma." A 2004 study by a child rights organization in Kathmandu says that 12,000 Nepali girls are trafficked each year, while 200,000 are already trapped in India's brothels.

The sex industry is fully entrenched in the four countries studied by the ILO and in all other Asian economies as well. Lim says that the increase in disposable incomes of a growing middle class has "meant an enhanced capacity and motivation of men to buy sexual services in a much wider and more sophisticated range of settings." The Internet has taken the sex business international and girls are now selected on the basis of video clips or from marketing CDs. The ILO says that "the virtual disintegration of the public sector, lack of viable employment, and the ghettoization of female workers into poorly paid jobs in the textile, garment, electronics and tobacco industries (all 90 percent female) means that they cannot earn enough money to survive." Neglect of rural development means that families sell their children into prostitution, or encourage one child to enter the trade. Tourist promotion policies, encouragement of urban-rural migration to provide cheap labor for export-oriented industrial growth, and lack of social welfare policies (safety nets, unemployment compensation, insurances, and the like) all contribute to the growth of the sex work sector.

The ILO warns that the growing scale of prostitution in Asia and its increasing economic and international significance have serious implications for public morality, social welfare, criminality, violation of human rights, sexual exploitation of children, and transmission of HIV/AIDS. Because sex work is not recognized as an official sector, and often operates contrary to local and national laws—although with the approval of corrupt authorities— it is not included in official statistics, government budgets, or development plans. More dangerous from the viewpoint of its largely female employees, the industry goes unregulated. Governments should at least begin to keep track of the sex work sector, says the ILO. Government recognition, legalization, and regulation would improve the lives of 1 million people in the four study countries alone.

---◆---

The case of the Philippines illustrates how economics, culture, religion, and politics—national and international—interact to fuel an incipient HIV/AIDS epidemic. A Spanish colony for almost three hundred years, the Philippines is overwhelmingly Catholic. They were discovered by Spain in 1521, when Ferdinand Magellan made landfall in the archipelago. A Portuguese who had distinguished himself in campaigns against Muslims in India, East Africa, and Morocco, Magellan was discredited and ridiculed with the nickname "clubfoot" by his King for a limp incurred in his service. He moved to Spain, married a friend's sister, and settled in Seville, where King Charles I agreed to fund his first expedition west. The route was unknown and very long—Magellan was the first to sail through the rough seas of the strait that bears his name at the base of South America—plagued by repeated mutinies, scurvy, boredom, and bad charts. Upon reaching the Philippines Magellan was killed by a chief who refused to convert to Catholicism, but his crew sailed on, past Ternate, through the Straits of Malaka, and back to Spain in 1522. After four unsuccessful tries, the Spanish finally conquered the Philippines in 1571 and established their capital in Manila.

Under the terms of the treaty of Paris in 1899, the United States gained control over the Philippines after it won the Spanish-American War, and immediately charted their path to independence. Independence was delayed until 1946 by the Japanese invasion in World War II and for twenty years the new country was beset with development problems. The dictator Ferdinand Marcos took over in 1965 and was driven out of power in 1986 by nonviolent protests. Peace returned in 1992 and economic growth has been solid ever since. The government has privatized industry, reformed the tax system, and promoted trade. Performance in social sectors is relatively good, with life expectancy close to 70 years.

In response to overwhelming international political and religious pressure, President Gloria Arroyo's government is now courting its worst development crisis since independence, an explosion of its HIV/AIDS epidemic. "In violation of the internationally recognized right to health," charges Human Rights Watch, "the Philippines both interferes with the delivery of effective

HIV prevention programs and invests in pubic health strategies that discourage condom use."[21] Until recently the government was pursuing "an exemplary strategy of condom promotion" and had a solid national AIDS prevention program in place. But Arroyo, influenced by the Philippines' Catholic hierarchy and Washington's abstinence-only policy, has blocked condom availability and promotion. The burden of the policy reversal is falling on the country's lower class, which relies on free government condoms. Those who can afford them still buy condoms through the commercial sector, "but for poor and marginalized populations, who are arguably at the highest risk of HIV," the supply is restricted.

According to Human Rights Watch: "It is a measure of the hypocrisy of the Philippine AIDS policy that the Department of Health admits the effectiveness of condoms against HIV/AIDS and yet refuses to supply them to local clinics or promote them aggressively" for fear of offending powerful conservative Catholics. Local health workers in some areas are pooling their own funds to buy condoms in bulk for resale at discount prices to the poor. The government also supports organizations that make misleading statements about condom effectiveness and has enacted local ordinances prohibiting condom distribution in public health facilities. School-based HIV education programs "met with stiff resistance from teachers and principals opposed to birth control." The curriculum includes sex education and HIV/AIDS education, but "you can't even begin to discuss reproductive health in any schools in Manila City," said an AIDS educator.

In a country that is 85 percent Catholic (9 percent Protestant, 4 percent Muslim, and 2 percent Buddhist), powerful bishops often oppose condom use for moral reasons. "More recently some have begun to buttress their moral arguments with false claims" about the ineffectiveness of condoms, including claims that condoms contain microscopic pores that are permeable by HIV pathogens, even though the World Health Organization has said they are "totally wrong." One male sex worker in Angeles City, confused by the Catholic campaign like many Filipinos, says: "I don't use condoms. I never have. I think condoms are not very effective." The government "also acts in ways that radically increase the likelihood of a rapid outbreak and spread of HIV/AIDS among populations at high risk, particularly sex workers." Sex work is extensive on the islands, which also have a historic problem of drug use. The police harass sex workers, using condom possession as evidence for arrest, and test peole without consent. "Before I got AIDS," says one young Filipino, "I used to say, 'I'm a Catholic. I don't use condoms.' It's what I learned in church— they are so stuck on procreation. I was on vacation in Dubai, and I took a girl into a hotel, thinking [AIDS] wouldn't happen to me. When I got home, I went for voluntary testing and that's how I found out."

———•◆•———

Women played a central role in Asia's early animist religions because of their superior ability to communicate with spirits. They helped cure disease, avert crop failures, and expand trade opportunities. In Mongol society, women were more independent than in neighboring Buddhist, Islamic, and Christian nations. They owned property, could use the courts, and were auxiliaries to the cavalry, joining the fight and helping dispatch captives. To this day, women engage as equals in riding and archery competitions. Marco Polo described the daughter of a khan who was a fearsome wrestler and amassed her fortune by challenging men and collecting portions of their flocks as her prize. She refused to throw a match with a potential suitor despite her father's plea, and claimed another 1,000 horses. She joined her father in every battle. Polo said, "There was never a knight more doughty than she. For many a time it happened that she plunged in among the enemy and seized a knight by force and carried him off into her own ranks."

Genghis Khan, who conquered in the name of his god, said his greatest pleasure in life was "victory: to cut my enemies to pieces, to drive them before me, to seize their possessions, to reduce their families to tears, to ride on their horses, and to make love to their wives and daughters." He was more than supreme ruler of the Mongol empire; he was the sky's representative on earth, whose mission it was to conquer—but not convert—the peoples of alien states. Tengri was the unity of all lesser gods of the earth, water, winds, and mountains. His spiritual leaders were shamans, traveling seers who kept mortals in line with the will of the universe by communicating with the spirits through trances. But subjects were free to keep their own religions, so segments of the Mongol empire that were predominantly Muslim at the time of conquest remained Muslim states under the khans. The empire was a mix of indigenous religions, Islam, Buddhism, Confucianism, and Christianity. Even the Mongol ruling class was a mix—Sorkhakhtani was a Nestorian Christian; Hulegu was educated by a Nestorian priest; and young Kublai was taught by a Confucian sage and in his later years by a Buddhist monk. All were Mongol at heart, and the main ideology of their states was secular—world hegemony and the perpetuation of the ruling dynasty.

Buddhism was the most important religion among the Il-Khans, who received monks and artists as missionaries from China, Tibet, and Uighur in

Central Asia. Their leader, Hulegu, was a shamanist but also a devotee of the Boddhisattva Maitreya. Hulegu's grandson Arghun brought Buddhist priests and yogi mystics from India, and the interaction of Buddhism and shamanism may have influenced later development of Islamic Sufi mysticism. At the same time, Hulegu's chief wife, Doquz-khatum, and at least one of his other wives were Nestorian Christians and prayed in a portable church-shaped tent while the armies were on the move. Once settled, she built churches throughout the Il-Khanate.Her mission was carried on by her niece, a concubine of Hulegu's. In 1281 the Nestorian church fathers elected a Chinese monk, Markus, waylaid at Hulegu's court on a pilgrimage to Jerusalem by Il-Khan-Mamluk battles, as their patriarch to please their Mongol masters. The modest little monk, who had just come for a visit, was suddenly head of his church. Patriarch Mar Yahballaha III never made it back to China.

Persian merchant missionaries had been carrying Christianity to Asia since the patriarch of Constantinople, Nestorius, was declared a heretic by the European branch of the church in A.D. 431 and fled the Roman empire (by then Catholic) for Persia. The eastern bishops adopted the heretical Nestorian version of Christianity in 486 because they, like Nestorius, simply "could not imagine God as a little boy" and declared that Christ's true nature was divine. Nestorians had been the target of Muslim riots in Baghdad as early as 1263 because of the preference shown to them by the Mongols. When Khan Ghazan made Christianity the Il-Khan's official religion in 1295, the Muslims' pent-up resentment was unleashed in persecution, killings, and mob violence. Mar Yahballaha was hung by his feet and beaten, but continued to lead a much smaller flock in Iran until 1317.

In 1368 the Chinese marched into Mongolia and burned Karakorum. Although the khan escaped, the Chinese vowed no "oceanic ruler" would ever control them again. Mongolia was tossed back and forth between China and Russia until 1691, when Outer Mongolia's rulers swore allegiance to the Manchu emperor. For the next few centuries, the country languished as a neglected Chinese dependency where secular institutions of any kind were virtually nonexistent. Generations of devout Mongols gave sizable tithes to the monasteries and as the lamaseries expanded, they absorbed more and more pasturelands and recruits. They were the only money lenders and had the only schools, craftsmen, and literacy in the country. Mongolia had only half a dozen settled towns, but 700 large monasteries and 1,000 or more smaller ones. Forty percent of its males were lamas or their serfs.

The chief lama was appointed by the Tibetans as a living Buddha, outranked only by Tibet's "Two Jewels," the Dalai (the Buddha of Compassion) and Panchen (the Buddha of Light) lamas. Mongolia's Exalted Revelation was going blind from syphilis, was paralytically drunk for weeks at a time, and enjoyed playing games with his male servant while his consort engaged in sexual capers with other lamas in the "oracle tent." Homosexuality was condoned, and senior monks selected "disciples" for their own use from children offered to the church. Nineteenth- and twentieth-century travelers claimed that wandering lamas, who begged and sold indulgences and fortunes to credulous herdsmen, had spread syphilis to 90 percent of the population.[22] Whether syphilis was that widespread will never be known, but between it and celibacy encouraged by the monks, the birth rate was so low that the population had fallen to 651,000 in 1925 and the extinction of the Mongols was predicted.[23]

The Mongolian People's Republic was proclaimed on November 25, 1924, as the world's second communist state and a satellite of the Soviet Union. The Mongolian Party mounted a massive education and indoctrination campaign that suppressed Buddhism. In 1924, when the Exalted Revelation died, the government declared the end of his reincarnation and a silent and nearly complete destruction of the holy city of Erdenzu was carried out. The Communists stripped the lamaseries of their land and privileges; they taxed the monks, who were made to pay a special fine to excuse them from military service. Four hundred lamas were expelled from one lamasery in a single day and since many evictions were done during the winter, many lamas died from the cold. Monasteries were bulldozed and the lamas were "reclassified" to work brigades and labor camps. Books were burned and sacred relics smashed. Only the Gandan monastery in Ulaan Baatar was preserved. In 1990 when the Party declared a moratorium on religious persecution, the lamas began to reappear, as if out of nowhere. Many had had been living with herders, practicing their religion in secret. They donned their wine-colored robes and yellow hats, brought out the long pencil boxes containing their sacred scriptures, and returned to Erdenzu, where several dozen ancient lamas took up residence again.

Mongolia is the fifth largest country in Asia by area but one of the smallest in terms of population, with only 2.6 million people. In recent years, autumn droughts and unusually cold and snowy winters have claimed a fifth of its 33 million livestock animals, destroying the livelihoods of thousands of families. The Soviet Union kept the Chinese out of Mongolia and never expropriated the land, but forced collectivization on the nomads, built schools, achieved almost 100 percent literacy, and set up a pension system and free healthcare. When they withdrew in 1990, they took with them the subsidies that made up a third of Mongolia's economy. Factories and schools closed, and many people returned to the nomadic life. Unemployment, alcoholism, commercial sex, and homelessness increased dramatically.

Prime Minister Nambaryn Enkhbayar plans to build a highway across the country, which he hopes will be 90 percent urbanized by 2030. "In order to survive," he says, "we have to stop being nomads." Many young people agree, unwilling to be "animal slaves." Although the nomadic life may look romantic to outsiders, one herder says, "The people who live it don't think it's romantic—it's a hard life. Mongolia gets a third of its money in foreign aid. Do we tell the World Bank that we want to keep our people migrating on oxen?" With the transition to a neoliberal economy, Asian experts say, "has come the transformation of the rural, primarily pastoral economy. With de-collectivization, households have been thrown into a highly insecure subsistence mode of production." Women enjoyed the equality shared in other socialist states in Asia. Steppe nomads are still more egalitarian than the hierarchical societies they conquered, but women are especially vulnerable to these neoliberal "political-ecological" changes, "manifested in increasing rates of poor reproductive health and maternal mortality."[24] This could contribute to the spread of HIV/AIDS. Currently, resources for surveillance are meager but a 2001 national survey of prenatal clinics determined that less than 1 percent of pregnant women had syphilis, and at the end of 2002, there was only one known case of HIV.

------◆------

Legend says that the first Tibetans were the children of a sacred monkey sent to the high plateau on a religious retreat and a female rock demon who seduced him. They were given permission to marry by the monkey's master, Avalokiteshvara, a disciple of Buddha, and had five children. In a later retelling by the fifth Dalai Lama, the monkey became Avalokiteshvara himself and the siren the Buddhist mother-savior, Tara, making the Tibetan kings their descendants. In some Chinese accounts, the mother goddess is a Han Chinese princess offered to the king of a nomadic warrior tribe who governed the inner plateau to keep peace along the boundaries of two empires. The legend may have been born in a real encounter; Tibetans smeared their faces with earth-based paint to protect them from the wind, which made them look a bit like monkeys to trespassers unwilling to come very close.

The first seven Tibetan kings were said to be attached to heaven by sacred ropes so that at their death their bodies could be pulled upward. The eighth king accidentally cut the rope while fighting with a rebel, and Tibet emerged from prehistory. Around A.D. 600, King Namri Songtsen united the warring tribes of the Yarlung Valley. Under his son, Songtsen Gampo, who moved the capital to Lhasa, the Tibetans began to expand into Central Asia. Tibet's formidable strength threatened Chinese control over the Silk Road oases. In 763 the Tibetan king, Trisong Detsen, sacked the Chinese capital of Chang'an. His empire encompassed half of modern China and extended west to include present-day Uzbekistan, Nepal, northern India, Pakistan, and Burma. Remnants of Tibetan rule and Buddhist manuscripts have been found in two forts in the Tarim Basin and in a fort in the western Taklamakan desert, but the greatest cache is from Dunhuang, western China, where many thirteenth-century Tibetan Buddhist and Mongolian manuscripts have been found in the sacred caves.

Trisong Detsen married the Nepalese and Chinese princesses sent to appease him but made Buddhism the state religion of Tibet in 779, displacing the traditional shamanistic religion. With the wealth and power of their new monasteries, the Buddhist monks came to challenge traditional rulers, and in 838 they killed the king. Lang Darma, the king's younger brother, was installed but assassinated five years later, ending the Tibetan dynasty. At the same time, Buddhist monks were persecuted, the monasteries were destroyed, and the Indian monks who had come as teachers were expelled. As warlords struggled for power, the collapse of the Tibetan empire began, and by 907 the Chinese had taken most of the land. Tibet's one final attempt to restore the empire ended with defeat by the Uighur in 966.

In the meantime, exiled Buddhists flourished outside the empire. Three Buddhist monks known as the Men of Khams had fled Lhasa during the early persecutions, settling at Amdo at the headwaters of the Yellow River. A second group settled in the western Himalayas, and in about 950, both groups of monks began to return to rebuild their monasteries and revive their religion. Tibet's most famous medieval scholar, Richen Zangpo, founded a monastic complex at Thöling that remained in use until it was destroyed during the Cultural Revolution in the 1960s. As Buddhism declined in India under Muslim pressure, Tibet became the chief inheritor of Indian Buddhism. Three schools developed—the Sakya, the Kagyu, and the Gelugpa—while older lineages were called Nyingma, "the old ones."

When Genghis Khan conquered Tibet in 1239, he was so impressed with the religion that he gave its monks his patronage. Kublai Khan granted supreme authority over Tibet to Sakya Pandit, leader of the Sakya order of Buddhism, and he became the imperial preceptor and a high official in the Khan's court. Tibet, like other lands brought under Mongol submission, was laid to waste by Mongke Khan so that "to the distance of twenty days' journey you see numberless towns and castles in a state of ruin," said Marco Polo when he visited the country as Kublai's emissary around 1280.[25] Merchants shackled their horses with iron bonds because "in consequence of the want of inhabitants, wild beasts, especially tigers, have multiplied to such a degree that merchants and other travelers are exposed there to great danger during the night." But travel through the country was worth the risk. Musk ox abounded in such quantity "that the scent of it is diffused over the whole country," and "in the rivers gold-dust is found in very large quantities . . . there are manufactures of camlet [fabric made of silk and camel's hair] and of gold cloth, and many drugs are produced in the country that have not been brought to ours." The merchants enjoyed the company of young women offered up to them by their families; women with the greatest number of gifts from travelers were highly esteemed for marriage. Polo said the shamans "by their infernal art perform the most extraordinary and delusive marvels . . . cause tempests to arise . . . with flashes of lightning and thunderbolts, and produce many other miraculous effects." But like his Chinese bosses, otherwise he found Tibetans to be "altogether an ill-conditioned race," although he knew that Tibet "was formerly a country of so much importance as to be divided into eight kingdoms, containing many cities and castles."

When the Mongul dynasty ended, Ming imperial patronage passed to the Kagyu order, and then in the fifteenth century to the Galugpa order. The third lama received the title of "Dalai," or "Ocean of Wisdom," from the Chinese. Threatened by the Buddhist-Chinese alliance, in 1611 the Tibetan king attacked the monasteries, sending the fourth Dalai Lama into exile. The Mongols retaliated in 1640 and executed the Tibetan king. When the fifth Dali Lama assumed power, he pacified Tibet with Mongol backing and peace lasted until his death in 1682. Under the sixth Dalai Lama, noted for his "unbridled licentiousness," the kingdom lapsed into disorder. He was deposed by a rival group of Mongols in 1717, but the Manchu Chinese threw them out, bringing the seventh Dalai Lama with them. They made Tibet a Chinese protectorate and appointed a king, but temporal rule reverted to the seventh Dalai Lama in 1750.

In 1788 the Gurkhas tried to invade from Nepal. The Chinese believed that the British were behind it, so they imposed a ban on foreign contact that lasted more than a century. In 1903 British diplomats, fearing Russian expansion into Central Asia, entered the country and found that the Dalai Lama had gone to Mongolia with a Russian "advisor." The British signed a protection agreement with the acting regent, but also signed a second agreement with the

Manchus in 1906 that recognized their suzerainty over Tibet. The British invaded but were turned out by the Chinese after the 1912 revolution. However, the Chinese were so distracted by internal problems that Tibet enjoyed virtual freedom for almost forty years until Chinese communists "liberated" the country in 1950 and instituted agricultural reforms that caused mass starvation. Widespread religious repression sent the Dalai Lama to India in 1959.

The Tibetan Autonomous Region was created in 1965. During China's Cultural Revolution, Red Guards sent to Lhasa brutally quashed all resistance. A 1977 fact-finding mission found that 1.2 million people had died or fled (one-third to one-half of the population), 6,254 monasteries and nunneries had been destroyed, 100,000 Tibetans were in labor camps, two-thirds of Tibet had been absorbed into China, and extensive deforestation had occurred. After negotiations for the Dalai Lama's return broke down in 1983, Tibet was targeted for mass resettlement, and more than 100,000 Han Chinese received financial incentives to move there. Chinese investment, continued Han migration, and exclusive use of Mandarin in higher education have marginalized Tibetans, but the Chinese believe they have modernized the country. In 2001 Tibet's puppet communist party secretary declared he would "never let Tibet split from the great family of the motherland and will also never allow Tibet to remain backward." The *Beijing Liberation Army Daily* declared that in the fifty years since "the peaceful liberation of Tibet . . . under the leadership of the Chinese Communist Party, earthshaking changes have taken place in the snowy highland. The former serfs, accounting for more than 95 percent of Tibet's total population, have become masters of the socialist new Tibet." According to travel writer Pico Iyer, "the Chinese would say that . . . Tibet is poor precisely because it devotes its time to gods and prayer and superstition. Many Tibetans might reply that karaoke parlors and industrial cranes look to them like what is truly barbaric."[26]

Tibet and Mongolia's parallel experiences with empire and Chinese conquest have yielded parallels between the experience of Tibetan women and women in Mongolia. The current reincarnation of Tibet's Pachen Lama—who technically has greater spiritual authority than the Dalai Lama because she is not also king—is a twenty-year-old political science student named Renji at Washington, DC's American University. Her father, the previous Pachen Lama, was publicly humiliated by Mao and imprisoned for eleven years. After seeing how Tibet had been destroyed by the communists, like many monks coerced to change their lives, he decided to marry. As the late Pachen Lama's only child, Renji was installed in the post by the Chinese government although she is a woman. In the meantime, the Dalai Lama picked a

Tibetan boy who was taken into custody with his family by the Chinese and has not been seen ever since. Many fear that China's manipulation of Tibet has left the country as marginalized as China's other autonomous regions, and that China's push to modernization has pushed the country into a major AIDS epidemic. Results are still out because HIV surveillance in Tibet is so poor.

———·✦·———

"Muhammed," says religious scholar Karen Armstrong, "was one of those rare men who truly enjoy the company of women." When asked who should be honored most, he replied three times, "Your mother," before he mentioned the other half. He was lenient toward his wives, who were free to speak their mind even when it did not please him. The Prophet "scrupulously helped with the chores, mended his own clothes and sought out the companionship of his wives." He took their advice to heart and often took them traveling with him. The emancipation of women "was a project dear to the Prophet's heart." The Quran gave women inheritance rights and the right to divorce "centuries before Western women were accorded such status." In the Quran, "men and women are partners before God, with identical duties and responsibilities," says Armstrong. The women of the first *ummah* took part in public life and even fought in battle, and the new religion brought great improvements in women's status. In the Prophet's new religion, women were not the source of sin, as they were in many other contemporary religions. The Quran makes it clear that Adam and Eve were equally at fault. The Quran also makes it clear that women should have access to education and retain control of their own property. The holy book does not require veiling, but only modesty in dress.

When the nomads began settling and their societies became more complex, Armstrong says, "as happened in Christianity, men would hijack the faith and bring it into line with the previous patriarchy." As the religion evolved, men derived authority over women from interpretation of two Quranic verses. The first says that in initiating divorce, men have precedence, and the second says that women suspected of ill conduct must be admonished, banished to their beds, and beaten (lightly or in a symbolic sense). "The history of Islam, like that of other great religions, is replete with contradictions between precept and practice. The vision and values communicated by the Prophet were all too soon confronted by the dynamic of conquest and the discriminating distribution of the spoils," says historian Ronald Segal. Female slaves were kept by the thousands in harems, guarded by male slaves who had been castrated without any painkillers on the way to market. Many harems were small armies; there were 6,300 women in Abd al-Rahman's harem in Cordoba in the mid-tenth century and the Fatimid palace in Cairo had 12,000. Special schools in Baghdad, Medina, and Cordoba trained musicians and dancing girls. Female slaves were also educated, an act which gained their masters merit. Unmarried female slaves could be enjoyed by their masters, but the privilege was ceded to their husbands when they married and masters were obliged to marry off their virtuous slaves.

One-fifth of humanity now follows Islam, the fastest-growing religion in the world, and the large majority of its practitioners are in Asia. In the course of Islam's development, an inevitable diversity of practice arose from centuries of change across the huge continent as the Prophet's words mixed with local religions and social systems that were in the process of solidifying their economics and politics. The diversity illustrates the extent to which religion interacts with its social and political context. A similar process is underway today as social mores change, prompting women to search for reconciliation of the Prophet's original intent for women and the trend in some societies toward their total subordination. In the 1990s, Islam attracted many new adherents from the young and the poor, who are drawn to the religion as they were during the days of European colonialization as a form of rebellion against the West and the upper classes. Religion is allied once again with rebellion, but in pursuing the lesser jihad of political power, militant Islam has abandoned its roots in community justice and the equal status of women. But the many problems entailed in returning to the authentically Muslim life of the *ummah* in a rapidly changing modern world have not yet been resolved, including the impact of HIV/AIDS on the status of women.

Differences of opinion are reflected in state responses to the epidemic and even within countries. In May 2004 a Malaysian Islamic cleric refused to bow to pressure from a health department official to ban marriages of HIV-positive Muslims. Reasoning that the ban would encourage non-marital sex, the cleric said under law only the father of a virgin could stop such a marriage. A cleric in southern Johor Province had set a precedent by requiring pre-marital testing for couples, following a program followed by the leaders of all religions in Uganda that led to declines in HIV transmission. Indonesian HIV/AIDS educators were forced to water down their messages when Islamic fundamentalist groups objected to the explicit information they were providing although only 10 percent of the ten million Indonesian men visiting sex workers each year use condoms. Moderate Muslims support sex education, but have objected to condom promotion campaigns. The head of Indonesia's highest Islamic authority said that, "in Islam, having sex outside marriage is forbidden. Since it is

an illicit act, the use of condoms by an unmarried couple is also proscribed."
He urged Muslim men to be more religious and closer to their families.

At the second international Muslim leaders' consultation on HIV/AIDS
in mid-2003—the first "non-woman" Islamic conference led entirely by
women—attendees, including Chief Kadis and ministers of Health, sorted
themselves into conservatives (men, on the right), and liberals (mixed men and
women, on the left). Held in Kuala Lumpur, Malaysia, the rector of the International Islamic University opened the meeting by urging Islamic leaders to
create a "caring *ummah*" and transform the response to HIV/AIDS. Malaysian
leader Amina Wadud attacked the simple moralizing underlying most Islamic
discussion of AIDS, telling fellow clerics and scholars that they must reduce
gender injustice and extramarital sex fueling the epidemic's spread, and that
Muslim men must stop denying the reality of HIV. Her presentation ended in
an uproar, with cries of blasphemy coming from delegates on the right and
support from the delegates on the left.

The feminine was celebrated in early religions as the source of life and the
gift of fertility. Over the past fifty years, more evidence has emerged that the
feminine, as Mother Goddess, was the first focus of primitive worship. However, once the male contribution to reproduction was understood, men began
to take more control over women's reproductive cycles by restricting the lives
of the women in their families. Social stratification increased as men took
control of other forms of social organization and their control over women
was carried over into the religious sphere. Even in India, where the feminine
is still central in worship, the feminine without the masculine is understood
to be destructive and fierce. It may be fear of women's sexuality and power
that leads to the perpetuation of severe subordination of women in modern
Hindu countries.

When Hinduism was emerging, women were believed to be unclean and
impure. At the same time, they were also recognized as the source of enormous power because they were capable of nullifying men's sacred mantras.
Since that power had to be contained, Brahmin priests had to keep women out
of their sanctuaries. To do this, the religion decreed that women must be totally dependent on men and cannot make decisions on their own. In childhood, a woman is subordinate to her father, in marriage to her husband, and at
his death, to her sons. The husband is the master or guru, no matter what his
personal qualities, his infidelities or cruelties, and a wife's devotion to her hus-

band is her highest good. If a woman fails in her duty to her husband, she is disgraced and may be subject to extreme punishments for even the smallest failing. Her husband can curse her and condemn her to permanent damnation. Women may not be divorced, no matter how unfaithful or ruthless their husbands are. By tradition, women cannot own property, can be murdered if their dowries are not paid, can be locked in their homes and not allowed to leave, and can be denied the right to read or get an education. In the context of the Hindu cultural system, women are comparable to or lower than the lowest of the castes. Since women are mere commodities—and not really human at all—their human and sexual rights can be continuously violated.

In India, "empowerment of women, leading to an equal social status in society hinges, among other things, on their right to hold and inherit property," says Dr. Sarala Gopalan.[27] Although legal reforms in some states give daughters an equal share of an inheritance, "equal status remains illusive. Establishment of laws and bringing practices in conformity thereto is necessarily a long drawn out process." In South Asia, women have trouble inheriting or owning property even where the law allows them to do so. Many women are not aware of their rights—thanks to their isolation from education and media—and lawyers often do not understand the law, especially if it involves HIV/AIDS. Women lose even the minimal rights they might have enjoyed before they became HIV-infected. The Positive Women's Network of South India says that women rarely inherit property shared during a marriage, and may even lose the property they brought into the marriage when their husbands die. The same is true in Bangladesh, where only one-third of women realize their rights under the inheritance law. HIV-positive women may be thrown out of their homes by their husbands or in-laws or returned to their parents without their dowry, even if the husband brought the infection home.

Some Indian feminists believe that despite limited advances in women's property rights, women's overall status is declining because of increases in female infanticide, *sati* (the obligation of a woman to die on her husband's funeral pyre, or widow burning), dowry-related murders, and crimes against women. "Indian feminism has not tackled the core of the evil, but has only squabbled about superficial aspects of the problem. Western feminism was merely transplanted onto the subcontinent," says Sita Agarwal. "The real reason for the sad state of Indian women is the continuation of . . . Brahmanism or 'astika' Hinduism."[28] Agarwal argues that "instead of wasting time attacking trivialities, the Hindu religion itself must be attacked by Indian feminism. If Indian women are to become free, it is this faith that must be tackled, and nothing else. No other religion . . . burns its women, or slaughters one-tenth of all women each generation except Hinduism. Indeed, Brahminism is nothing but the legitimized genocide of women."

Thanks to intensive pressure from women's groups in the primarily Hindu state of Nepal, the civil code was amended in 2002 to allow daughters to inherit property equally with sons (the property must be returned to the other heirs when daughters marry), and parents are required by law to provide the same care and protection to daughters as sons. Now a woman can initiate divorce proceedings if her husband is abusive or has an STD, including HIV, and the new law increased the punishments for rape and polygamy, declared illegal in 1975 but still rampant in Nepal. Abortion under limited conditions is also allowed, making Nepal the first South Asian country with this provision. Despite this progress, the guarantee of equal rights to women under Nepal's 1990 constitution is far from being fulfilled. A March 2004 report showed that less than 1 percent of women legally own their land, homes, livestock, or other assets, and only 16 percent have some kind of regular income. Although 55 percent of women are economically active, most work in fields or tend to household chores. Hundreds of thousands of women are "suffering silently," dependent on their fathers, spouses, or sons, and "there are still dozens of legal provisions that are discriminatory to women," says Sapna Pradhan Malla, president of Nepal's Forum for Women, Law and Development. "It is absurd that even in the 21st century, a citizenship certificate is provided only to women whose fathers' or husbands' citizenship is known. Mothers and wives do not count," says Dr. Durga Pokharel, chair of Nepal's National Women's Commission. The Badinis of western Nepal—traditional prostitutes who work in temples—are especially disadvantaged because the mother has to identify her child's father.

———◦•◦———

Sometime around 500 B.C., the Buddha rejected his wealthy family in favor of his search for enlightenment. Just as Buddha was about to abandon his quest, frustrated with his lack of revelation about the nature of suffering, the god Brahma descended from heaven to plead with him to continue. He said that humanity needed the Buddha's teachings, urging him to "look down at the human race which is drowning in pain and to travel far and wide to save the world." The religion was founded on the conviction that "where a bestial man or women puts self-interest first, a spiritual person learns to recognize and seeks to alleviate the pain of others."[29] But Buddhism was an animal of its time, born from a Hindu culture that reviled women. Not surprisingly, all of Hinduism's beliefs about women prevailed except one. The Buddha took the radical position that women could become completely enlightened just like men if they followed the path of renunciation, the same path he advocated to men.

His decision on women's potential was influenced by his maternal aunt, Pajapati Gotami, who was also his foster mother. She had raised the Buddha from his birth, and when he left, he had persuaded her own son to join him. Miserably lonely, she asked the Buddha if she could establish an order of nuns. When he turned her first three requests down, she shaved her head and donned a yellow robe, as did 500 women who had become her followers, and they walked 357 miles by foot to the monastery where the Buddha was. As they progressed, curious onlookers joined the procession. Persuaded by her determination when she reached the gates, the Buddha approved her request to start a nunnery. In his conditions for approval, he decreed eight ways in which nuns were subordinate to monks and also said that his teachings, which were to be eternal, would last only 500 years because women could be nuns. When she was 120 years old, Gotami still looked like a girl of 16, and when she achieved enlightenment, the sky opened, thunder rent the air, and deities came to the earth to rejoice.

Modern interpretations suggest that the Buddha made nuns subordinate to monks so that they would be more acceptable to the society of his day, and that because women could extend Buddhism to the other half of the human race, it would only take 500 years to enlighten the entire world. Many women soon became nuns, especially women who had been widowed, orphaned, or who needed security for other reasons. The families of women who did not want to marry also saw the religious life as an appropriate alternative, and the nunneries grew for many of the same reasons they did in the Christian world. Wealthy women also gave the new religion financial support, bringing money and property to the temples. In the first seven or eight centuries of Buddhism in India, nunneries were patronized by wealthy queens.

As Buddhism grew, the monks became involved in politics because they controlled their own patrons as well as those of the nuns. If they supported local regimes, they provided manpower for education and crafts and, more importantly, justified the rule of the elite and secured peasant acquiescence. However, their compliance could change, and the Buddhist hierarchy could turn on a ruler and encourage rebellion. Historian John Keay says that by the ninth century A.D., Buddhism in India "was a Buddhism far removed from that preached by the Enlightened One, indeed as remote from it in both time and spirit was medieval Christianity form the New Testament. Although originally a rationalisation of the human condition and a code of ethics, both of which largely ignored the deities and rituals associated with conventional religion, Buddhism had been steadily assuming the trappings of orthodox religious practice ever since the Buddha's death." At first sympathetic advocates of the needs of the poor, large monasteries gradually became a political force in their own right and accumulated wealth at the expense of the peasants.

In China, in a reaction against the wealth and power that had been accumulated by Buddhist monasteries, thousands were destroyed in the ninth century, opening the way for neo-Confucianism. Zhu Ti synthesized Confucian thought with ideas drawn from Buddhism, Taoism, and other religious philosophies. Incorporated into the mandarin examination system, however, it became increasingly rigid, "stressing the one-sided obligation of obedience and compliance of subject to ruler, child to father, wife to husband, and younger brother to elder brother," says University of Maryland sinologist Leon Poon.[30] "The effect was to inhibit the social development of premodern China, resulting both in many generations of political, social, and spiritual stability and in a slowness of cultural and institutional change up to the nineteenth century. Neo-Confucianism doctrines also came to play the dominant role in the intellectual life of Korea, Vietnam, and Japan."

Despite Gotami's saintly example, women to this day are viewed as polluted and inherently unclean by some modern Buddhists. They are the temptresses men must resist if they are to attain enlightenment. Some experts believe this view has vilified women, branding them as inherently evil beings that stand in the way of enlightenment. Certainly, monks still enjoy more community support than nuns, although the women perform valuable services as teachers, nurses, and moral exemplars. Early in the morning in the streets of any Buddhist country, it is women who kneel at the curbside, filling the monks' begging bowls.

In August, 2003, 60 monks, nuns, and government officials from Cambodia, China, Myanmar, Thailand, and Vietnam met in Bangkok to discuss the religion's response to the growing HIV/AIDS crisis. Supreme Patriach Somdech Tep Vong, Cambodia's Buddhist leader, said, "It is part of the traditional role for monks and nuns to provide a refuge for the people. By taken the Buddha as our example, we can bring an end to the suffering caused by HIV and AIDS." Buddhist ideas of compassion and self-discipline "are central to effective HIV prevention and care." National efforts, including the Cambodian law that supports Buddhist clergy and institutions in HIV/AIDS prevention and care programs, were discussed. The Sangha Mehta movement, begun in the mid-1990s among monks in northern Thailand, has spread to Bhutan, Cambodia, Laos, Mongolia, Myanmar, southern China, and Vietnam. The monks, who were horrified by the suffering of human beings drowning in the pain of AIDS, broke centuries-old traditions and began to help the residents of surrounding communities organize themselves as caring communities for adults and children living with the disease. The monks also spread a message of compassion to those who are not HIV-infected to reduce discrimination against people who are, and help families who are caring for AIDS orphans. The spiritual impact of the movement on people who were dying alone, rejected by their families and loved ones and isolated from their communities by fear of contagion, is only matched by its spiritual impact on those who are not.

————•◦•————

In Southeast Asia's first societies, women had a central religious and cultural role that was stronger than in contemporary Indian and Chinese societies because the region's cultures were not patriarchal like their northern neighbors. Men were so willing to submit to the will of women that they underwent the "excruciatingly painful male practice of implanting penis balls to heighten female pleasure," say experts Barwise and White.[31] In modern times, demographers say that Southeast Asia is still distinguished from East and South Asia by the relatively higher status of its women.[32] Before the Bronze Age, women maintained their status because they produced pottery, which they bartered for jewelry, and were given prestigious burials. In the islands, women kept their status through their role as merchants until the seventeenth century and also exercised control in the political realm, where succession and inheritance were not exclusively through the male line. "The freedom and enhanced position enjoyed by women only began to erode with the spread of world religions to the region after 500 A.D.," according to Barwise and White.

When AIDS was first emerging, orthodox thinkers in most major faiths denounced those who fell ill and said that their fate was divine punishment for immoral behavior. The 1994 International Conference on Population and Development in Cairo was typical of early reactions because most religious delegates opposed measures like condom distribution to stop the spread of HIV. As more people fall ill and the destructive effects of blocking condom promotion and encouraging discrimination against HIV-infected individuals are becoming evident, even orthodox leaders are rethinking their stance. At a December 2003 meeting in Kathmandu, representatives of all South Asia's major faiths surprised HIV/AIDS activists because they have become more open and thoughtful about the meaning of disease and its challenge to religious simplicity.

Many religions are going back to their roots to call on deep traditions of caring and humanitarian support both to help those suffering with the disease and to prevent further spread. Buddhist monk Ven Phra Tuangsit of Thailand told the Kathmandu gathering of imans, priests, and pundits that "At first people were worried that it was inappropriate for a Buddhist cleric to work with condoms and things, but now people realize that I'm practicing Buddhist compassion and helping people avoid painful, humiliating illness. They listen and respect us because we are monks. So much has changed." To fully respond, religions must also rethink their positions on other very fundamental issues, including gender inequities that lie at the heart of the epidemic's spread. And they must examination the contradictions in their moral positions, such as that which allows the Catholic church to stand in the way of condom distribution while advocating for increased access to HIV/AIDS drugs.

Cataloging the extent of human rights abuses against women related to the HIV/AIDS epidemic, Human Rights Watch says, "Every day, in every corner of the world, women and girls are beaten in their homes, trafficked into forced prostitution, raped by soldiers and rebels in armed conflicts, sexually abused by their 'caretakers,' deprived of equal rights to property and other economic assets, assaulted for not conforming to gender norms, and often left with no option but to trade sex for survival. Some are 'inherited' by male in-laws when they become widows, often becoming wives in polygamous families. These acts of discrimination and violence are conduits for HIV infection. Women living with AIDS confront not only stigma, but also the deprivations caused by violations of their rights. Relative to the scale and severity of these abuses, laws, policies and programs to combat HIV/AIDS by protecting the rights of women and girls are negligible."[33] Over the past five years, international human rights organizations, alert to the "feminization" of the HIV/AIDS pandemic that stems from women's low status, have begun to take up the issue. Amnesty International has said that violence against women is "the greatest hidden human rights issue of our time."

UNAIDS says, "Our understanding of what needs to be done is substantially more evolved than our understanding of how to do it. The institutionalization of gender," the report continues, "has long been problematic."[34] Because gender is so embedded in the social fabric, not simply manifested in individual behavior, making changes challenges all social institutions. The international CEDAW Committee has urged governments to become active in passing laws and implementing measures that protect women. Governments are expected to go out of their way to ensure that poor rural women, especially, have the assistance they need to realize their rights. As we have seen with the drug industry, governments pursue "control" policies that punish sex workers instead of their clients or refuse to go after the businessmen and politicians behind the scenes will fail. These policies only make the sex workers and their clients more vulnerable to infection. In Bangladesh sex workers faced extensive abuse and discrimination, including abduction, rape, gang rape, beatings, arbitrary arrest, and extortion by the *mastan*—"powerful thugs who sometimes act as musclemen for Bangladesh's political parties"—in exchange for tolerance of their racketeering and other criminal activity. Sex workers report repeated abuse rather than law enforcement by the police who are often connected with the criminal gangs.

In Asia as in other world regions, sex workers are a major vector for spread of the HIV/AIDS epidemic. They have been at the heart of the epidemic in every Asian country, serving as a conduit for the virus from high-risk populations to populations thought to be less at risk. Two Asian countries, Thailand and Cambodia, have faced this issue squarely and, by providing protection for sex workers through their legal system, have managed to stem the growth of HIV prevalence rates. All other countries in the region, because of social and religious sensitivities, have failed to take a strong protective stance and the epidemic has spread rapidly. In some Asian countries, the plight of women in the sex trade has been ignored, and those who contract HIV have been doubly punished. Even where the government takes a hands-off position and sex workers are less stigmatized, the epidemic has grown rapidly.

Although in their early years Asia's great religions and ethical systems argued for moderation and humanistic self-interest by governments in state affairs, they also at the same time played an important role in the subjugation of women. Confucianism and Buddhism encourage filial piety and the notion that children are indebted to their parents, and while male children can fulfill this obligation with work in other labor sectors, women are often stuck. Religion is one of the earliest forms of social control and manipulation, and a key goal was replication of the social group, including sex and care of children. Women are viewed as subordinate to men in all the world's religions, as naturally and innately weaker, and as the source of earthly temptation for men. Once legitimized in religion, their subordination in economics, politics, and law is assured. Religions, from this point of view, are merely subconscious expressions of genetic strategies and a profound fear of the danger surrounding sexuality, a fear that led to separation of women and men in worship and other aspects of social organization.

From a demographic perspective, women may have the "last laugh" in another twenty years. They already live longer than men in all Asian societies, even the poorest. Nicholas Eberstadt says that the deep-rooted preference for males in Asian cultures, seen all over Asia, is getting stronger and promises unusual demographic imbalances and severe social problems in the future.[35] "In ordinary human populations, about 103, 4, 5 or 6 boys are born for every 100 baby girls. China has broken this natural law," according to Eberstadt. The ratio in 2000 census lists 120 baby boys for every 100 baby girls. Eberstadt found the same pattern in South Korea, Taiwan, Hong Kong, Singapore, India, the Punjab, Armenia, Azerbaijan, Georgia, and the Caucasus. The combination of declining fertility rates, strong preference for boys, and technologies that permit gender discrimination before birth have combined in a misogynist's dream.

Eberstadt predicts many future problems when these skewed gender ratios are combined with higher death rates from AIDS among females, such as those occurring now in Africa. He forecasts an unprecedented "marriage squeeze" in the decades ahead, when large proportions of men in countries with these birth ratios, at least 15 percent, will be forced to remain unmarried. In China, "the expectation of universal male marriage has prevailed, and where Confucian tradition stresses the son's obligation to marry and honor his ancestors by continuing the family line,"[36] the pressure will be extraordinary. While the world has no precedent for understanding what the reverberations might be, "this 'surplus of males' will make for a 'deficit of peace' pushing China toward a more martial international posture." Even if regional peace is not at risk, "rise of this phenomenon may occasion an increase in social tensions in China—and perhaps social turbulence as well. The government may find it difficult to 'socialize' future cohorts of young men who cannot settle into married life and have no tradition of 'honorable bachelorhood.'"

As Emmeline learned from her work, it may take a war, or at least some very violent demonstrations, before women claim their rights, especially the right to health and freedom from HIV/AIDS infection and death.

SEVEN

FULFILLING HEAVEN'S MANDATE

The Impact of AIDS on Children

MOLLY SMILED ENCOURAGINGLY AT PHET, whose serious face had become ashen as Rageena told her story. "We never gave Phet a chance to finish his story," she told the others. "Let's do that now." I've had quite enough misery for one day, she thought to herself as Phet prepared himself to speak. But they don't seem to be able to get enough.

Phet spoke as if he could read her thoughts. "I've never been able to tell anyone what happened to me. It is such a relief to know that I am not the only one, that I wasn't evil or bad, but that the rest of you have suffered, too." The others were nodding. He laughed. "What I mean to say is that I can now see that the problem spreads beyond me and beyond Laos and beyond Thailand, the countries that I know. I am beginning to wonder where the end of the problem can be found."

"Not in Russia," Vladimir quipped. "I know personally that it goes as far as Estonia, because I carried drugs there once." The others laughed.

Phet looked at his hands nervously. "The rest of my story is so hard to tell." He heaved a big sigh. "I wasn't as pliant as the rest, or as humble. I was bigger, and after a while I was more disgusted than afraid about what he was doing to us. At first he liked that. But then it began to get on his nerves. He wanted me to dress in women's clothes—"

"You weren't a *katoy*, were you?" Geeta asked, incredulous. "I read about them on the net. Some of those boys are as beautiful as any women I've ever seen."

"No," Phet answered. "Those boy-girls can be beautiful, but I am afraid I am a little too big to be convincing." He gestured helplessly at his own body. "No. I refused, so he sold me to a brothel owner in Bangkok. I learned how to be a bartender, but I also learned how to do sex for money. In Laos, where I came from, men will sometimes love other men, and it is the same in Bangkok. Every Wednesday there was a sex show, and I learned how to take off my clothes to music. It disgusted me, but my owner said I owed him money for food and rent, and he would turn me over to the police if I didn't do what he said. Since I had no visa and I knew he paid off the police regularly, I was afraid that if I refused I would end up on the side of a road with my face burned off with quicklime. When I went back in my village after my first visit to Thailand, I learned that one of the girls who had gone to Thailand to work had been badly hurt. She defied the factory owner and asked for more money. He forced her girlfriends to beat her with electrical cords, pour acid on her, tie her in a garbage bag, and lock her in a closet. It took her girlfriends a day to convince the police there was something wrong, and by that time, you could not recognize her face. When I visited her mother and she told me the story, she could not stop crying.

"So I did what they said and eventually earned enough money to get back to Laos. After I returned to my village, my money ran out quickly, so I went to work in Vientiane, the Lao capital. Factory jobs paid so little that I eventually slid back into bar work." He looked at his hands, and Molly could see that everyone else was looking at theirs. "I wasn't strong enough. I hope I will not be evil forever. I have tried to get a job where I could go back to villages like mine and work with young people to warn them what it's really like, but so far no one has the money to support me."

———◆———

"In your minds you are saying, 'Woman Suffrage is sure to come; the emancipation of humanity is an evolutionary process,'" she told crowd overflowing New York City's Cooper Union on October 21, 1913. "'How is it that these militant women are using violence and upsetting the business arrangements of the country in their undue impatience to attain their end?'" "Why," she asked them rhetorically, "Why are we militant?[1] The answer is simple," she went on. Through experience, British suffragettes had learned that "people who are patient where mis-government is concerned may go on being patient forever." Women in Britain had allied themselves with the Labour Party only to be disappointed time after time that some other issue, like minimum wages for men, always took precedence over women's rights. Year after year, they had presented petitions with hundreds of thousands of signatures to parliament and been ignored. On March 18, 1901, over 29,000 women working in the Lancashire cotton mills signed in a single day. But they had been ignored.

After 50 years of patient waiting, women's violence was now in order, and it was time for "good girls" to act. Britain's upper classes had withheld the vote from men and only extended it when they were threatened by large-scale violence, Emmeline told the crowd. In 1832 the Reform Bill was passed after there was "arson on so large a scale that half the city of Bristol was burned down in a single night." In 1867 the franchise was expanded again after "rioting went on all over the country," and in 1884 agricultural laborers earned the right to vote after their leader threatened to march on parliament from Birmingham with 100,000 men. Rioting, demonstrations, and civil disobedience were feared by "mis-governments," and when the older suffragettes decided to take the advice of younger women in the movement to "pull down the Hyde Park railings" they began to be heard.

On a speaking tour of the United States five years earlier Emmeline had told the 3,000 women gathered at Carnegie Hall that "I am what you call a hooligan." But "you cannot make omelets without breaking eggs. There comes a time in the life of human beings suffering from intolerable grievances when the only way to maintain their self-respect is to revolt against that injustice." Patience was no virtue unless the people in power—the men of the world—were ready to acknowledge the rights of the other half of humanity. "All my life I have tried to understand why it is that men who value their citizenship seem to think citizenship ridiculous when it is to be applied to the women of their race," she told the New York crowd. "A thought came to me in my prison cell"—where she had been locked innumerable times for leading women's attacks on private property and hunger strikes—"that to men women are not human beings like themselves." Men, she said "think us sub-human; they think we are a strange species unfortunately having to exist for the perpetuation of the human race. They think that we are fit for drudgery, but that in some strange way our minds are not like theirs, our love for great things is not like theirs, and so we are a sort of sub-human species."

To the men in her New York audience she said, "You know perfectly well that if the situation was reversed, if you had no constitutional rights and we had all of them, if you had the duty of paying and obeying and trying to look pleasant, and we were the proud citizens who could decide our fate and yours—because we knew what was good for you better than you knew yourselves—you know perfectly well that you wouldn't stand for it a single day, and you would be perfectly justified in rebelling against such intolerable conditions." In 1911 she had urged that British women boycott the census, "to refuse to be numbered" until they could vote. "Men have no right to make laws affecting women until women are free and have the power to voice their opinions." Understand our militancy, she asked the New York crowd, realize "that we are women fighting for a great idea; that we wish the betterment of the human race, and that we believe this betterment is coming through the emancipation and uplifting of women."

While she was in New York, she visited the Night Court for Women, a shocking experience that "was heart-breaking. All the women were charged with solicitation. It all seemed so hopeless, and it was clear they were victims of an evil system." Women, she told a crowd at her next stop in Cleveland, Ohio, "are cheap. Because they are not paid enough to keep body and soul together . . . Give us the vote and there will be no such thing. The women will eradicate it." The debasement of women unable to support themselves and their children in Britain was profound. In 1913 Visiting Australian suffragette Vida Goldstein wrote of 300,000 women in London earning 2 pence a day, and of "25,000 people in London earning a living by the proceeds of the white slave traffic. [Our] laws for destitute children and mothers are far in advance of the laws [in Britain] and I can see the influence of the women's vote in Australia."[2]

Goldstein defended the violence of Britain's suffragettes, saying "we must remind critics that the choice for suffragettes lies between broken windows and the broken lives of helpless women and children." Christabel Pankhurst's passionate outcry against male promiscuity, the double sexual standard, and the resulting spread of venereal diseases, *The Great Scourge and How to End It*, had not yet been published in England, but her *Plain facts about a great evil* had been published in New York to extreme public outcry. Speaking in New York's Carnegie Hall on November 24, 1913, Emmeline described the "white slave traffic" and the need for an equal moral code for men and women. "The English government," she said, "is the greatest white slaver there is. It is engaged directly in the white slave traffic in the miserable army of native women it provides for its army and navy in the east," referring to practices in the British colonies of Asia. "A broken window is a small thing when one considers the broken lives of women, and it is better to burn a house than to injure little children. This is a holy war." As Emmeline's steamer approached its English harbor a month later, two women hailed her from a fishing dory. "The Cats are here, Mrs. Pankhurst," they cried. "They're close to you!" Her feet never touched ground because she was immediately carried to prison. On her release a few days later, she went directly to Paris. Faced with three years imprisonment, she decided to remain there, in exile.

What she did, Emmeline often said, was as much for her children, their children, and the children of the world as for herself. Emmeline and Richard had taken the lead in setting up Manchester's Committee for the Relief of the Unemployed and found temporary housing for them all. They made additional changes to improve the condition of workhouse children and spearheaded the establishment of a summer home for them in the country. She once observed that her contact with the degraded and despised girls and women of the workhouse were "potent factors in my education as a militant."

With the outbreak of World War I, the suffragettes put their grievances aside to support the war effort. During the early months of 1915, Emmeline was fired by discussions in the press of "war babies" being born to unmarried mothers made pregnant by British soldiers. "There is among [these illegitimate children] an appalling death rate & of those who survive I should think the majority become criminals & prostitutes. I want these children saved & made useful citizens," she wrote a friend. Unable to raise enough money for an orphanage—the British public was uncomfortable with advertising the delinquency of their soldiers—Emmeline adopted four female babies. Although she was 57 years old, she adored young babies and told a friend, "I wonder I didn't take forty." She raised the children in Canada, where she lectured extensively after World War I and eventually became a citizen. Ten years later, however, she became so impoverished that she was forced to send two of the girls back to England for adoption by parents who could afford to keep them.

———◆———

One of the saddest long-term social and economic impacts of the HIV/AIDS epidemic is its effect on children. "HIV/AIDS is having a devastating impact on the world's youngest and most vulnerable citizens," says the U.S. Agency for International Development.[3] Children are being orphaned in unprecedented numbers, are being infected in the womb or as young children and adolescents through sexual and drug activity, and millions are caring for parents, siblings, or other relatives who are ill or dying from the disease. In China's AIDS-affected central provinces, where villagers who contracted HIV from donating blood ten years ago are now becoming ill, "the condition of the families made [Beijing-based AIDS activists] weep."[4] Chung To, founder of the Hong Kong-based Chi Heng Foundation and one of the few outsiders allowed into Henan villages, said he watched an eight-year-old boy taking his father out for a walk in a creaky wooden cart. The man was too weak to walk, and the boy hoped some fresh air would bring him back to life. "It was an unforgettable scene," To said.

In Henan alone, 200,000 children may have already been orphaned. The local hospital had only two doctors caring for more than 1,000 HIV-positive patients, and they had been trained by To's group. "In heavily affected provinces like Henan, Hebei and Shangxi, an entire generation is vanishing in the shadows of AIDS," says reporter Alice Park.[5] Because AIDS takes the most active and productive members of a population, villages are devastated, left with only old people and children. The elderly are forced to borrow money or sell off their assets to care for their dying children and have nothing left to care for their grandchildren. In July 2004 Beijing announced the establishment of the first orphanage in Hubei, for which it promised financial assistance. It also announced that it was making AIDS prevention education mandatory for all high school students.

The epidemic is creating catastrophic numbers of orphans in Asia. The proportion of children under the age of fifteen who have lost one or both parents will increase precipitously as the epidemics worsen between now and 2025, when the world will face the worst orphan crisis ever known. Asia already has 65 million orphans according to official estimates, enough for the children to form their own country, but new projections are needed to take account of the rapid rise in infections expected in China, India, Myanmar, and Russia over the next two decades. When infection levels and deaths begin to approach the levels predicted by Eberstadt of several hundred million in 2025, the current number of orphans will skyrocket. Some countries in the region, such as India and Vietnam, are already struggling to care for these children. In China, deaths from the blood scandal are now leveling entire villages.

When orphaned children are asked about their problems, the first one most mention is that they miss the love of their parents and family. Orphans are traumatized by loss of care and protection as badly as children traumatized by war and other violence. Denied the basic closeness of family life, they lack love, attention, and affection. They are segregated and isolated at mealtimes and suffer harsh treatment and abuse from step- or foster parents. Orphans receive less attention and care when they are sick, and they have higher death rates than biological children. Preyed on by relatives and neighbors, they lose property and inheritances. Children can be resilient even when their lives and roles are changing radically, acting as household heads, making decisions, and supporting siblings at great cost to themselves. They often help other children who are vulnerable by providing them food, shelter, counseling, and friendship, and are active members of orphan committees in Africa's AIDS-affected villages.

Experience in Africa has shown that countries with rapidly worsening AIDS epidemics and the seemingly sudden growth in orphans, like China right now, go through four stages in their response once they are finished denying the problem entirely.[6] In the first stage, orphanages begin to sprout up like mushrooms, started first by local communities and then by an influx of kind-hearted strangers. Many governments react like China has, welcoming growth of these orphanages, because they do not understand the extent of the problem and do not understand that it is impossible to build institutions for millions of children. In the second stage, orphanages begin to overflow and thousands of children are still without care, prompting someone to estimate the size of the problem and the costs of an institutional solution. In the third stage, governments recognize the ways in which communities are responding to care for large numbers of orphans and begin to seek models of community care from outside. Finally, the government develops a national strategy that integrates the community's own responses with a national system of benefits, including poverty relief, food supports, and measures to expand access to healthcare and education for guardians of orphans so they are able to keep children in the community without becoming absolutely destitute.

The first European orphanages were built in Renaissance Europe to house children whose parents had died from the plague. Florence's Innocenti Center was built in 1445 as a "foundling hospital" to house the overflow from three other hospital orphanages using the bequest of Francesco Datini, whose own illegitimate daughter, Ginerva, had been secretly placed in a similar hospital in Florence. A large, revolving lazy Susan was set into the thick wall just to the left of Innocenti's front entrance. Compassionate nuns created the "baby catcher," where desperate women through the centuries had gently placed their rag-swaddled infants. With a brief and tear-soaked prayer, mothers could turn the shelf and swing their babies into the safety of the orphanage. Innocenti accepted 200 children the year it opened, but by 1500 the orphanage was accepting 900 children a year, most of whom were born to parents of "disparate status" (slave mothers and unidentified fathers). Half to three-quarters of the children died within a year of their ride on the orphan wheel, victims of plague and other infectious diseases that swept unmercifully through institutions like Innocenti. Fostered children were returned in charnel carts from homes of their "parents," dumped by families who had taken them to work as household laborers, never officially adopting them and unwilling to pay the cost of their burials. Orphanages established as knee-jerk reactions to the AIDS epidemic in

Africa worked no better and they also required considerably more resources than the community care, leaving a few children with some care and lots of children with none.

Most African governments began going through the four stages of response in 1989. Today many are just now entering the last stage. In most countries in Africa, as in Asia, denial played a strong role in delaying responses until the late 1990s. Still, 39 percent of countries around the world with widespread epidemics have no national plans or policies in place to support orphans and other vulnerable children. A few told UNAIDS that they were starting, but a quarter were not even thinking about it. Most of those were in Asia. In Africa, many countries with the rudiments of social welfare systems left over from their colonial period had to catch up rapidly by revising adoption and fostering laws and changing their education and health policies from the private-sector models introduced by World Bank reforms that limited access for the poor. Due to financing problems, most of these countries, which are extremely poor, cannot implement adequate social supports for AIDS-affected families, and the results have been catastrophic. With inadequate budgets, most African countries are now entering a fifth stage, where they stand by helplessly and watch while chaos develops in hard-hit rural areas and poor urban neighborhoods.

———•◦•———

The Chinese government has another alternative that was not available to governments in Africa: to provide dying parents with antiretroviral therapy (ART) that slows the growth of the AIDS virus, keeping them alive and productive long enough for their children to grow to the age where they can take care of themselves. Antiretroviral treament has advanced so much in the past few years that is cheap enough to administer to large numbers of people. China is manufacturing its own drugs, but up until 2004, these were sold abroad rather than being distributed at home. Now China is distributing the drugs to its badly-infected provinces. This policy is the least costly approach to the orphan problem a country can adopt over the long term from an economic and social perspective, although it requires cash up front. It is also the most humane, but the government faces a major challenge in rebuilding its public health system to deliver the drugs safely on a large scale. Right now, China's government is courting the disaster of large-scale drug resistance by providing too few drugs with no instructions to facilities that lack the laboratory facilities to manage them.

China may find a suitable model in Brazil, where the government began providing antiretroviral therapy to any citizen who needed it in the mid-1990s. Brazil's courage in providing treatment despite the World Bank's objections and constant harassment by the United States and the World Trade Organization (WTO) for its manufacture of generic drugs not only saved the lives of thousands of Brazilians, it was the only way the world community could learn that providing treatment drastically cuts new infection rates. Brazil's progressives staunchly defended their right to provide drugs. Not only have they slowed their orphan crisis to a manageable level and reduced suffering and chaos, but it also has reduced hospital costs, increased human productivity, extended people's working lives by keeping them well, and reduced the burden on health and social services of long-term illness and death. Vietnam also manufactures the antiretrovirals and began universally introducing them in 2004. In Thailand, the drugs are provided as an essential medicine by the national healthcare system.India's government is only beginning to respond. Manufacturers in developing countries have led the way in improving the drugs and their administration by developing single-pill fixed-dose combinations of standard regimens that can be taken once or twice a day. Until mid-2004, fixed-dose combinations were not approved in the United States because no U.S. drug company manufactured them. HIV-positive people had to take massive numbers of more expensive pills that were cumbersome and less effective.

The discovery of antiretroviral therapy (ART) in 1996 revolutionized the care and treatment of people living with HIV/AIDS. While ART is not a cure for AIDS, it dramatically improves longevity and quality of life and reduces mortality and morbidity from AIDS and related infections. It also transformed the perception of HIV/AIDS from a plague-like disease into a chronic but manageable illness, reducing the fear factor that helped contain its spread. Third-world manufacturers have taken the mystique out of ART by making the drugs much less expensive, so they are more affordable in developing countries. Despite these advances, as of December 2003, only 400,000 people in developing countries had access to these treatments—2 percent of Africans and 7 percent of Asians who need them—and 25 percent of Brazilians.[7] In September 2003, at the UN General Assembly High Level Meeting on HIV/AIDS, the World Health Organization (WHO), declared the lack of access to HIV treatment a global health emergency. This declaration has not, however, motivated rich countries to donate the money needed for treatment in poor countries, so millions of fathers and mothers continue to perish and the orphan population grows.

Antiretrovirals (ARVs, also called anti-HIV drugs and HIV antiviral drugs) work against HIV infection by slowing down the virus's reproduction in the human body. Because HIV can mutate rapidly, for the treatment to be effective and to reduce the rate at which drug resistance develops, infected individuals take more than one antiretroviral drug in combination with others. It is now recommended that a minimum of three drugs be taken at once, a treatment called highly active antiretroviral therapy (HAART). HAART, or ART for short, involves taking drugs every day and also requires some form of monitoring by a healthcare professional to determine how the drugs are affecting the person taking them. Although so much of the international debate has been focused on delivery of ART, drugs are only one component in a comprehensive package of care for individuals living with HIV and AIDS that includes care for opportunistic infections, nutrition programs, social and economic support, home care, palliative care, and psychosocial support.

ARVs are grouped into four classes according to the way they affect HIV. Nucleoside reverse transcriptase inhibitors (NRTIs, also called nucleoside analogues, or nukes) slow down the production of the reverse transcriptase enzyme so that HIV is unable to infect cells and duplicate itself. Nonnucleoside reverse transcriptase inhibitors (NNRTIs, non-nucleosides, or nonnukes) stop HIV from infecting cells by intervening with the trancriptase of the virus. They bind to the cell's reverse transcriptase in a different way from NRTIs to block the duplication and spread of the virus. Protease inhibitors (PIs) slow the process whereby immature noninfectious virus becomes mature and infectious. HIV uses protease, a digestive enzyme contained in almost every living cell that breaks down protein, to reproduce itself. PIs stop the protease in HIV from breaking long chains of enzymes and proteins in healthy cells into smaller pieces so they can infect new cells. The NRTIs and NNRTIs only have an effect on newly infected cells. PIs, on the other hand, slow down the reproduction of the virus in newly infected cells or those that have been infected for a long time. The fourth class, Fusion or entry inhibitors (ENFs), stick to proteins on the surface of healthy cells and prevent HIV from attaching itself to the cells. They are currently undergoing clinical trials in the United Kingdom and the United States. ENFs must be injected—if taken orally they are digested by the stomach—and are also very costly. For these reasons they are not currently recommended for use in developing country settings.

Close to twenty ARVs have been approved for use in humans, and a number of effective combinations of these ARVs, or treatment regimens, have been identified for use in developing countries. When adopting regimens for national treatment programs, country regulatory and public health authorities consider a number of factors. WHO recommends specific regimens of drugs and clinical monitoring procedures for HIV-positive pregnant women, children and infants, and people with tuberculosis. Injecting drug users can tolerate the medications, but they have to be monitored to make sure they stick to the treatment. Co-blister packs wrap the necessary combination of drugs together so it is easier for a patient to stay organized. Fixed-dose combinations include two or more drugs in one pill, simplifying patient compliance, which must be 95 percent or better to avoid development of drug-resistant strains of HIV.

CD4 is a protein found on the surface of T-helper cells, the main cells attacked by HIV. The more HIV reproduces itself, the fewer number of these cells, and the lower the CD4 count. According to international guidelines, HIV-infected individuals should start ART when their CD4 count is between 200 and 350, or if their disease has reached Stage III or Stage IV. These stages are WHO symptom-based descriptions of HIV/AIDS severity, such as wasting, chronic diarrhea, prolonged fever, and recurrent opportunistic infections. Patients are classified by stages when CD4 testing is unavailable.

Despite ART, some HIV continues to replicate in an individual's body. With each new generation of HIV, there is the possibility of mutations, and some of the new HIV strains may be unaffected by the ARVs being taken. This is drug resistance, and if CD4 counts rebound or do not respond to a particular drug combination, usually the drug regimen has to be changed. Combination therapy and compliance help reduce the incidence of resistance. A person who cannot tolerate the side effects of certain drug regimens has to try different treatments. For all these reasons, clinical assessments are needed after treatment has begun to watch for signs and symptoms of drug toxicities and side effects; adherence; response to therapy; and weight gain or maintenance. Laboratory monitoring of CD4 counts is also necessary and varies depending on the drug regimen being used.

WHO recommends a public health approach to providing ART, whereby treatment regimens are standardized and simplified so everyone in need of treatment can get it (called universal access). Everyone should be given the same drugs when they start treatment, called the first-line treatment regimen. A second-line treatment regimen is also selected by a country to give to patients who cannot tolerate the side effects or have HIV that is resistant to the first-line regimen. Most countries providing treatment chose a first-line regimen of two NRTIs and one NNRTI. WHO's recent treatment guidelines describe potential regimens using six criteria (toxicity, use in pregnant women or patients with tuberculosis, availability as a fixed-dose combination, laboratory monitoring required, and price).

Persons living with HIV/AIDS are more vulnerable to other diseases, known as opportunistic infections, because their immune systems are weakened by HIV. Prevention and treatment of opportunistic infections can significantly reduce morbidity and mortality and result in dramatic gains in life expectancy and quality of life among people living with HIV. In fact, opportunistic infections are so dangerous that some experts feel that even in the absence of ART, high-quality treatment for opportunistic infections and provision of nutritional support can help patients live a normal life for many years. When newly infected with HIV, individuals often develop TB, malaria, pneumococcal pneumonia, shingles (herpes zoster), staphylococcal skin infections, and septicemia; people with more advanced HIV disease or AIDS are prone to pneumocystis, toxoplasma, and cryptococcus. All are diseases that people with normal immune systems also get, but individuals with HIV are more vulnerable to them and will take longer to recover because their immune systems are compromised.

From the viewpoint of public health, one of the most dangerous opportunistic infections is TB, which had been in decline worldwide for forty years but is now increasing as the global HIV/AIDS pandemic grows. It is the leading cause of death for HIV-positive people, accounting for about one-third of all AIDS deaths worldwide, and is the only HIV-related opportunistic infection that poses a major epidemic risk to other people. One-third of the 40 million people living with HIV/AIDS at the end of 2001were thought to be co-infected with mycobacterium TB. Even in well-run TB programs, the current TB diagnostic tool detects the disease in only half of HIV-infected patients. TB progresses faster in HIV-positive people. Drug interactions can make TB treatment in HIV-positive people more difficult and they must be monitored to prevent drug-resistant forms of TB from spreading.

———————◆———————

Only the richest Asian governments are able to provide AIDS-affected families and orphans with the complete range of services they will need to avoid major and lingering social problems. They need the support of their communities and governments, but experience in Asia and Africa shows that most policymakers are slow in responding until a state of emergency sets in. The task facing Asian countries in developing adequate systems of care for AIDS-affected children and their parents is simply enormous. So far only Thailand and Vietnam have begun putting larger-scale systems of care into place, borrowing models of community care developed in Africa. Most Asian countries are still in the denial stage, not even providing adequate prevention services, so it is not likely that they will be able to provide even more complex HIV/AIDS and orphan care.

Child-headed households and vulnerable children will be a social fact of life in societies with high infection levels for many years to come. Supporting children on their own requires an enlightened social welfare system, creative thinking, and financial resources. Interventions must be targeted directly to children, not just families and communities, and must enable children to stay in school or allow working children to attend alternative schooling. Orphaned children benefit psychologically if they can stay with their siblings in their own homes and communities. In such cases they are also more likely to be able to retain their family property if they are not put in orphanages. However, countries must create systems to make these "child-level" interventions possible. Changes are required in child law, child welfare systems, and property law. Support is needed from trained community members and from health, education, and social workers sensitized to children's needs.

In Africa, lack of social services and outside support has left families and communities to provide the bulk of care to children affected by HIV/AIDS. This traditional approach accords well with economic realities and with African value systems. However, good monitoring systems are critical to determine if these systems of care are providing adequate support. Numerous studies of exploitation and abuse demonstrate that children are at risk in these settings if there are no regular monitoring systems in place, even when parents or guardians have the best intentions. Psychosocial support is also essential to help families deal with discipline problems associated with children's grief. Children in female-headed households are significantly more disadvantaged compared to children from two-parent or male-headed families, largely because women have less access to property and employment. Female-headed households are larger and poorer than male-headed households everywhere.

The extended family system is not infinitely elastic, nor is it an unconscious response. In private, grandparents express dismay at having to restart families late in their lives, both in terms of their loss of personal freedom and in their anxiety about meeting the needs of small children financially, physically, and emotionally. They are also frustrated by the behavioral problems of children and young people who have been traumatized by events surrounding their parents' deaths. Guardians are usually traumatized themselves by repeated deaths within their families. In some areas of Africa, fostering had become less common before AIDS and families feel they are returning to a more traditional—and less advantageous—way of life. Families are very poor in many heavily infected countries, and families with orphans and elderly and disabled members—or with a female head—are more likely to be so. Traditional poverty studies have focused on work and income generation from the man's point of view, treating women and children's poverty as derivative. As a result, few countries identify female household heads as targets for special programs, even when they comprise 30 to 50 percent of the total.

In most African countries surveys show that the capacity and willingness of households to support orphans is limited only by their poverty. Economics also plays a role in psychological adaptation. Abuse grows with increasing economic and social pressure. More orphans per family mean less care for each child, household crowding, and pressure on resources, all of which contribute to psychosocial stress. A one-room house may also be the hospital room for someone dying of AIDS to whom the family can provide little physical or medical assistance. Fostering families face increased workloads, reduced ability to socialize with other adults, and increased need to supervise and care for children because there are fewer adults and more children in their households. Their productivity declines and they lose remittances when migrating members fall sick or die. Foster parents may be unable to absorb additional children, even when they are wanted, because of poverty and lack of access to resources.

Sadly, children in Africa and Asia who have lost parents to HIV/AIDS are migrating, dropping out of school to look for work in the city or to take care of sick relatives. According to U.S. senator Bill Frist, African children growing up in the shadow of AIDS with little or no guidance from adults constitute "a pool of recruits for terrorists."[8] Many live in situations of profound abuse because they have lost parental protection. "When my father and mother died, I lived with my uncle," said a child in Malawi. "Then my uncle also got sick and died, so I went to live with my granny. She could not manage to send me to school [so I] ended up on the street to work." Sexual abuse and HIV infection of young children is on the rise in many African countries as more parents die. According to the South African Law Commission, of the 1.6 million rapes that occur yearly in South Africa, a country of 42 million people, 20,000 involve children. "Survival sex" for rent, food, or money is a fact of life for growing numbers of girls living on the streets and for many working as domestic servants or in marginally paying jobs. Unprotected vaginal and anal sex is common among street boys and girls as a form of initiation, play, or to establish dominance, and it can be rough. "You don't go halfway," said one street boy in Tanzania, "if you want to show them what's what."

Asian epidemics will produce social problems that are very different from those confronted in Africa. Because many of the epidemics in the region are based in injecting drug users and sex workers, providing treatment and care for the HIV-infected individuals and their children presents an entirely different set of issues than in countries where the major transmission route is heterosexual. Also, the impact of AIDS on children will be different in Asia because in most countries, fertility levels have dropped substantially and there are vastly fewer children as a proportion of the total population.

In China's central provinces, where AIDS was transmitted by the blood donation system, communities may be entirely wiped out by the disease, and a great deal of movement and social unrest may rise. The country may face a major decline in agricultural productivity similar to the one that has been experienced in Africa since the late 1990s, when a substantial number of farmers, mostly women, started dying. In Africa, too, the loss of women created problems in community-based systems of care that are resulting in massive lost productivity, malnutrition, and decline in children's health. In African communities affected by HIV/AIDS, local power structures changed radically in the initial stages of the epidemics when more men were dying, leaving more room for the participation of women and young people in decision making. Communities that received some coaching and support became more open and stronger as they were trained in self-governance and mutual assistance through these programs. They accepted development programs and inputs in agriculture, education, and health faster, and as a consequence, the productivity of available labor increased. Although there have been many success stories, in urban communities, extremely poor areas, and areas with frequent civil disturbances, these systems of care work less well.

The death of key personnel in all areas of social infrastructure in Africa has severely affected care. Teachers, healthcare, and social welfare workers are being lost at the rate of one per day in many heavily infected countries, and those who are left are burning out from the stress of serving ever-growing populations in need. Community-based care programs have also suffered from these losses. Communities face burn out as their surviving members try to care for increasing numbers of sick adults and orphaned children, and also experience the collapse of social institutions, loss of traditions, and dissolution and loss of identity when a sufficiently large proportion of their population dies. In Uganda, too few skilled government workers are surviving at the district level to undertake new bureaucratic and organizational responsibilities. Most community-based projects work through traditional structures, also losing personnel to the epidemic.

Millions of orphans and people living with HIV/AIDS are a crushing responsibility for poor governments in Africa, but much has been done by governments that are ready to think outside the box. Many African governments have spent considerable time and effort designing and building social welfare systems that provide services and support to the elderly, the disabled, and the needy. These systems originally were designed and budgeted to help several thousand beneficiaries, mostly the elderly, and have had to rapidly expand to accommodate hundreds of thousands of vulnerable adults and children. Several problems are common to governmental responses. As AIDS increases poverty, budgets become insufficient for benefits promised, and there are too few people to distribute benefits. Most African countries have social worker-to-population ratios of 1 to 100,000 or greater, but until recently relied on an individual casework approach to benefit distribution that required a great deal of paperwork. African adoption and fostering laws and systems were outmoded. Lack of free universal primary education meant that social welfare benefits were used to pay school fees or health charges. Governments are overrun by well-intentioned donors needing strong direction. Many people, for example, want to donate to or develop orphanages, but as mentioned, such institutions are costly, inefficient, and less acceptable than community care on a large scale.

In Asia, social welfare systems are similarly underdeveloped, so notions of family welfare systems will have to be completely reoriented, as they have in Africa, in the face of growing AIDS epidemics. As in Africa, lack of data on AIDS-affected families and children contribute to development of unrealistic strategies of assistance or to a general lack of preparedness in many countries. Social welfare systems built to address much smaller populations of needy children and the elderly are now overwhelmed by families and children newly vulnerable due to HIV/AIDS. Massive increase in demand for social welfare services have created bottlenecks or denials of entitlements to persons living with HIV/AIDS and vulnerable children. Support goes to self-identified families and is urban-biased. Many social welfare departments or ministries still assume that existing social welfare mechanisms can provide care for families and children affected by HIV/AIDS on a case-by-case basis. Coverage of existing social welfare is very low, constrained by poor budgets and lack of personnel. When coupled with lack of information on seroprevalence, the ability of government ministries to articulate targeted strategic plans is minimal.

There are several important exceptions. Thailand has provided a comprehensive system of care through its sophisticated healthcare and health insurance systems, and has also led Asia in helping communities organize other services to address the needs of AIDS-affected individuals and their children. Vietnam, known for its stalwart commitment to reducing poverty and improving the health, education, and care of its children, is expanding community-based care through volunteer groups organized by the communist party's Women's Unions and Youth Unions. It is in the planning stages for implementing universal antiretroviral treatment on the Brazilian model. Malaysia and Singapore, rich countries with small epidemics, also provide good care. One of the most important limits on government action in other countries is widespread poverty. Cambodia and Laos, for example, are also organizing community-based assistance, but resources for the programs are much lower.

Poverty is also the principle constraint on households affected by AIDS. According to many studies in many sub-Saharan African countries and a few Asian countries, persons living with HIV/AIDS—even those who are receiving home care—report that their biggest problem is lack of food. Many who could have lived longer even without HIV/AIDS drugs were going as long as a week without food. AIDS-care expenses can absorb as much as one-third of a household's monthly income. As in Asia, some are purchasing AIDS drugs using income that was allocated to purchase of food, pay rent, and buy other essentials. Burdens like these are shared by the children, as evidenced by the pervasiveness of malnutrition. Since poverty is so widespread in Asia, the same results are likely. In Chiang Mai, Thailand, 41 percent of AIDS-affected households have sold land and 24 percent are in debt. ART, TB treatment, and nutritional assistance can help these households preserve or recover their income and assets. The property of women in Africa and Asia is commonly seized by relatives, and legal reform, coupled with strong local enforcement, is urgently needed to secure their tenure and right to inherit land.

In 2002 United Nations Children's Fund (UNICEF) delegates from twenty-two African countries with high orphan levels from AIDS demanded more help, saying that the crisis threatened to cause child labor, homelessness, and prostitution to skyrocket. By 2010 the total number of children orphaned is expected to double in Africa. Because their situation leaves them thoroughly traumatized, they may fall into prostitution and crime and are likely to become HIV-positive themselves, sending the epidemic in Africa into another upward spiral.[9] In 1990 Kenneth Kaunda, then president of Zambia, told a visiting U.S. congressman that he did not know what he would do when the population of street children in that country's capital reached 500,000 because the roaming bands of uneducated and unsocialized orphans would become uncontrollable. Recent reports say child trafficking is spreading across the southern African region, where it was formerly quite rare.

In its fourth annual *Trafficking in Persons Report* released on June 3, 2004, the U.S. State Department said that 800,000 people worldwide are forced to cross international borders and work against their will each year. Many more children and adults are trafficked within borders, or are brought across porous national borders with no one's knowledge. Reports of child slavery among northern Thailand's Hill Tribes are common, and the children are also trafficked within the country's borders. The State Department report, which surveyed trafficking activities in 140 countries, places fourteen Asian countries with badly deteriorating conditions on the watch list, including India, Japan, Laos, Pakistan, the Philippines, Russia, Thailand, Vietnam, and many states in Central Asia and Eastern Europe. Bangladesh, Myanmar, and North Korea were already on the bottom of the State Department's list.

In addition, the International Labor Organization (ILO) reported in July 2004 that there are 250 million child laborers under the age of fourteen, more than half of whom work in Asia "under appalling conditions, facing sexual abuse and even slavery."[10] Twenty percent of the children employed as domestic laborers, mostly girls, are "often heavily exploited. Away from their families, often laboring long hours, with little or no pay, these children are routinely denied their right to attend school and are vulnerable to physical, emotional, psychological and sexual abuse at the hands of their employers." When they get too old, they end up on the streets because they have no idea who or where their families are. The problem is "mostly ignored" by countries in the region. ILO's senior specialist on child labor in the region, Panudda Boonpala, said the situation was "depressing" and will get worse if urgent steps are not taken. The children include increasing numbers of AIDS orphans. Because families are too poor to support children themselves, they view their children's bosses as benefactors and do not question their motives or follow up on the children's working conditions. "The problem is very serious, and international governments need to take more concerted action," the ILO report said. Afghanistan, Australia, India, and Myanmar were among the countries that refused to sign the 1999 accord to eliminate forced work or slavery, prostitution, pornography, or hazardous work for children.

Of Nepal's 2.6 million child workers (40 percent of Nepali children), 127,000 are involved in hazardous work. Their working conditions are similar to those of millions of Indian children working as bonded laborers in India's factories. Most are Dalits or untouchables, imprisoned by a caste system that says they are condemned to the work by actions in their past lives. The same Hindu belief system that condemns women to permanently lower status provides a convenient philosophical underpinning for economic extortion of India's youngest citizens. Human Rights Watch says "one of the foundations of bonded labor is the caste system, through which a traditional expectation of free labor, lack of land, and the threat of violence and social and economic boycotts from upper castes conspire to keep many so-called untouchables, or Dalits, in bondage and a perpetual state of poverty."[11] Vimali, a fifteen-year-old girl in Tamil Nadu bonded by her parents to a silk loom owner for $167, says "this is the thing that God blessed me with, so I have to do work like this. It is written on my head. I don't want to go to the looms, but there is no other way." These children work 14 hours a day, sleep in the factories between the looms, rarely see their families, are beaten if they make mistakes—and because of scurrilous accounting systems, they always stay in debt no matter how much they earn.

Between 60 and 115 million children work in India. A 1996 Human Rights Watch Report concluded that "the Indian government has failed to study, accurately report, or acknowledge the incidence of bonded labor, child labor, and bonded child labor." With the same negligence that has led to India's scandalous blood supply problem, the government failed to enforce its own laws, prohibiting use of bonded child labor or to implement the policies it had adopted to address the problem. So the Supreme Court of India set forth a detailed framework to punish law-breaking employers and ordered India's National Human Rights Commission to supervise implementation by the state governments. Instead of addressing the issue squarely, the state governments underestimated the practice and only a few high profile cases were prosecuted. The money allocated to rehabilitate bonded child laborers goes unspent, says a 2003 Human Rights Watch update, which advocated widespread government and police reform.

Developing social welfare systems adequate to the task of averting the social disasters promised by growing HIV/AIDS epidemics takes a massive investment in health, education, and poverty relief. For that to happen, Asia's avaricious social elites will have to feel sufficiently threatened by the epidemic to reverse their current thinking about their responsibilities to the poor. Although poverty is growing rapidly, most governments keep taxes and business costs low by not requiring social security measures or safety nets such as unemployment or health insurance for workers, old age pensions, or allowances for families taking care of orphaned or fostered children. Their failure to create safety nets has already created the crushing and "depressing" conditions of child labor evident in the ILO report, which works to their advantage by absorbing the 65 million or more orphans that already exist in these countries and keeping the cost of living lower. Their failure to do so also contributes to the rapid growth in many countries' sex sectors, victimizing women and children alike. Their failure to do so leaves millions of their citizens suffering the punitive consequences of addiction to harmful drugs and has left billions of people living in horrendous conditions of poverty. Their failure to create safety nets to catch families and children falling into degradation for other reasons—despite the ILO's persistent urging—provides little reason to hope that they will be motivated by the fast-approaching social catastrophe of HIV/AIDS.

———◆◆◆———

Children in Asia are affected by HIV/AIDS in many other ways besides being orphaned. Like AIDS-affected children in Africa, they suffer terrible discrimination and psychological problems and receive very little support. In fact, they are often stigmatized and drop out of school because their families, drained by the costs of AIDS care, cannot afford school fees. Parents dying of AIDS often try to get their children adopted, but stigma against the family gives them little hope of succeeding. In Henan, China, when a program to help AIDS-affected village children with their school fees was publicized, local administrators shut it down. Government assistance is promised but often not received. Some children live alone because their relatives are too afraid of infection to take them in, and they have to look for jobs when they are as young as ten years old. In Cambodia, one-fifth of children in AIDS-affected families had to start working to support their families, and one-third provided care or took on major household work. All of them suffered stigma and psychosocial stress.

"In regions affected by the epidemic," says the Human Rights Watch report on China's blood scandal, "tens of thousands of children, if not more, may face catastrophic economic and social problems."[12] In Hindu cultures, such as India and Nepal, becoming an orphan carries the additional stigma of having very bad karma. While African communities do not attribute bad karma to orphaning, stigma is still sometimes attached to losing a parent to AIDS because it is associated with promiscuous sexuality. Differences in family totems sometimes constrains adoption, but often stigmatizes survivors. Most orphans are welcomed into the homes of relatives who share what little they have as best they can. Hindu culture, by contrast, openly reviles orphans for having brought on the death of their parents; they are called *ama tokwa* or *babu tokwa*, mother eater and father eater, or just plain *mulya*, bad luck. They are ejected from their families, isolated by their communities, even spit on in the streets.

HIV-positive children suffer severe illnesses and almost-certain childhood death unless they are given treatment. Children who are HIV positive are also stigmatized. In China, these children are often refused school admission. Song Pengfei, infected at age sixteen by a blood transfusion during a surgical procedure in Shangxi Province, was expelled from school. His neighbors demonstrated against his family, calling them offensive names, and eventually hounded them out of their home town. One-third of children born to HIV-positive mothers are infected. In 2003 worldwide, 700,000 additional children became infected with HIV, most through mother-to-child transmission (MTCT) during pregnancy, labor and delivery, or breastfeeding. Three million children are battling the negative effects of HIV infection or full-blown AIDS contracted in this way, but this number does not include complete estimates for most of Asia. Since the beginning of the pandemic, close to 7 million children have been infected, but the number of new infections has been dropping over the past few years thanks to prevention programs. In the absence of any intervention, rates of MTCT can vary from 15 to 30 percent without breastfeeding and up to 30 to 45 percent with prolonged breastfeeding. Interventions in developed countries since the mid-1990s have reduced HIV transmission from an infected mother to her child to 2 percent or less with the introduction of counseling and testing, short-course ART, elective cesarean delivery, and the safe use of infant formula instead of breastfeeding.

Because of low official infection rates, many countries gave MTCT prevention low priority, but enthusiasm for the program is increasing as more children are infected. Thailand, with a national program, is demonstrating how effective it is in reducing the overall size of its epidemic. The fact that the prevalence of prenatal HIV is still relatively low in most of Asia makes MTCT prevention programs easier to run, even in poor countries, but most are only beginning to implement it. The continent's most populous countries—China, India, and Bangladesh—are implementing programs in a few states. Vietnam and Cambodia are moving to full-scale implementation, but most other countries have yet to start. Higher-income countries, such as Malaysia and Singapore, have no trouble with this low-cost intervention because of their size and their robust healthcare systems. A country's ability to implement such programs depends on a number of factors, the most important being the sophistication of the healthcare system. In countries where the healthcare system is poor and a large proportion of children are not born in hospitals, implementing even these simple programs will be a formidable challenge.

A 2003 evaluation of UN-sponsored MTCT prevention pilots in eleven countries shows that the benefits of PMTCT far exceed individual impact on mothers and children and reduction in overall infection rates. Such programs improve the outlook of HIV-positive women, their health and the health of their children; increase male involvement in family health and interest in HIV prevention; and increase access to treatment and resources for physical and mental health that improved quality of life for women with HIV and their families. MTCT prevention also had very positive effects on healthcare provider attitudes toward AIDS. Acquiring the skills and tools to help women and their infants empowers providers to do something about HIV/AIDS and makes them more supportive of their clients. Although health workers had to greatly expand their responsibilities and workload in pilot programs, usually with no additional compensation, they were highly committed because the program made them feel more effective and useful. Community HIV/AIDS education was expanded, increasing the proportion of women who know how to protect themselves and their babies from HIV transmission. Most communities in which the pilots took place lacked the full array of care and support services, but providers developed an intricate web of referrals for antiretrovirals and psychosocial and home-based care.

Since the thirteenth International AIDS Conference in Durban, South Africa, in 2000, there has been a dramatic increase in global political and programmatic commitment to MTCT prevention worldwide. The Global Fund to Fight AIDS, Malaria, and Tuberculosis funds pilot programs in many developing countries, including implementation of national PMTCT prevention programs in Thailand, Botswana, and Uganda. Because of the importance of expanding access to PMTCT around the world, four other large-scale international initiatives have been started, but coverage is still very low. In Africa, infant and child mortality has increased sharply over preepidemic levels in all countries with severe HIV/AIDS epidemics. Not only do more children die of AIDS, but others die because their mothers are too sick to care for them, because there is no one to care for them when their parents die, or because community support for them and their parents collapses.

Another way Asian children will be affected by HIV/AIDS is by catching it themselves through injecting drug use or sex, which in young girls is often forced, usually by people they know, including family members. The latest craze in Asian pornography is *Deep Love*, the story of a teenage girl named Ayu who dabbles in prostitution. Yoshi, the book's author, first published the book in installments as downloadable text files and plied high school students with promotional flyers. When the serialized story was compiled as a book, it sold 1.8 million copies, and a film adaptation hit the theaters in April 2004.[13] Japan's adolescent girls even have their own magazines—two, *Egg* and *Cawaii!*, have readerships of more than 30,000—that celebrate their independence, impertinence, and self-confident sexuality. Young women all over Asia copy

Japanese fashions through magazines, television, and books. *Candy*, Mian Mian's tale of teenage prostitution and drug addiction in Guangdong Province has become an international literary sensation. Tolerance of sexual diversity is also increasing. Young transvestites at the Chiang Mai Technology School in northern Thailand lobbied their school for a "Pink Lotus Bathroom" where they can attend to personal care matters without harassment.

In 2000 UNAIDS estimated that six people under the age of twenty-four were being infected with HIV every minute. In countries with infection levels over 15 percent among adults—a level foreseen in Asia's not-to-distant future—one-third of fifteen-year-olds will also become infected sometime in their lives. Half of all people who are now infected got the disease before they are twenty-five-years-old. Two-thirds of Asia's young people are "alarmingly ignorant about HIV/AIDS," says a 2004 UNICEF report, and more than half say they know nothing about drug use.[14] "Even where HIV/AIDS is high, unsafe sex and drug use can still be common." Many young people who know how to avoid infection are unwilling to use condoms or receive voluntary counseling and testing services to learn their HIV status. Often girls are unable to negotiate the terms of their sexual relations, including condoms, while young injecting drug users are often aware of the risks but fail to protect themselves because of low self-esteem.

The world's largest-ever generation of adolescents faces increasing disease risks, unwanted pregnancy, and poverty. Besides getting more than half of all new HIV infections, each year they acquire more than one-third of the world's 333 million new curable sexually transmitted diseases. Young girls face teen pregnancy, early marriage, and violence. Because only 17 percent of women between fifteen- and forty-nine-years-old in developing countries have access to contraception, they account for one-fourth of the 20 million unsafe abortions performed each year. But their governments are doing very little to help. Of 104 countries surveyed in 2003, forty-four did not include AIDS or sex education in their curricula and many, such as the United States and the Philippines, are cutting back on sex education and becoming even more insistent that "good" young people will "just say no." HIV spreads fastest in conditions of poverty, powerlessness, and lack of information, conditions in which most young people now find themselves. Human Rights Watch says that abstinence-only education programs threaten the lives (and human rights) of young people because they exclude information on condom use and other ways to prevent HIV transmission.

On average, young girls are likely to be infected with HIV ten years earlier than men, leading the U.S. Census Bureau to project a sustained imbalance in the number of men and women that will lead men to seek even younger women, further increasing infection in female adolescents. Many men around the world believe that younger girls are less likely to be infected with HIV, while others hold the mistaken belief that having sex with a virgin can cure AIDS. Because they were recently infected, HIV-positive young people are highly infectious. HIV is most infectious when viral loads in the blood are highest, resulting in HIV shedding in many body fluids. Viral loads are high for a few months immediately following infection. Informed behavior could help prevent the young people from infecting their partners.

The problems faced by adolescents are universal. Young Americans are having sex at increasingly younger ages and have more partners by the time they reach twenty than their parents dreamed of in a lifetime. The average six-teen- to twenty-year-old has already had five partners, gaining ground quickly on twenty-five to thirty-four-year-olds with eight partners, and those over forty-five who report an average of nine. The University of Minnesota's Center for Adolescent Health and Development reports that 34 percent of ninth graders in the United States have had sexual intercourse. A seventeen-year-old who has had seven partners says that pregnancy is a more immediate concern than HIV, although "the anxiety [about AIDS] never leaves me. But I still have sex. And I know I can always get oral sex without getting too emotionally involved." Only African teens have sex more often than American teens. At least one-third of young African women are married by eighteen, and half have had sex. Of these, half want to use birth control but can not get it, so the rate of unintended pregnancy is 20 percent. Like teens in the United States, over half of the Africans do not think they are at risk for AIDS.

The age of puberty has dropped continuously since 1900 due to improved nutrition, so some of the explanation for the rapid increase in teen sex may be physical. But for teenagers, sex is more than a way to satisfy raging hormones. It is part of broader exploration of the world and a way to separate from their families and form new social bonds. The new relationships may require rebellious and even destructive or copycat behavior such as injecting drug use or suicide, a common cause of death among young people worldwide. Many of their coming-of-age behaviors put them at risk of HIV infection. More than 5 million U.S. teens, 23 percent in a 2002 survey, said they had unprotected sex because of alcohol or drug abuse, cross-over behavior that contributes to rapid HIV spread. The National Survey of Family Growth, which interviewed 1,280 teen girls between fifteen and nineteen, found that adolescents using birth control were no more sexually active than nonusers and were more likely to use protection when they had sex. Government programs had little effect, but they found that the quality of family and community life is critical in shaping young people's behavior.

In the few African countries in which the epidemic is declining or slowing down, the most important factor has been a change in teen sexual norms. In the late 1980s, young Ugandans began delaying their first sexual experience because of AIDS; by 1995 the proportion who had intercourse before their twenties was halved. Change in teen norms is vital to stop HIV spread because the majority of new infections occur among young people. HIV infection in teens will continue to define the epidemic and global population structure for the next three decades. Between 1960 and 1990, when HIV/AIDS took hold, the proportion of young people in the world doubled; today more than half of the world's population is under twenty-five. By 2025, the average age will increase only five years, to thirty. The world is young and will not get much older until the middle of the century, especially the developing world, where 85 percent of young people live and where close to 95 percent of persons living with HIV/AIDS are concentrated. High infection rates among young people mean that epidemic's global drag will be even greater. Young people get sick just when they reach their prime productive years, wasting their society's investment in education and job training. They also live longer and need more care than older people with the virus. The United Nations Development Programme claims that, "never before in history have death rates of this magnitude been seen among young adults of both sexes and from all walks of life."

"I'm an orphan," the twenty-something Nepali leaned toward me and whispered. "My mother died when I was six." Like many Asian orphans, Surendra had been schooled by years of poverty and desperation to feel ashamed of himself and his family, as if he had somehow brought the condition of being an orphan on himself. "She was a prostitute," Surendra told me, lowering his eyes and choking on the words. When his father abandoned the family, his mother had done the only thing she knew to put food on the table, but Surendra refused to recognize her heroism because he had suffered too much for having had a mother in the world's oldest profession. "She died of AIDS," he continued—not surprising in a country and a continent where many sex workers carry the HIV virus. Surendra lived with his father's brother for a while and, by working very hard, put himself through all but two years of secondary school. But his uncle drank and beat Surendra frequently, so he left their rural home and came to Nepal's capital city, Kathmandu. He was living on odd jobs, sleeping where he could and getting by, but barely.

Nepalis are buoyant, friendly people who enjoy telling a good yarn when they get the chance, but Surendra's culturally patterned behavior was merely a thin patch over a very deep psychic crack. As he talked, his hearty confidence dwindled. His face hardened and his jaws clenched so tight the facial muscles in his thin cheeks twitched. Like many children of his generation orphaned by AIDS, he had toughed it out, but he was showing the strain, his toughness worn thin each time he felt obliged to repeat his sad story. How else to get a job or a donation, or any help at all on a continent when one-third of the population is malnourished and unemployment is astronomically high?

After his mother died, Surendra received little love or kindness from any of the human beings charged with his care. Alone in the world since he was old enough to fetch firewood, carry water, and work in the fields, he, like so many bright kids under these circumstances, had become an opportunist, a chameleon, and an entertainer. What he had achieved was remarkable in the context of Nepal's economic and social systems, but it was tenuous. Surendra was on a slippery slope; at any minute, a stroke of bad fortune—or losing an opportunity like the one he had with me right now—could mean a plunge back into truly desperate living conditions. Surendra would somehow go on, but he could never completely relax and he would probably never trust anyone fully. He was affectless even when he smiled, the deadness in his eyes unrelieved by the dimpling of his cheeks or his jocularity. Staying one step ahead of imminent privation and cruelty had damaged this young man badly.

Surendra's relentless self-exposé was the compulsive litany of a person grown used to seeking support from strangers, the song of a shattered childhood held together by a frightening level of self-control. This was the same boy I had met in the Ugandan banana field that I had visited fifteen years ago, the sixteen-year-old who had taken care of five brothers and sisters in a broken-down, two-room mud shack with no water or latrine and utterly no help from his family because there was no family left to give it. This was the boy whose three-month-old sister had died in his arms because he did not know what to feed her and there was no one there to tell him. This was the boy who silently prayed beside the stone cairns marking his parents' graves every day for strength, their deaths forgotten by everyone else. Except in his memories, they had disappeared from the world without a trace. These were the children whose parents' bodies came home in the back of pickup trucks, in buses, or as corpses propped on old boards sticking out from the backs of bicycles, wrapped in sienna-colored bark-cloth shrouds.

Surendra had been lucky. He was alive, after all, surviving the brutal existence that had taken many other orphaned boys and girls over the past decade. On the strength of his exceptional intelligence, he had created himself by an act of will from the shreds of turmoil and despair that were his life. Surendra had learned how to survive on his own in the households that gave him shelter, with the on-again off-again affection of poor relatives burdened by his presence. When he was older, he had learned to survive with no shelter or protection of any kind because those households were no longer able to provide for him and the state was too poor to help.

Many orphans are in the care of their grandparents, who are frustrated by discipline problems. "The children care about nothing," one old man said. "They run away when food is low, or when they think we've been unfair," or when other children in the family got preferential treatment. "With five children of my own and three orphans to feed," one woman said, "I have to choose." The old man sighed. "There's just not enough for all of them. They go to the towns to do casual jobs, where they are victimized" by Fagans to this new generation of Oliver Twists. "Growing up without school or vocational education, they are becoming juvenile delinquents and potential rebels. What future do they have? What future have we?"

Many of Africa's child soldiers are taken at an early age from the ranks of street children and orphans and intentionally brutalized to become killers. For years now, the press in South Africa has been full of reports of increasing violence and robberies, some of it attributed to the growing number of street children due to AIDS. South Africa is one of the few countries on the continent with a social welfare system that provides benefits to disadvantaged children—when the national budget allows. Needy children are guaranteed a $5 monthly allowance. With the end of apartheid, the beneficiary list was opened to millions of poor blacks, so the budget is often insufficient and benefits do not come regularly. Botswana and Namibia, the other countries in Africa rich enough to consider social welfare, face similar problems. All three countries have temporarily brought demand for assistance under control by creating strategic bottlenecks in the welfare application process.

Surendra is Asia's future for the next thirty years or beyond: driven, haunted, just a wee bit wild. Clenching his jaws and his entire psyche, predatory and primitive in his vigilance. Growing up in an uncertain environment, Surendra was never able to develop a consistent template to predict what might happen or what he can expect. The same behavior may have provoked completely different responses, ranging from physical beatings to mental abuse to tender loving care. His mother had died of AIDS and he had been the caregiver in their relationship. If she was a sex worker, Surendra may have been handed from family member to friend or been on his own without care very early in his life. Orphaned and adopted children do not experienced open warmth and unconditional love, the kind of love associated with the biological and genetic bonds of parenthood. With no model for this behavior, a child does not understand it as a possibility. The closer you approach them, the more uncomfortable they get. When they receive love, they rebel against it, testing it in the same way they test all the other responses they elicit in their lives. Surendra has developed a condition known as reactive attachment disorder—emotionally guarded, constantly wary, restricted, blunted, and exuding mistrust although he was outwardly normal and friendly.

Martin Maldonado-Duran of the Menninger Clinic's Department of Psychiatry says that children develop templates, or working models, of relationships based on their relationship with early caregivers. If their models are positive, they learn to trust other people, but if they are negative, children will learn that there is no one to trust and that they are alone in the world. The National Adoption Center reports that 52 percent of adoptable children in the United States have symptoms of attachment disorder, and the older the child when adopted, the higher the risk of social maladjustment. A child adopted at one week of age has a much better chance at a normal life than one adopted at the age of ten. Attachment develops when a child receives consistent responses from the caregiver, and the infant can be confused if the caregiver is moody or angry. If the caregiver is suddenly replaced or removed, the child's basis for future attachments is threatened. Six months appears to be the cutoff point; during the first six months of a child's life, the infant needs a warm and boundless relationship with the mother or another permanent caregiver. After six months, the baby begins to explore and separate, but returning to a caring base is still critical for reinforcement and emotional refueling. The theory of attachment disorders was developed by American psychoanalyst John Bowlby in the 1950s, who also recognized that children whose mothers or fathers were insensitive to their internal emotional states and who failed to respond to them warmly and sensitively suffered from similar problems.

Children with attachment disorders may be unable to respond to social interactions appropriately, and will either withdraw (inhibited reactive attachment disorder) or will be indiscriminately sociable, accepting anyone as a caregiver as though the relationship is intimate and lifelong (disinhibited reactive attachment disorder). Children resort to psychological defense mechanisms, relying only on themselves and not expecting to be soothed or consoled by adults. Or they may suppress their sense of fear and develop a "pseudocomfort" or "undifferentiated closeness" with anyone who is available. Attachment can also be confused if the caregiver is present and the relationship is strong but angry, so the child develops an angry pattern of behavior with anyone who is close but behaves normally with other people.

Villagers in Laos polled in a recent study were evenly divided in their opinion of the life prospects of orphans, reflecting the opposing manifestations of attachment disorder. Orphans are the most pitiable children alive, some thought. They are quiet, withdrawn, and depressed. No, others protested. Orphans are tougher and more resilient because they learn at an early age to deal with life's difficulties by themselves. The orphan of today, a famous saying goes, is the general and statesman of tomorrow. That is, if they do not die miserably or become psychologically disfigured in the meantime.

Maldonado-Duran says that 35 percent of middle-class American children have insecure attachment styles that affect them throughout their lives. Children with inhibited reactive attachment disorder can fail to thrive, appear bewildered, unfocussed, and blank, and not respond to familiar social signals. Children with disinhibited reactive attachment disorder, the most common form, exhibit "excessive familiarity or psychological promiscuousness," giving hugs indiscriminately and going off with strangers or asking them for comfort, food, and toys. Children with the severe form of the disorder often show signs of physical maltreatment and undernutrition, have rashes from unchanged diapers, and the backs of their heads may be flattened from lying in bed too much. Children who have been in several foster homes sometimes have excessive appetite and thirst.

Although many children begin showing symptoms by age five, middle childhood and adolescence is the most difficult risk period for many. At this point, children are searching for their own identities, and the absence of a biological bond with adoptive parents may create grave issues of trust. Adopted children do not have a stable sense of who they are, and often have incomplete information about why they were adopted and their biological and cultural roots. At any point, children with the disorder can become cold, cruel, and emotionally abusive to their caregivers, and destructive, self-abusive, or dangerously and overly friendly with strangers. They have trouble establishing eye contact, lie, steal, have poor impulse control, engage in cruelty to animals, and seem to lack a conscience. Adoptive parents often do not have the skills to deal with their special needs and have difficulty finding professionals who do. In 2001 a desperate attempt to "cure" an attachment disorder in a ten-year-old U.S. girl resulted in her death when inexperienced therapists smothered her while trying to "rebirth" her. One Colorado mother beat her two-year-old adopted Russian son to death when her self-control broke; many adoptive parents have relinquished or "unadopted" children whose behavior was too difficult for them to handle.

Dana E. Johnson, an expert in adoption medicine from the University of Minnesota, says that a child raised in an institution has virtually zero chance of developing normally. Children in orphanages are high risk, especially those from poor countries, he claims, because of the circumstances of their abandonment (parents who drink, do drugs or abuse them—or nursing a parent who is dying from AIDS) and because of the impact of neglect while in the orphanage. Johnson says orphanages are "a terrible place to raise an infant or young child" because of the lack of stimulation and of consistent caregivers, the poor nutrition, and the physical and sexual abuse. A 2003 study of the Kenyan orphanage deaths, which have popped up in response to increased HIV/AIDS, documented rampant physical and sexual abuse.

Often, as Surendra knew, the orphan's fate depends on the kindness of strangers. Harry Potter would still be living in the cupboard under his aunt and uncle's staircase were it not for the determined protection of wizards who needed his strength to defeat evil in the world. Indisputably fearless, Henry Morton Stanley, the great African explorer, was sheltered by the Louisiana merchant from whom he took his name. A cruel opportunist who unabashedly promoted himself, Stanley was unable to form loving relationships with any of his prospective brides. Charles Dickens, who created the most famous paradigm of the worthy orphan before Harry Potter, was not an orphan but was sent to a work house at the age of twelve when his family's fortune ran thin. Oliver Twist triumphed like Dickens himself did because he had enough self-esteem to ask for more (literally and figuratively) and resisted the pressure of adults bent on corrupting him for their own evil purposes.

While fictive Oliver struggled with the vicissitudes of London life, between 1854 and 1929 troubled city fathers in New York and other east coast U.S. cities sent real-live "Street Arabs" from impoverished homes to rural America on "orphan trains." The total may have been as high as 400,000; 100,000 were sent to Missouri alone. From 1820 to 1860, more than 5 million English, Irish, and German immigrants swelled the ranks of the poor in New York, followed by Eastern Europeans after the Civil War. The vast majority were dirt poor, looking for opportunity in a city that had relatively few jobs. The flood of workers meant low wages, dangerous working conditions, no labor unions, no sick leave, and no insurance. The children of these families suffered terribly, and in the 1850s, tens of thousands of working children roamed city streets searching for money, food, and shelter, selling matches, rags, and newspapers, engaging in petty theft and banding together to protect themselves from criminals and policemen.

Charles Loring Brace, an ordained Methodist minister from a Hartford, Connecticut family that educated him at Yale and New York's Union Theological Seminary, transformed his mission for these children into the Children's Aid Society of New York. Because it was impossible to build enough institutions to house all of them, he hit on the idea of sending homeless children to farm families in the West, secretly believing that if the children were removed from "depraved" urban Jewish and Catholic families and placed in "upstanding" Anglo-Protestant homes, they would be properly Americanized. "The cheapest and most efficacious way of dealing with the 'Dangerous Classes' of large cities," orphan trains would provide "the influences of education and discipline and religion for the abandoned and destitute youth of our large towns," drawing them "under the influence of the moral and fortunate classes that they may grow up as useful producers and members of society, able to aid in its progress." Declaring that every American community, especially those in the West, had "many spare places at the table of life," his orphan trains were born.

"WANTED: Homes for Children" read the advance advertising for one such train. "A company of homeless children from the East will arrive at TROY, MONTANA ON FRIDAY, FEB. 25TH, 1910." Two Children's Aid Society agents worked with a local committee to "distribute" the children at each stop. The poster declared them "well disciplined, having come from the various orphanages," but the majority were temporarily "placed" by resourceful immigrant families with more able middle-class "child savers" who provided them a home and an apprenticeship until their own parents could reclaim them. Children as young as a few months old were sent to midwestern and western states, Canada, and Mexico, and displayed at local train stations, where families arrived at the appointed hour to inspect them and make their choices. Some children were lucky. Irma Craig Schnieders arrived in Osage City, Missouri, a few days before her third birthday. She found a loving home with German immigrants, became her high school's valedictorian, graduated from teacher's college, and married and raised eight children of her own. Adopted at five months by a couple in St. Louis, Mary Ellen Pollock discovered her adoption papers when she was ten but never told her parents. "Back then, children were seen and not heard," she said. "No one in the family mentioned it, though they must have known. It didn't bother me. I had a good life."

Street boys Andrew Burke and John Brady grew up to be governors of their adopted states of North Dakota and Alaska, but not all adoptive families were subject to the same oversight as those in Troy, Montana, where prospective adopters were instructed to "treat the children in every way as a member of the family, send them to school, church, Sabbath school and properly clothe them until they are 17 years old." Many children labored as field hands, abused and neglected by their adoptive families. In 1927, twelve states still allowed indentured labor of institutional charges and children turned over to county authorities or poor farms. Taken from his alcoholic father when he was eight years old (his mother had died when he was two), shoeless Elliot Bobo boarded the orphan train with a cardboard suitcase containing one change of clothes. "I had the whole future ahead of me," he said, recalling his past at eighty, "and I didn't know what to expect." Elliot's first train station parade was a fiasco. When a farmer came up, felt his muscles, inspected his teeth, and decided to "adopt" him, Bobo bit and kicked him. Young Bobo soon learned from his mistake and was adopted at the next station by a loving family.

Orphan trains were banned in Missouri and Kansas in 1901 because they encouraged wholesale dumping of children. The Kansas State Board of Charities scrutinized all organizations and institutions placing children in the state and ruled that no homeless child could be brought in without a certificate of good character and $5,000 security bond. "We cannot afford to have the State made a dumping ground for the dependent children of other states, especially New York," declared the state's then governor, William Stanley. "Baby farms" that sold ("placed out") the children of unwed mothers, sex workers, and destitute or deserted wives had gained in popularity; similar operations have thrived in many countries around the world before they banned international adoptions.

Little Orphan Annie, born in 1924 in a U.S. newspaper, rarely had time to sing wistfully of "tomorrow" from the top of the orphanage's broad staircase because she was too busy fighting with adult villains (in one strip she is beaten to a pulp offstage by Mr. Mack). She became a World War II plane spotter. Harold Gray said that his brainchild "is tougher than hell with a heart of gold and a fast left who can take care of herself because she has to." In the Wednesday, October 23, 1935 strip, Annie, the on-screen double for a spoiled child actress named Tootsie, is called to jump off a cliff. Tootsie walks off bawling while Annie enters right, musing "Gee, she is scared. I guess some folks just can't help it, and we hadn't ought to blame 'em. I can't help feelin' sorta sorry for th' poor kid." She strides to the cliff edge in her bobbed black wig and Tarzana costume and executes a perfect swan dive into the river below. Harold Gray chose an orphan as his feature strip's lead character even before he decided to make Annie a female—she started as Little Orphan Otto—because "she'd have no extraneous relatives, no tangling alliances, and the freedom to go where she pleased." Shortly before he died in the 1960s, Gray hoped that after his death, "Annie would continue to sell the idea that life is a battle, with victory for the brave and strong hearted alone. Probably she'll never grasp complete victory, but she'll get a few tail feathers now and then!" One hopes that Asian children orphaned by the AIDS epidemic will live long enough to "catch a few tail feathers," too.

Three of Asian history's most pivotal figures—Muhammad, Genghis Kahn, and Chu Yuan-chung—are also three of the most famous orphans in history. If you survive, orphaning makes you tougher, faster, stronger, and smarter. Chu Yuan-chung, the peasant who threw the Mongols out of China in 1356, founded the Ming dynasty as Emperor Hung Wu. He was, like Genghis Kahn, "an orphan of humble origins who rose to command a rebel group through sheer force of personality and ability in the doubtful arts of intrigue," says Colin Mason.[15] Like the great Khan, his authority was "direct, brutal, and decisive." He had a furious temper and "imposed the death penalty more or less on whim." He beat offending mandarins who dared to cross him "with bamboo clubs, to death," says Mason.

Born between 1155 and 1167, Temuchin (the future Genghis Khan) was named after a Tartar chief recently slain by his father. He was born gripping a clot of blood, an auspicious sign that the Fates had their eyes on him. When the Tartars took revenge and poisoned his father, Temuchin, as eldest son, became head of his family at nine years old. Too young to assume command of his father's followers, the clan abandoned him with his mother and five brothers in the Kentai Mountains, where they lived in abject poverty, eating berries and marmots and avoiding the rival chieftains who seized control of his clan. He was tough from the start, and the hardship made him tougher. He and his younger brother Qasar killed their half-brother Bekter when they caught him stealing a fish and small bird Temuchin had trapped. Their distraught mother cursed them: "Except for your shadows you have no companions. Except for your horses' tails you have no whips, and you can not even regain leadership of your father's clan." Temuchin slowly improved the family's fortunes by stealing horses and other livestock. He managed to escape the rival Tiichi'ut clan by cracking his guard's skull wide open. When he reached his majority, he inherited blood feuds with the other Mongol clans, including the Merkits, from whom he stole the bride promised to him while his father was still alive. The Merkits stole Borte back, but Temuchin escaped the raiders and fled to the highest peak in the Kentai, where he prayed to Tengri, the Everlasting Blue Sky. He soon recovered Borte in another raid, but the son she bore nine months after her recapture was never allowed to play a leading role in the Khan's affairs.

Muhammad ibn Abd Allah was born in 570 to the Banu Hashim family in the tribe of Quraysh after his father had been killed in a desert raid. His grandfather took him in and at an early age he was visited by two angels whom he said "opened his chest and stirred their hands inside." This was the first of several spiritual experiences that led the young boy to begin his search for the truth of God. In adolescence, he began working with his uncle, a trader, who became his guardian. Employed by a widow, Khadijah, to take a trading caravan north to Syria, he met Christians and Jews and a monk named Bahira who recognized in him the signs of a new messiah. Muhammad learned much about the Jewish and Christian faiths and the respect he gained was embodied in the Quran's insistence that "there shall be no coercion in the matter of faith." His experiences also gave him a yearning to start a religion for Arabian nomads that could be the equal of those he had seen. When he returned, he cultivated his visionary abilities in periodic retreats to a cave where he meditated alone on the social problems of his people. His reports back to the tribe became the basis of the Quran, which gave the nomadic tribesmen a vision for their own destiny. He christened the new religion *Islam*, or "surrender." Converts set about building a community, the *ummah*, that was inspired by practical compassion. Wealth was equally distributed so all could be comfortable enough to seek spiritual perfection. It was their duty, the Prophet said, to create a just community in which all members, even the most weak and vulnerable, would be treated with utmost respect. The Quran is the only holy book in the world that states the specific entitlements of orphans and widows, and the Prophet's command is respected in most Islamic communities to this day.

Prior to the AIDS epidemic, African censuses showed that 5 percent of children under fifteen were missing one or both of their parents. Although this proportion is shockingly high when compared to less than 0.1 percent orphaned in developing countries, it was manageable. Families and communities were used to high adult death rates, and orphans were so well absorbed that their identity as nonbiological children was virtually erased in normal day-to-day social activity. As AIDS continues to accelerate, orphans increasingly stand out in communities and families overburdened by poverty. No longer can they be easily absorbed into extended families. There are no signs that the orphan crisis will diminish before 2020 or 2030. A World Bank report released in

2003 speculated that social and economic collapse in Africa is imminent unless more help is provided to slow the spread of the virus and prolong the lives of those who are already HIV positive. In this way, at least, children will not be orphaned until they are old enough to fend for themselves and have some education. Treatment can avert the routine social exclusion children suffer as they care for desperately ill parents on their own, attempting to keep them clean and alleviate their suffering while they fend off human predators who are trying to take their land and what is left of their homes and furniture. Unlike previous human disease disasters, it is children that stand to pay the greatest price with HIV/AIDS.

Children of the epidemic are entering a world that is increasingly hazardous for all children, no matter what their infection status. "The global scandal of violence against children is a horror story too often untold," says Human Rights Watch.[16] "With malice and clear intent, violence is used against the members of society least able to protect themselves—children in schools, in orphanages, on the street, in refugee camps and war zones, in detention, and in fields and factories." All over the world, the organization "has found a disturbing but persistent theme—in almost every aspect of their lives, children are subject to unconscionable violence, most often perpetuated by the very individuals charged with their safety and well-being." In country after country, perpetrators go unpunished and governments take no action, leading Human Rights Watch to conclude that "these acts of violence are [a] global phenomenon demanding a concerted international response." HIV/AIDS promises to make this situation worse.

Before he died, orphan train veteran Elliot Bobo mused that "When a child of the streets stands before you in rags, with a tear-stained face, you cannot easily forget him. And yet, you are perplexed what to do. The human soul is difficult to interfere with. You hesitate how far you should go." The social and economic crisis AIDS is causing in many Asian countries suggests that the time of hesitation is past.

EIGHT

AS ASIA GOES, . . .

"NO ONE HAS ENOUGH MONEY FOR AIDS PREVENTION in Bangladesh, either," Safia said, fingering the long scar on her arm. "No one is interested in protecting children. They just want to protect the criminals like the ones who did this to me." The others nodded. "The first time I asked one of my clients to pay me more so he wouldn't have to use a condom, he sliced me with a broken beer bottle. I was a sex worker for twelve years, and only one of my clients ever used condoms because they are too expensive for most people. He was a schoolteacher who had a wife and two small children and enough education to know he didn't want to kill them."

"I wish my husband had been so careful," Kamilika cried. "There he was, a high-paid chemist, much needed by our country. And yet, to be a 'man' he endangered my life and our children. I tried ignored what he was doing—after all, I am a Hindu. Our husbands are our gods, no matter what they do. I found out I was HIV positive when my youngest child was born. When I learned the results of the test, my heart was broken. And my youngest is HIV positive, too, because the Sri Lankan government, which can well afford it, was not providing HIV treatment when she was born." She looked apologetically at Safia. "I am so sorry for interrupting." The group laughed in understanding. "I am still so angry!"

"I am angry, too, and I don't know when I will ever get over that feeling," Safia said. "I was only eighteen years old when my father's younger sister sold me across the border to Assam. I was kept in a shed on the border, waiting for a buyer, and eventually they got about $1,000 for me because I was very pretty then. They once got almost $5,000 for a woman who was smuggled from Karachi in Pakistan because she had light skin and green eyes. Like Phet, I was repeatedly threatened by the bosses, who said they would hand me over to the Indian immigration authorities if I didn't do what they told me. Neither government did anything to protect us, or to stop the trafficking. Finally, when I was twenty-four and pregnant, my boss put me out on the street. He didn't give me any money, so I sold myself even though I was pregnant so I could buy a bus ticket home and pay off the border officials so they would let me across."

She sat back. "When I got home no one would talk to me. My baby was HIV positive and died because he was so small." She started to cry, wringing her handkerchief. "There are so many like me. Even though my own relatives sold me—my aunt used the money she got to buy a house, and my little brother is now in secondary school because of the money I sent back—no one knows me. They cross to the other side of the street when they see me. I am so happy that the people at the clinic sent me to an AIDS organization, where I have met so many other young women and men who are infected. They are my family now. We are helping each other making traditional Bangladeshi crafts." She reached into the bag at her side. "I have brought you each a beaded AIDS ribbon that we made."

Molly smiled. Almost every African she knew who had anything to do with HIV/AIDS had a little beaded ribbon just like the ones Safia was passing around. They had become signs of futility as well as hope. So many groups were making crafts that no one would buy to raise money for their children. Well, she thought. At least it gives them hope. She cleared her throat. "I think these ribbons are so beautiful. I think of each of the small and beautiful lives they represent. The poor mothers and fathers. And the little children with no one to care. When I lost poor Pauline to AIDS, it made me realize that each life that's lived is a precious jewel that can never be replaced. We may be poor farmers, black and brown and women, young people who are sex workers or injecting drug users, but whoever we are there will never be anyone like us again." The group nodded, smiling now. Safia's tears had saddened them all. When I was their age, Molly thought, I never had a care. What has happened to this world, that these children suffer so?

"Maybe we can help each other, despite the differences in our ages and colors and backgrounds," she said. "If no one else will help, we have to stick together and help ourselves!" The group was smiling. "How many of you belong to an AIDS group like Safia's?" she asked. Phet raised his hand with the others and said, "Our friendships help us to remember to have compassion for those who reject us. The monks help us meditate and pray and learn how to eat right so we can stay healthy. For some, it's the only way they can get AIDS drugs, because our group was started by Médecins Sans Frontières—you know, Doctors Without Borders."

"I started the first group for HIV-positive people in my country," Kamilika said proudly. "We have helped so many people like us!" Safia looked up. "It is the only place I know where people care."

San nodded. "In Myanmar our groups are being supported by the Nurses Association. We are helping them distribute food donated by the World Food Programme to families with this disease. Many would starve without the food, or the children would be forced to sell themselves like their parents did to help feed the family. Because of the food, some of the children have gone back to school. I am one of many volunteers that help families care for their infected loved ones. Most people die at home, and the strain it causes is terrible."

The young African man stirred in his chair. "This epidemic will change a lot of things, I think, and as volunteers we can help make the changes needed at the grass-roots level," Zacharia told the group. "In my village in Zimbabwe, the AIDS support group first did an exercise with the older women. An old woman who could neither read nor write stood up at a village meeting to present the findings to the chiefs. She explained that the women had realized as they talked with one another that they were facing starvation. Because they were caring for so many orphans, they no longer had the capacity to tend their fields and their crops were being swallowed by weeds. The elders were shocked, as the women had been. Each one had thought the problem was hers alone, until they started talking. At that meeting, the chiefs decided that the boys and young men had to help these women tend their fields so the women could feed their families. As we talked, we realized that the problem belonged to all of us."

The group was quiet. Molly leaned down and pulled a book out of her purse. "I got this in the airport," she said. "It's by the Dalai Lama. One thing he said really struck me. Let me see if I can remember it. Ah, yes. It goes something like this: 'My work is not done. As long as one human being is suffering, we are all suffering. I cannot be happy if even one other person suffers.'" The words caught in her throat, but she took a deep breath. "If there is any blessing to be had from this terrible epidemic, and from the suffering we have all had, it will be that the world learns what our churches have tried to teach us for a long time. We are all bound together by our sins and our strengths. As unique as each individual is, there is no life that is not affected by every other life on earth."

<hr />

Imprisoned for the first time in 1909, Emmeline sent a petition to the home secretary, Herbert Gladstone, asking that she and the other feminist inmates be treated as political prisoners instead of common criminals. This would give them the right to get the books and newspapers that they wanted and carry out correspondence related to their work as suffragettes. From time to time she had thought about Gladstone's earlier words, and wondered if he had actually been giving the suffragettes advice when he scorned them for not being more vocal, violent, and masculine in demanding their rights.

Herbert was the fourth and youngest son of the distinguished Liberal, William Gladstone. Emmeline knew that William had been a religious man who worked fourteen hours a day but still found time to volunteer three evenings a week to help London women quit prostitution. He was a moving spirit behind the founding of the Anglican Church's Association for the Reclamation of Fallen Women, which collected donations to build safe houses where the women could stay while learning other trades. William had started a similar refuge in Soho Square and the St. Mary Magdalen Home of Refuge in Paddington, and served on the Management Committee of Millbank Penitentiary, where his wife Catherine volunteered to work with prostitutes who had been arrested. Their love match had lasted more than a half-century, until he died in 1898.

Emmeline also knew that the older Gladstone had started his political career as an archconservative member of the Tory Party—in his first speech to parliament he supported slavery, claiming that his father's slaves were healthy and happy—but he had gradually let his heart lead him to the forefront of Britain's liberals. He was a famous opponent of Benjamin Disraeli's every effort to raise income taxes, fought the government's increasing military allocations, locked horns with Britain's most powerful groups to improve government schools for the working class, pushed through reforms that improved the position of Irish peasants, and advocated tirelessly for the expansion of the franchise to working-class men. He'd been outspoken against the Britain's Opium War in China, and for twenty-five years consistently opposed Disraeli's aggressive and expensive expansion of the British Empire on the grounds that it increased the deficit and raised the taxes of the lower classes for whom it provided no benefit.

Emmeline knew that while Herbert had been in Parliament, he had been a critical force in securing worker's compensation, protection for coal miners, and a minimum wage for the "sweated" industries. He had also forwarded the 1908 Children's Act that called for registration of foster parents, made incest a matter for state jurisdiction, and set up juvenile courts. Emmeline appreciated his work on behalf of poor women and children. Having served as a poor Law Guardian, she had frequently headed community drives to collect food for soup kitchens and personally spent many days cooking meals for the indigent. Most of the unemployed refused to go into the workhouses, where conditions were severe and inhumane, but there were never enough other places to house needy men, women, and children.

Gladstone refused the feminists' petition, so Emmeline continued her hunger strike. On Sunday, November 1, she broke the prison rule of silence, walked up to Christabel in the exercise yard, linked arms with her, and spoke. Her daughter had been ill and she had been refused the right to see her. Emmeline was immediately thrown into solitary confinement.

Through the window of her cell, she could hear the faint singing of "La Marseillaise," the French national anthem and revolutionary freedom call for all human kind. It cheered her. The suffragettes had arranged a grand parade, led by a large brass band, and it circled the prison twice. The thousands-strong procession of supporters was a half mile long. A few days later, another demonstration was held and protestors yelled out "Emmeline" and "Christabel" through their megaphones when they found that the roads to the prison were blocked by 1,000 police. The processions eased her pain and loneliness. Confronting society's most ingrained prejudices and the political and economic forces that kept them in place was not only backbreaking work, but sometimes it took all the courage she could muster.

Gladstone finally allowed Emmeline and her daughter to meet once a day for an hour. Pressure against his harsh policies toward the women was building in the House of Commons and causing many public outcries of sympathy. After one month's imprisonment, when Emmeline was allowed to write one letter, she told her followers, "it is a great joy and support to me to know that although I am withdrawn from active work for a time, you are working harder than ever." The suffragettes and their supporters were planning a demonstration to mark Emmeline and Christabel's release from prison, but the government learned of it and let them out early. Several days later, after a victory breakfast, they were paraded through London's streets in a flower-covered wagon drawn by four white horses. The band played the French revolutionary anthem again.

At a meeting that evening, thousands filled the hall. When Christabel rose to speak, she was greeted with frantic cheering and shouting from the galleries and stalls. When it was Emmeline's turn, the cheering became exultant. As she strode toward the podium, someone stepped forward and presented her with a replica of a medal struck to commemorate the storming of La Bastille, the notorious French prison where thousands of poor enemies of the state had languished and died before the Revolution. With tears in her eyes, she thanked the crowd, touched that they had remembered how special the anniversary was to her. It was her birthday, and the birth of liberty for all humankind.

Although she had been called a "pariah of humanity," she knew her struggles would not be in vain. Emerging liberalism, which had ostensibly sought equal participation for all, would not leave women behind. The death of aristocracy had brought "an absolute tyranny of men," but she knew in her heart it would not last forever. By 1917 Emmeline's WSPU had overcome every obstacle placed in their path and won the right to vote. In 1919 the Sex Disqualification Act enabled them to enter professions and become magistrates, lawyers, policewomen, and top civil servants. In an article that year she rejoiced, saying, "What a change from the time when to be healthy and active, to be intelligent and intellectual, to be ambitious and take part in the world's work, was to be unladylike and unwomanly and unsexed." She also observed that women could now finally grow up instead of spending the entirety of their lives as dependent as infants.

The women's movement, which went through a "second wave" in the 1960s, has effected many changes in Western society, including women's suffrage (the right to vote and hold office); property rights; changes in language use; more equitable wages; the right to marry and divorce; and the right of women to control their own bodies (medical decisions, the right to safe abortion, and birth control use). Some beliefs that are now mainstream in the West, like women's rights to buy, own, and inherit land, were radical in Emmeline's day and still are radical in many parts of the world. A third wave of feminism emerged in the 1990s, and the major goal of the feminist movement in the twenty-first century is to improve the situation of women in non-Western countries. For the majority of women in the world, the tyranny of men is an everyday reality that binds us all in the unrelenting upward spiral of HIV/AIDS. "A threat to justice anywhere is a threat to justice everywhere," said U.S. civil rights hero Dr. Martin Luther King, Jr.; where women and children lose, the battle is lost for all of us.

———————◆◆◆———————

The injustice that is HIV/AIDS pervades the AIDS establishment itself. As if it were not enough that women and young people are becoming infected faster than men, their participation in HIV vaccine clinical trials has been low or nonexistent and they are also being sidelined by antiretroviral treatment programs. At an August 2004 meeting of international vaccine experts in Geneva, Dr. Catherine Harris, Chief Scientific Advisor for UNAIDS, told the group that "women and girls are particularly vulnerable to HIV infection for biological, social and economic reasons. In spite of the epidemiological reality, women and adolescents, especially girls, have often had minimal involvement in clinical trials of HIV vaccines as compared to men. This is in spite of the fact that they would be major beneficiaries of a future HIV vaccine."[1] The exclusion is critical, because earlier trials have resulted in rejection of vaccines that were not effective overall but offered some degree of protection to nonwhites and women. Similarly, men have had more access to antiretroviral treatment than do women because they have more access to healthcare overall. Many antiretroviral treatments that are currently available are also not tailored to the regular hormone shifts that women experience and their impact on the fetus during pregnancy is not well understood. Lack of information about long term effects on children whose mothers have accepted antiretroviral treatment to avert mother to child transmission of HIV infection in their newborns has led some women to refuse the therapy. In many countries, ensuring equitable access to treatment for women and girls means changing attitudes and removing discriminatory laws and practices. Proactive measures must also be taken to ensure that injecting drug users, and sex workers, who are predominantly female, are not denied access because by discriminatory screening.

The story of AIDS in Asia today is not a pretty one, and so far the plot suggests that the ending will not be happy, either for the continent or the rest of the world. Commentator Bruce Sterling says that failure to confront AIDS is creating a global problem that "will make Iraq look like Disneyland."[2] Peter Jennings of *The Australian* says that governments are facing "the most turbulent Asia-Pacific outlook since the mid-1960s."[3] The "decline of effective government" in the region works "hand-in-hand with corruption, crumbling infrastructure, AIDS and ethnic violence." More and more countries in Asia are teetering on the brink of violent explosion resulting from their inability to resolve the demands of tradition with the realities of the new world order, and the outcome may be an epidemic the likes of which has never been seen in world history. While some have called it a "silent epidemic," the sounds of weeping are growing louder. "No inspectors are needed to find this weapon of mass destruction," says Dr. Mervyn Silverman, head of the American Foundation for AIDS Research.[4] "HIV can be found in virtually every country in the world and in every major city. To defeat this enemy, we have to be unified in purpose," across genders, age groups, cultures, regions, religions, political powers, and economic might.

Reports of growing distress from the AIDS epidemic are coming in daily from sub-Saharan African countries, which are falling apart in the face of mounting deaths. "The HIV/AIDS pandemic is an economic time bomb that poses major threats," said South Africa's second largest financial group, Sanlam.[5] "AIDS has put Zambia into unchartered territory," declared the U.S. ambassador to the east African republic where HIV infection levels have settled in at 20 percent. "HIV/AIDS is the most important obstacle on the road to Zambia's future, but there is no map to show the way past it."[6] A 2003 UN Development Program's report says that "the impact of HIV/AIDS . . . has been conspicuous . . . including decreasing life expectancy, the slowing of economic growth, increasing extreme poverty, and a multiplicity of other factors that compromise development. The pandemic is forcing families, communities, businesses and governments to invest less in productive activities as people fall sick and die and resources are shifted to care for them. Societies are losing human and social capital, and often the seriousness of the situation is not recognized, let alone remedied."[7]

Although the relationship between AIDS and the resurgence of tuberculosis is well known, recent reports of new sub-Saharan plague and polio epidemics are completely unnerving. Infectious diseases are not the only things that are multiplying as sub-Saharan Africa's soft underbelly becomes more and more exposed by its AIDS epidemics. A 2004 report says that AIDS has amplified cancer cases in Uganda, the east African country that has been so successful in turning its epidemic around. Over the past two years, cancer cases have doubled, the nation's cancer institute recently reported.[8] The loss of human potential due to premature death and active illness reduces productivity and well-being. A sense of these changes can be gained by looking at the drastic loss in productivity from declines in life expectancy anticipated in all heavily infected countries. With no antiretroviral programs, life expectancy in Swaziland, Zambia, and Zimbabwe will drop by 30 years to levels not seen since the nineteenth century. Without treatment, 60 percent of Africa's fifteen-year-olds will not reach their sixtieth birthdays. While many of the most productive, educated, and innovative members of society are being lost before they can make their full contributions, the AIDS epidemic is also claiming ordinary farmers, laborers, and urban and rural workers who contribute on a daily basis to the lives of their families, their communities, and their countries. Southern Africa's famines over the past several years have been attributed in part to deaths from AIDS. Gains in child health and life expectancy realized in the 1970s and 1980s in most eastern and southern African countries have already been eroded. Losses such as these take years to recover from.

"In the end," says International AIDS Vaccine Initiative director Seth Berkley, who cut his teeth as an epidemiologist in Brazil and Uganda in the

1980s, "only a vaccine will matter" because "we are still fooling around on the edges" of prevention.[9] Two things work against making a vaccine a reality: insufficient investment, which Berkley tries to address through the Vaccine Initiative, and scientific ability to apply knowledge of molecular genetics to the problem. At least thirty AIDS vaccines are in various stages of development, but the virus's ability to hide in white blood cells eludes standard vaccine technology. Most experts agree with National Institute of Health physician Anthony Fauci, who believes "it will eventually happen. But there are many problems we need to solve in order to produce [a vaccine]. I would have to say the virus is winning, not us."

World Bank AIDS expert Martha Ainsworth thinks that governments are reluctant to take responsibility for AIDS prevention because it requires honest talk about sex. "Nearly half of the 4.8 billion people in less developed countries live in areas where HIV infection is not yet widespread," she says, and argues rightly that intelligent action by policymakers could "spare them the ravages of the epidemic." Talking about sex is indeed a problem, but claiming that it is the main problem is nothing but a cover-up for more deeply rooted elitism and the stranglehold of the uninformed and undesirable on socially oriented decision making. In Asia, most governments are clearly choosing to align themselves with their countries' conservative religious establishments, corrupt local party members, foreign aid partners and investors, the military, and even the criminal lords of their underworld sex and drug sectors, instead of adopting policies that will alleviate poverty and control the spread of HIV in their young, poor, and marginal citizens.

Even when poor countries are committed to providing effective interventions, they still have to find the money to intervene. Developing countries had steadily increased their funding to $2 billion in 2002, which is about 6 percent of total AIDS expenditures worldwide. Most of the total is spent in developed countries, where the problem is least acute. Spending per HIV-positive person in the United States is 35 times that of Latin America, and 1,000 time that of Africa. As of early 2004, $2 billion had been pledged to developing countries for ART, leaving a shortfall of $3.5 billion, a shortfall that grew as the United States deferred the $15 billion it pledged before the Iraq war. Global spending on HIV/AIDS in 2002 was $2.2 billion, less than one-third of what is actually needed. In 2007 prevention will require $20 billion, and by 2015, $25 billion. We can afford more. Currently, the United States spends less than 0.5 percent of its gross domestic product on all foreign aid, the lowest of any developed country, and most of it goes to military aid and support, programs to fight terrorism and the illicit narcotics trade, and ill-advised abstinence-only education programs. Poor countries must also fight global economic rules that have placed many of them into intractable debt, so that many of them pay out more to rich world creditors in debt service than they receive in foreign aid.

AIDS activists have had to push most transnational corporations to provide HIV/AIDS prevention and care for their employees. Twenty-nine of the world's top 100 economic entities are companies, and their value has grown faster than countries over the past ten years. Exxon, for example, is comparable to Chile or Pakistan in value; Nigeria ranks between DaimlerChrysler and General Electric; and Phillip Morris exceeds Tunisia, Slovakia, and Guatemala. Many companies in Africa, such as British American Tobacco, De-Beers Diamonds, and Anglo American Mines (which estimates that 20 percent of its workforce in forty countries is HIV positive) began providing prevention, diagnosis, and treatment for African workers after studies showed how high their replacement costs would be for deaths from AIDS. Coca-Cola, one of the largest private-sector employers in Africa, was providing full medical coverage for 1,500 direct employees and family members and free advertising space and marketing know-how for HIV prevention, but activists wanted more. After fifteen months of badgering via international e-mail campaigns and live protests, Coke, which made $630 million from cola sales in Africa in 2001, agreed to provide care for another 98,500 workers who are bottlers, canners, and distributors under contract arrangement with the company. By 2004, only 21 percent of the top transnational corporations had workplace AIDS programs of any kind, although the Global Business Coalition on HIV/AIDS is encouraging greater responsibility in the private sector.

Finally, poor countries have had to fight the pharmaceutical industry, backed by the World Trade Organization (WTO) and the U.S. government, for the right to manufacture or purchase low-cost AIDS drugs.[10] In 2000 the United States allied itself with the pharmaceutical industry to threaten economic sanctions against Brazil, South Africa, Zimbabwe, and other countries using cheap imported or home-made generic versions of anti-AIDS drugs to reduce treatment costs for an individual from $10,000 per year to $300. After a media and e-mail campaign led by Médecins Sans Frontières, public indignation was so intense that pharmaceutical giants dropped their lawsuits.

In 2001 the UN Commission on Human Rights declared that access to medicine was an essential human right and asked member states to "refrain from taking measures which would deny or limit equal access" to HIV/AIDS drugs and to actively "facilitate access" of poor countries to drugs, including their manufacture. Drug factories in African and Asian countries produced generic AIDS medicines, anticipating a successful legal challenge to WTO prohibitions. African drug companies have made generic copies of many different drugs for decades, paying royalties to western drug companies with patented formulas. In March 2002 the World Health Organization (WHO) included generic AIDS drugs on its approved list and the European Union and United Nations Children's Fund (UNICEF) agreed to finance generics, but big drug companies still refuse to accept the idea that they should not be the only ones making life-or-death decisions about access to these drugs In March 2004, U.S. government officials called the Botswana government to task for using generic medications, which it has been providing to all of its HIV-infected citizens free of charge for over two years. When Botswana refused to switch to U.S.-branded antiretroviral treatments, the U.S. government moved its regional offices out of the country.

In the meantime, pharmaceutical companies remained the most profitable sector of the U.S. economy for the third decade, ranking at the top of all of *Fortune Magazine*'s measures of profitability. Frank Clemente of Public Citizen's Congress Watch was prompted to remark that "during a year in which there was much talk of sacrifice in the national interest, drug companies increased their astounding profits" by 32 percent in 2001; other industries declined by 53 percent. Clemente attributed this to "advertising some medicines more than Nike shoes" and lobbying campaigns that keep U.S. congressmen safely in drug company pockets, extending "lucrative monopoly patents. Sometimes what's best for shareholders and chief executive officers isn't what's best for all Americans, particularly senior citizens who lack insurance coverage for prescription drugs." In early 2003 Swiss drug maker Hoffman LaRoche announced a new AIDS drug with a record-breaking price of $20,000 per year, more than double the cost of any other drug on the market, which the firm concedes will definitely put it out of the reach of anyone in developing countries.

The same U.S. administration cynicism that brought us the war on Iraq is now bringing us a quiet jihad against Africa, young people, and people of color everywhere. This lesser jihad is finding collaborators in some Asian governments and demonstrating that corruption is not limited to the East. On both fronts of the global struggle to contain AIDS, prevention and care, the Bush policy constitutes nothing less than a catastrophic attempt to turn back the clock on science while handing his supporters a bonanza in cash and control. In an insane policy switch that ignores everything learned about preventing HIV/AIDS since the epidemic began in the 1980s, the administration is forcefully promoting a "Just Say No (to Sex)!" approach on domestic and international fronts that harkens back to the "Just Say No!" days of Reagan's war on drugs and will be just as unsuccessful. On the treatment side, Bush is saying an emphatic "Yes!" to pharmaceutical giants, who will be awarded no less than half of the $15 billion in taxpayer funds in AIDS assistance he promised in his 2003 State of the Union address. What could not be accomplished through the United States shameless support of its pharmaceutical companies' unsuccessful demands that access to life-saving drugs be restricted in developing countries through the World Trade Organization's TRIPS restrictions will be accomplished by placing foreign aid subsidies in their pockets.

Not only will both approaches do little to stem HIV's relentless spread, but they will cost U.S. taxpayers huge amounts of money now and in future health-care costs incurred for the AIDS-related hospitalizations and drugs of young people catching HIV because they just could not say no. They also will cost the lives of millions of people around the world and in the United States, too, largely dark skinned and youthful lives sacrificed to a president interested in little else than his own reelection, pandering to his right wing Christian supporters, and lining the pockets of his already-wealthy cronies. To cover his tracks Bush has ostentatiously declared "his fairly radical belief" in the "human rights" of AIDS orphans in Africa and is taking up a stance against sex trafficking. Such righteousness is sardonic at best in a president who ignores the fact that access to AIDS drugs is a UN-declared human right. Although the president acknowledges that AIDS orphans apparently have human rights that are in the same league as his own, his policies have denied their parents the right to avoid HIV infection by using condoms and the right to treatment once they get it.

Bush got elected on the back of righteous Christians—40 percent of his vote came from white evangelical Christians in the 2000 election. On the second day of his administration, he reinstituted the 1981 Mexico City Rule that prohibits provision of federal support for institutions that provide abortion, discuss it with their clients, or refer them to abortion counseling services. Bush pulled the plug on UN Population Fund monies, which provide condoms, voluntary family planning, nutrition and AIDS prevention education to millions of young women living in poverty. Venerable institutions invaluable in the war on AIDS and in providing safe reproductive health services to women around the world like the International Planned Parenthood Federation and Marie Stopes stood up to Bush and were rewarded with crippling funding cuts that forced them to close vital services in the most vulnerable areas of the world. But at least they stood up. Many of America's Christians are unknowing lambs lying down with the lion in a largely ideological jihad that amounts to a death sentence for young people and people of color everywhere. Human Rights Watch says that abstinence-only education programs threaten the lives (and human rights) of young people because they exclude information on condom use and other ways to prevent HIV transmission. In May 2004, the Bush administration cut funds for the Global Health Council's work, which focused on sex, health, and young people, and also reduced support for the fifteenth international conference on AIDS, the biannual meeting where policymakers and scientists from around the world learn about the latest advances in AIDS control.

Perhaps worst of all, Bush's scientists are willing to support this folly. In a letter to Health and Human Services secretary Tommy Thompson, twelve Democratic House members protested agency actions, concerned that "scientific decisions making is being subverted by ideology." National Cancer Institute findings that abortion did not increase a woman's risk of breast cancer were removed from the National Institute of Health's web site, and the Institute and Centers for Disease Control both removed information about condom and sex education effectiveness from a list of "Programs that Work" on their web sites. A White House-appointed committee of experts sent to see what worked against HIV/AIDS in Uganda quit after the Bush administration attempted to bribe them to say condoms did not work when their findings showed just the opposite. Bush's Food and Drug Administration advisory committee appointee Dr. David Hager is an obstetrician-gynecologist who opposes abortion rights and condemns oral contraceptives as a "convenient way for young people to be sexually active outside of marriage."

Some leaders in the Catholic Church have jumped on the anticondom bandwagon, spreading misinformation, confusion, and death among their parishioners worldwide. Although some highly-placed members of the church hierarchy reaffirmed the safety and importance of condom use, the message that condoms are dangerous had already reached far too many Catholics in developing countries. The damage had already been done. It is true that some religious leaders are standing up to this assault on reason and science, but they are not being rewarded with the same large U.S. programming grants given to right-to-lifers and Christian advocates opposed to any form of birth control but abstinence. The Bush administration spends $135 million annually on abstinence-only education that condemns sexual activity outside of marriage and limits contraceptive information, and is busy channeling a huge chunk of the $15 billion not going in pharmaceutical company pockets to FBOs—faith-based organizations opposed to condom use. This is "bad theology based on bad biology," says lay Catholic leader Jim FitzGerald. The Bush administration is silent about the reality of sexuality and its commercial importance in America today, even among righteous Christians. How can hormone-hyped teens learn to say no when the need for commercial gain overrides morality, and sexually explicit prime-time TV programs are interrupted only by Viagra ads?

————•◦•————

Because many countries in Asia are unable or unwilling to take up the cause of HIV/AIDS, international human rights organizations are doing it for them. Over the past few years Human Rights Watch has done a superb job pushing government into policy changes that they should have made a long time ago on their own. Amnesty International and UNIFEM are also holding up bright lamps in the darkness created by violence against women and the growing injustices they are suffering from unmitigated HIV epidemic. In the face of repeated criticism from the United Nations and from other groups, Bangladesh, China, Kazakhstan, India, and Indonesia are beginning to curb the worst of their abuses, but it has taken constant watch-dogging from the outside to change repressive government approaches.

In *Pathologies of Power* Harvard's Paul Farmer tells us that ill health invariably derives from lack of power, which in turn always originates in the violation of human rights.[11] So, for example, in Haiti, where Farmer has worked unstintingly to bring antiretroviral treatments to the poor, many have died from AIDS, tuberculosis, and other treatable conditions because their poverty makes them invisible and takes away their ability to end repression and demand their rights. Sex expert and Brown University professor of biology Anne Fausto-Sterling says that the power differentials arising from gender bias put many more women into poverty than men and makes the suffering of poverty even worse. These violations of women's human rights invariably lead to ill health—including inordinate exposure to HIV and AIDS—and other indignities, lost opportunities, abuse, and suffering that may be even worse than death.

Human rights violations are increasing across Asia as governments struggle with separatist movements and the threat from Islamic militants and the criminals with whom they are associated. The rights of those who are preyed on—ordinary Muslims—are also violated in the most fundamental ways. Instability serves the interest of militants and the interests of crime, drug trafficking, and the trade in women and children. It serves the interests of HIV/AIDS. The enslavement and trafficking of children is the worst indictment of government inaction, delivering a clear message that governments are perfectly willing to compromise honor and sacrifice self-respect as they bow to the interests of their avaricious elites. No emperor or conqueror ever exacted such a mean-spirited toll, and its consequences may be as dire as the Great Khan's own dead earth strategy.

———————◦•◦•◦———————

The plot of the HIV/AIDS story is a bit more interesting than a typical sci-fi disaster movie because the signs of hope are beginning to emerge. Developed nations are slowly loosening the strings on their change purses. Funding prevention and care for Asian countries, which consume more in western products than all the development aid they receive in any given year, is a no-brainer. Asian countries, on their part, can do a few things quickly that will radically change the endings of their AIDS stories. The first is to develop zero tolerance for the abysmal safety levels of their national blood supplies and ensure that their hospitals and health facilities have the syringes, lab equipment, and test kits to stop spreading the virus. China is taking steps to do just that; when India wakes up, it just might follow suit. India's pharmaceutical company, Cipla, took on the international legal drug cartel single-handedly and set off a chain of events that has modified the way AIDS drugs are delivered, making compliance possible and delivery cheap. It has even done what no U.S. politician could do: it embarrassed U.S. drug companies badly by making cheaper drugs available to the HIV-infected and elderly. Thailand has demonstrated that preventing mother-to-child transmission is only a small pill away for pregnant women, and has pioneered national systems of antiretroviral treatments, home care, and first-rate epidemic monitoring. Malaysia and Singapore demonstrated long ago how to stop government involvement in the drug industry and radically reduced the number of drug addicts in their populations. Middle-of-the-road Muslims in Indonesia are leading the way toward a reason-based society on the principles of the greater jihad. And if someone buys Gloria Arroyo a new and very fashionable set of glasses, the plot in the Philippines will begin to look a lot less like *The Titanic*.

In the meantime, real epidemic management goes on in the villages, as it always has, giving the story of the epidemic a surprising bunch of heroes: ordinary men and women of all ages, like the ones you have met in this book, who have struggled with HIV/AIDS, preserved their dignity and enlarged their compassion to give and give again. Most of the key responses to this epidemic were created locally by a few committed people upset at the suffering they were seeing among their family and friends. They were created by a few leaders who wanted to help people in their community crushed by the manifestations of this unforgiving disease. They were created by a few professionals who were distressed at the rejection of AIDS sufferers by their relatives and friends and the exploitation of the surviving widows and children, and pitched in to provide care and services. And they were created by a few enlightened government servants with the vision to anticipate what an AIDS epidemic can do to everyone in a country, poor and elite alike. Through their work, heaven may decide it is not weary of China yet.

NOTES

CHAPTER ONE

1. Burma's name is now officially Myanmar. Both names are used in this book depending on whether what is being discussed took place before or after the name change. Burmese is still commonly used as an adjective.
2. J. Purvis, *Emmeline Pankhurst: A Biography* (New York: Routledge, 2002), p. 104. Purvis' reexamination of Pankhurst's life resuscitates a legend that had been tarnished for half a century and is the principle source for the material on Pankhurst in this book. Other sources include I. Noble, *Emmeline and Her Daughters: The Pankhurst Suffragettes* (New York: Julian Messner, 1971); and P. Romero, *E. Sylvia Pankhurst: Portrait of a Radical* (New Haven, CT: Yale University Press, 1987).
3. "AIDS Rate Surges in People 50+," *Bulletin of the American Association of Retired People* (May 2004): 2.
4. "HIV/AIDS Cases Increasing at Southern Universities," *WRUF News*, March 11, 2004, www.am850.com.
5. R. Jablon, "Porn Industry at Standstill after Stars Test HIV Positive," *The Scotsman*, April 17, 2004.
6. D. King, "Number of New HIV Cases up 20%," February 13, 2004, www.news.scotsman.com.
7. UNAIDS, "AIDS Threat Growing Throughout Europe," February 23, 2004, www.unaids.org.
8. K. Bradford, "Canada: STD Rates Soaring," *Edmonton Sun*, April 13, 2004.
9. This number is slightly lower that the total quoted in *Black Death: AIDS in Africa* (New York: Palgrave Macmillan, 2003) because at the end of 2003, UNAIDS made the controversial move of lowering its estimates of infections.
10. N. Eberstadt, "The Future of AIDS," *Foreign Affairs* 81, no. 6 (November/December, 2002): 22–45.
11. UNAIDS, 2002, "AIDS Epidemic Update," (Geneva, December 2002), p. 29; predictions of a vaccine by 2007, such as that made by J. McHugh in "The Cure: Nanobombs, Microbots, Vaccine Pills. A Report from the Medical Frontier" (*WIRED*, May 2004, pp. 172–173) are purely fanciful.
12. J. Lederberg, "Pandemic as a Natural Evolutionary Phenomenon," in *In Time of Plague: The History and Consequences of Lethal Epidemic Disease*, ed. M. Arien, (New York: New York University Press, 1991), pp. 35–36.
13. R. Parker, "Administering the Epidemic: HIV/AIDS Policy, Models of Development, and International Health," in *Global Health Policy, Local Realities: The Fallacy of the Level Playing Field*, eds. L. Whiteford and L. Manderson (Boulder, CO: Lynne Reinner Publishers, 2001), p. 40.

14. D. Morens, "Certain Diseases, Uncertain Explanations," *Science* 294 (2001): 1658–1659.

15. T. McMichael, *Human Frontiers, Environments, and Disease: Past Patterns, Uncertain Futures* (Cambridge: Cambridge University Press, 2002), p. 28.

16. T. McMichael, 2002, p. 27.

17. "Daily HIV/AIDS Report," March 16, 2004, www.kaisernetwokk.org.

18. K. Stanecki, *The AIDS Pandemic in the 21ˢᵗ Century* (Washington, DC: U.S. Agency for International Development and the U.S. Department of Commerce), p. 21.

19. Palgrave Macmillan, 2003.

CHAPTER TWO

1. Literally, *aunt;* in this case a familiar word for the brothel's madam or manager.

2. *Rog* means a serious illness.

3. Many of these stories were gathered during fieldwork I did in Asia from 2001 to 2003. Other sources for Nepal include D. Beine's excellent study, *Ensnared by AIDS; Cultural contexts of HIV/AIDS in Nepal* (Kathmandu, Nepal: Mandala Book Point, 2003), and S. Samuha, *Mother Sister Daughter: Nepal's Press on Women* (Kathmandu, Nepal, 2002).

4. The World Health Organization's estimate of global deaths from the first wave of the plague is 60 million (see WHO, "Report on Global Surveillance of Epidemic-prone Infectious Diseases," 2000, www.who.int/emc). This is a conservative estimate which I revised based on Laurie Garrett's estimate that the plague killed one-quarter to one-third of all human beings alive in the fourteenth and fifteenth centuries (see L. Garrett, "Amplification," in *Epidemic! The World of Infectious Diseases*, ed. R. DeSalle (New York: New Press, 1999), p. 193). Historical evidence suggests she is correct. Plague recurred up until the twentieth century in Asia and Europe during frequent periods of collapse or chaos. The major plague center in the world now is sub-Saharan Africa, where it is likely to worsen as the devastation of HIV/AIDS mounts.

5. M. White, "Source List and Detailed Death tolls for the Twentieth Century Hemoclysm," 2002, at www.users.erols.com/mwhite28/warstat1.htm. White is also the source for the remainder of the death tolls cited in this paragraph. He compares multiple sources and estimates and provides solid justification for each of his estimates, plus a wealth of other information on societies and government. Related areas of his web site compile estimates of death tolls for wars of previous centuries.

6. J. Mann and D. Tarantola, eds., *AIDS in the World II: Global Dimensions, Social Roots, and Responses* (New York: Oxford University Press), p. 60.

7. Sources for AIDS include UNAIDS, the 2002 *Report on the Global HIV/AIDS Epidemic*, and the 2001 and 2003 editions of "AIDS Epidemic Update" (December 2001), which can be accessed at www.unaids.org, Also see the World Health Organization, *The World Health Report 2001* (Geneva: 2002); M. Merson, J. Dayton, and K. O'Reilly, "Effectiveness of HIV Prevention Interventions in Developing Countries," *AIDS* 14, Supplement 2 (2002): 68–84; A. Vakhovskiy, "Winning the War on AIDS, Brazil Style," *Dartmouth Free Press*, August 10, 2001; "Hope for the Best. Prepare for the Worst," *The Economist*, July 13, 2002, pp. 66–67; UN Fund for Population Activities, "Advances in New Technologies

and Issues, Male Circumcision," *Strategic Guidance on HIV Prevention* (New York: 2003), www.unfpa.org/hiv/strategic/; AIDSMark and USAID, "Male Circumcision: Current Epidemiological and Field Evidence, Conference Report" (Washington, DC: Population Services International, 2002); E. Preble and E. Piwoz, "Prevention of Mother to Children Transmission of HIV in Asia: Practice Guidance for Programs" (Washington, DC: USAID and AED/Linkages, 2002), www.linkages@aed.org; M. Ainsworth and W. Teokul, "Breaking the Silence: Setting Realistic Priorities for AIDS Control in Less-Developed Countries," *The Lancet* 356 (2002): 55–60; P. Alagiri et al., "Global Spending on HIV/AIDS in Resource-Poor Settings," part 3, *Spending on the HIV/AIDS Epidemic* in Kaiser Family Foundation and Ford Foundation (2002), www.kff.org; S. Ramsay, "Global Fund Makes Historic First Round of Payments," *The Lancet* 359 (2002): 6; J. Laurence, "It Isn't Over," *AIDS Patient Care and STDs*, 12, no. 1 (1998): 3–4; J. McGeary, "Death Stalks a Continent: In the Dry Timber of African Societies, AIDS Was a Spark," *Time Magazine* 157, no. 6 (2001): 36; K. Stanecki, *The AIDS Pandemic in the 21st Century* (March 2004), (www.usaid.gov/pop_health/aids/publications); UNAIDS, UNICEF, USAID, *Children on the Brink 2002: A Joint Report on Orphan Estimates and Program Strategies* (Washington, DC: TvT Associates/The Synergy Project, 2002), www.synergyaids.org; M. Greene, "What Will Become of Africa's AIDS Orphans?" *New York Times Magazine*, December 22, 2002, pp. 49–55; World Bank, *Education and HIV/AIDS: A Window of Hope* (Washington, DC: World Bank, 2002), www.worldbank.org/hiv_aids/publications; UNFPA, "HIV/AIDS and Poverty," *State of the World's Population* (New York: 2002), www.unfpa.org; Food and Agriculture Organization, "HIV/AIDS Devastating Rural Labour Force in Many African Countries," Rome, press release, January 30, 2001 (www. fao.org archives); International Labour Organization, "ILO Says HIV/AIDS Impact on African Development 'Underestimated,'" Rome, press release, July 11, 2002, (www.ilo.org); American Public Health Association, "HIV/AIDS Worsens Hunger Crisis in Southern African Countries," *The Nation's Health* (November 2002): 12; R. Swarns, "Meager Harvests in Africa Leave Millions at the Edge of Starvation," *New York Times*, June 23, 2002, p. 1; S. Booker, "IMF and the World Bank Blamed for Worst Health Crisis in History," *Foreign Policy in Focus*, May 16, 2002 (www.fpif.org); "SA Cemetery Crisis," *African Business* (April, 2002): 6; American Public Health Association, "AIDS, STDs Continue to Hit Hard in Southern United States," *The Nation's Health* (June/July 2003): 9.

8. L. Garrett, *The Coming Plague* (New York: Farrar, Straus and Giroux, 1994); N. Boyce, "New Plagues of Monkey Viruses?" *U.S. New and World Report*, April 8, 2002; A. Fettner, *Viruses: Agents of Change* (New York: McGraw-Hill, 1990); K. Bellenir and P. Dresser, eds., *AIDS Sourcebook*, vol. 4, 1995; D. Ward, *The AmFAR AIDS Handbook: The Complete Guide to Understanding HIV and AIDS* (New York: W.W. Norton and Company, 1999); M. Klesius, "Search for a Cure," *National Geographic* (February 2002); G. Garnett and E. Holmes, "The ecology of emergent infectious disease," *BioScience* 46, no. 2 (1996); C. Zimmer, *Evolution: The Triumph of an Idea* (New York: HarperCollins, 2001).

9. Condom material comes from "Birth Control," *Encyclopedia Britannica*, vol. 15, (2002): 113–114; "Condoms: History, Effectiveness, and Testing, " AVERT.org, 2002; J. Fowles, "Notes on the History of the Condom," Planned Parenthood Federation of America, 2002; D. Nelkin and S. Gilman, "Placing the Blame for

Devastating Disease," in *In Time of Plague: The History and Consequences of Lethal Epidemic Disease*, ed. M. Arien (New York: New York University Press, 1991): 39–56.

10. See, for example, Edward C. Green's take on condoms in *Rethinking AIDS Prevention: Learning from Successes in Developing Countries* (Westport, CT: Praeger, 2003), pp. 93–122.

11. For more information on sexually transmitted diseases, see in my earlier book, *Black Death: AIDS in Africa* (New York: Palgrave Macmillan, 2003). See chapter 6 for sexually transmitted diseases and chapter 7 for the impact of diseases on evolution.

12. References on STDs include the World Health Organization, *The World Health Report* (Geneva, 2001), pp. 144–145; C. Turkington and B. Ashby, *Encyclopedia of Infectious Diseases* (New York: Facts On File, 1998); P. Ewald, *Plague Time: The New Germ Theory of Disease* (New York: Anchor Books, 2002); P. Ewald and G. Cochran, "Catching On What's Catching: Some Infections Are Slow to be Recognized," *Natural History* 108, no. 1 (1999); R. DeSalle, ed., *Epidemic! The World of Infectious Disease* (New York: New Press, 2001); American Health Consultants, "Check STD Screening: Room for Improvement?" *Contraceptive Technology Update* (2003); J. St. Lawrence et al., "STD Screening, Testing, Case Reporting, and Clinical and Partner Notification Practices: A national Survey of U.S. Physicians," *American Journal of Public Health* 92, no.1 (2002); M. Hogben et al., "Sexually Transmitted Disease Screening by United States Obstetricians and Gynecologists," *Obstetrics and Gynecology;* Centers for Disease Control, *Sexually Transmitted Disease Surveillance Report, 2001* (Atlanta:); A. Crosby, Jr., *The Columbian Exchange: Biological and Cultural Consequences of 1492* (Westport, CT: Greenwood Press, 1972); B. Hoff and C. Smith III, eds., *Mapping Epidemics: A Historical Atlas of Disease* (New York: Franklin Watts, 2000); E. Kolbert, "The Lost Mariner: The Self-Confidence that Kept Columbus Going Was His Undoing," *The New Yorker,* October 14–21, 2002; W. McNeill, "Unlike AIDS, Says a Historian, Ancient Plagues Swept the World Scythelike and Suddenly," *People Weekly* vol. 28 (1987); A. Speilman, "Emergence of New Diseases," in R. DeSalle, ed. (2000): pp. 39–56; S. Andreski, *Syphilis, Puritanism and Witch Hunts: Historical Explanations in Light of Medicine and Psychoanalysis with a Forecast about Aids (sic)*, (New York: St. Martin's Press, 1989); S. Watts, *Epidemics and History: Disease, Power and Imperialism* (New Haven, CT: Yale University Press, 1997); HERE: A. Brandt, *No Magic Bullet: A Social History of Venereal Disease in the United States since 1880* (New York: Oxford University Press, 1985); C. Quetel, *History of Syphilis* (Baltimore, MD: The Johns Hopkins University Press, 1990); B. Wandrooij, "'The Thorns of Love': Sexuality, Syphilis and Social Control in Modern Italy," in *Sex, Sin and Suffering: Venereal disease and European society since 1870*, R. Davidson and L. Hall, eds. (New York: Routledge, 2001); "Roots of Black Syphilis Epidemic in World War I," *New York Amsterdam News* 88, no. 18 (1997): 13; J. Knowles, "Notes on the History of the Condom," Planned Parenthood Federation of America, 2003; J. Cutler and R. Arnold, "Venereal Disease Control by Health Departments in the Past: Lessons for the Present," *American Journal of Public Health* 78, no. 4 (1988): 372–374; D. McBride, *From TB to AIDS: Epidemics among Urban Blacks Since 1900* (Albany, NY: State University of New York Press, 1991); H. Dibble and D. Williams, "An Interview with Nurse Rivers," and B. Roy, "The Tuskegee Syphilis Experiment: Biotechnology and the

Administrative State," in *Tuskegee's Truths: Rethinking the Tuskegee Syphilis Study*, ed. S. Reverby (Chapel Hill, NC: University of North Carolina Press, 1991); P. Levine, "Public Health, Venereal Disease and Colonial Medicine in the Later Nineteenth Century," in *Sex, Sin and Suffering: Venereal Disease and European Society since 1870*, eds. R. Davidson and L. Hall (New York: Routledge, 2001); K. MacPherson, "Health and Empire: Britain's National Campaign to Combat Venereal Diseases in Shanghai, Hong Kong and Singapore," in *Sex, Sin and Suffering*, eds. Davidson and Hall; M. Vaughn, "Syphilis in Colonial East and Central Africa: The Social Construction of an Epidemic," in *Epidemics and Ideas: Essays on the Historical Perception of Pestilence*, eds. T. Ranger and P. Slack (Cambridge: Cambridge University Press, 1992); A. Fausto-Sterling, "Why Do We Know So Little About Human Sex?" *Discover* (June 1992); H. Wardlow, "Giving Birth to Gonolia: 'Culture' and Sexually Transmitted Disease among the Huli of Papua New Guinea," *Medical Anthropological Quarterly* 16, no. 2 (2002).

13. AIDSMark, *Male Circumcision: Current Epidemiological and Field Evidence* (Washington, DC: USAID Office of HIV/AIDS, 2002).

14. J. Badger, "Worldwide Male Circumcision Rates," 2003, www.circlist.com/rites/rates/html.

15. N. Eberstadt, "The Future of AIDS," *Foreign Affairs* 81, no. 6 (2002).

16. D. Gordon et al., "The Next Wave of HIV/AIDS: Nigeria, Ethiopia, Russia, India and China" (Washington, DC: National Intelligence Council, September 2002), ICA 2002–04D.

17. M. Wilson, *A World Guide to Infections: Diseases, Distribution, Diagnosis* (New York: Oxford University Press, 1991), pp. 6–8.

18. UNAIDS includes the United Nations Children's Fund (UNICEF); the United Nations Development Program (UNDP); United Nations Fund for Population Activities (UNFPA); United Nations Educational, Scientific, and Cultural Organization (UNESCO); the United Nations Office on Drugs and Crime (UNODC); the World Bank, the World Health Organization (WHO); the International Labor Organization (ILO), and the World Food Program (WFP).

19. The same is true in many countries outside of the region. When HIV first hit the United States, its victims were members of what was sardonically called the "4-H club": homosexuals, heroin users, Haitians, and hemophiliacs. Largely because of its aggressive "migration" into minority populations through bisexuals and injecting drug users, it was the top killer of men and women ages eighteen to thirty-four and now infects almost as many women as men. Aggressive treatment for AIDS has cut deaths from HIV in the United States by 70 percent since 1994, but it is still the sixth leading cause of death between ages twenty-five and forty-four, hitting blacks and Hispanics in this age group disproportionately. New infections can increase rapidly and unexpectedly. Over the past few years, AIDS has also migrated into rural populations in the Southern United States, where seven of the states with the top ten AIDS case rates are located. For more information on inter-country variability, see *Black Death: AIDS in Africa* (New York: Palgrave Macmillan, 2003).

20. J. Farquhar, *Appetites: Food and Sex in Post-Socialist China* (Durham, NC: Duke University Press, 2002); UNAIDS, *Report on the Global HIV/AIDS Epidemic 2002*, p. 29.

21. In the year since *Black Death* was published, this has increased from 4 percent reported there.

22. For behavior, see "Study Indicates Americans place themselves at Risk," *MMR*, March 24, 2002; S. Dube, *Sex, Lies and AIDS* (New Delhi: HarperCollins India, 2000); M. Seshu and J. Csete, "India's Voiceless Women Are Easy Prey for AIDS," *Los Angeles Times*, December 1, 2002; S. Maman et al., "HIV-Positive Women Report More Lifetime Partner Violence," *American Journal of Public Health* 92 no. 9 (2002); Centers for Disease Control, "CDC Reports the Health-Related Costs of Intimate Partner Violence Against Women Exceeds $5.8 billion Each Year in the United States," April 28, 2003, www.cdc.gov; C. Blackden and C. Bhanu, *Gender, Growth, and Poverty Reduction: Special Program of Assistance for Africa*, 1998 Status Report on Poverty, World Bank Poverty Technical Working Group Paper No. 428, 1999; L. Van Gelder, "The Beauty of Health: AIDS," *Ms. Magazine* (May 1983); E. Brown, "Crystal Ball," *New York*, April 29, 2002; J. Levi, "Ensuring Time Access to Care for People with HIV Infection: A Public Health Imperative," *American Journal of Public Health* 92, no. 3 (2002); G. Herek et al., "HIV-Related Stigma and Knowledge in the United States: Prevalence and Trends, 1991–1999," *American Journal of Public Health* 92, no.3 (2002); M. Burford, "Girls and Sex: You Won't Believe What's Going On," *O Magazine* (November 2002); K. Mojidi, "Repositioning Family Planning in Africa: A Call to Action," *USAID in Africa* (Fall 2002); D. Carr et al., *Youth in Sub-Saharan Africa: A Chartbook on Sexual Experience and Reproductive Health* (Washington, DC: Macro International, 2001); M. Lytle, "Better Prostitution Through Technology," *WIRED* (December 2002); M. Gladwell, *The Tipping Point: How Little Things Can Make a Big Difference* (Boston: Little, Brown, 2002); "Substance Abuse, Alcohol Linked to Unprotected Sex," *The Nation's Health* (April 2002): 15; C. Wright, "Programs Don't Affect Teens' Sexual Activity," *The Nation's Health* (December 2002/January 2003): 21; UNAIDS, *A Measure of Success in Uganda: The Value of Monitoring Both HIV Prevalence and Sexual Behavior* (Geneva: UNAIDS, May 1998); UNICEF, UNAIDS, and WHO, *Young People and HIV/AIDS: Opportunity in Crisis* (2002); U.S. Census Bureau, *World Population Profile 1994 and 1996*.
23. A. Mozes, "Tainted Blood Supply Spread HIV/AIDS in Poor Nations," Reuters Health, 2002, www.rense.com; J. Chamberland et al., "HIV Screening of the Blood Supply in Developed and Developing Countries," *AIDS Review* 3 (2001): 24–35.
24. L. Lim, ed., *The Sex Sector: The Economic and Social Bases of Prostitution in Southeast Asia* (Geneva: International Labour Office, 1998).
25. L. Murthy, "Illegal Sex Business Adds to National Incomes" (New Delhi: Indian Press Service, 1999).
26. H. Miletski, *Understanding Bestiality and Zoophila* (Bethesda, MD: East-West Publishing Company, 2002), p. 61; D. Beers, "You Sexy Animal, You," Alternet.org., 2001; A. Fausto-Sterling, "Why Do We Know So Little About Human Sex?"
27. R. Shilts, *And the Band Played On: Politics, People and the AIDS Epidemic* (New York: St. Martin's Press), p. 83.
28. References on migration include A. Kroeber, "The Hot Zone," *WIRED* (November 2002); J. Wojcicki, "'She Drank His Money': Survival Sex and the Problem of Violence in Taverns in Gauteng Province, South Africa," *Medical Anthropological Quarterly* 16, no. 3 (2002); B. Ehrenreich and A. Hochschild, eds., *Global Woman: Nannies, Maids and Sex Workers in the New Economy* (New

York: Metropolitan Books, 2002); S. Chantavanich et al., *Mobility and HIV/AIDS in the Greater Mekong Subregion* (Bangkok: Asian Development Bank and United Nations Development Program, 2000); K. Jochelson, *The Colour of Disease: Syphilis and Racism in South Africa, 1880–1950* (New York: Palgrave Macmillan, 2001); T. Sowell, *Migrations and Cultures: A World View* (New York: Basic Books, 1996); S. Rajagopalan and R. Nagarajan, "Nurses, Teachers Chasing the American Dream," *Sunday Hindustan Times* (New Delhi) February 16, 2003; UN Population Division, *International Migration Report 2002* (New York: UN Publications, 2002); World Tourism Organization, *Tourism Highlights 2002* (Madrid: 2002).

29. Healthlink Worldwide, *Combat AIDS: HIV and the World's Armed Forces* (London, 2002).

30. H. Epstein, "The Hidden Cause of AIDS," *New York Review*, May 9, 2002, pp. 43–49; see also pp. 1–12.

31. Poverty references include World Bank, *Partnerships in Development: Progress in the Fight Against Poverty* (Washington, DC: World Bank, 2004); D. Narrayan et al., *Voices of the Poor: Crying Out for Change* (Washington, DC: World Bank, 2000); D. Narayan and G. Pennushi, *Poverty Trends and Voices of the Poor* (Washington, DC: World Bank Poverty Reduction and Economic Management Group, 1999); R. Parker, "The Global HIV/AIDS Pandemic, Structural Inequalities, and the Politics of International Health, *American Journal of Public Health* 92, no. 3 (2002); D. Bloom et al. "AIDS & Economics," Working Group 1 of the WHO Commission on Macroecnoomics and Health; UNDP, 1998, *Human Development Report* (New York: UN Development Program, 1998).

32. H. Epstein, 2002, p. 48.

33. Commission on Macroeconomics and Health, "Health, Economic Growth, and Poverty Reduction," 2002, www.who.int.org.

34. B. Rau and J. Collins, *The Impact of HIV/AIDS: A Population and Development Perspective*, UN Population Fund. Population and Development Strategies, No. 9, 2003.

CHAPTER THREE

1. Molly, Pauline, and Robina's story is told in detail in S. Hunter, *Black Death: AIDS in Africa* (New York: Palgrave Macmillan, 2003), so I have omitted her full narrative here.

2. C. Mason, *A Short History of Asia: Stone Age to 2000 AD* (New York: Palgrave Macmillan, 2000), p. 6.

3. Australia and New Zealand are not included in this book because they have substantially smaller AIDS epidemics and greater means of control than most of the countries considered here.

4. A. Waley, *The Secret History of the Mongols and Other Pieces* (New York: Barnes & Noble, 1963), p. 224.

5. T. Abercrombie, "Ibn Battuta, Prince of Travelers," *National Geographic* (December 1991): 30.

6. Sources on the Mongol invasion and Mongol life include Time-Life Books, *The Mongol Conquests: Time Frame AD 1200–1300* (New York: Time-Life Books, 1989); D. Nicolle, *The Mongol Warlords* (Dorset, U.K.: Firebird Books, 1990); T. Severin, *In Search of Genghis Khan* (New York: Atheneum/Macmillan, 1991), and

Tracking Marco Polo (New York: Peter Bedrick Books, 1986); C. Dawson, *The Mongol Mission: Narratives and Letters of the Franciscan Missionaries in Mongolia and China in the Thirteenth and Fourteenth Centuries* (London: Sheed and Ward, 1955).

7. K. Armstrong, *Islam: A Short History* (New York: Random House, 2000), p. 27.
8. B. Hoberman, "The Battle of Talas," *Saudi Aramco World* 33, no. 5 (September/October 1982).
9. T. Abercrombie, "Ibn Battuta, Prince of Travelers," *National Geographic* (December 1991): 21–22.
10. J. Man, *Atlas of the Year 1000* (Cambridge, MA: Harvard University Press, 1999), p. 66.
11. P. Curtin, *Cross-Cultural Trade in World History* (Cambridge: Cambridge University Press, 1984), pp. 104–105.
12. The Khan set up a postal system for his empire, the *orto*, with a chain of relay stations extending 5,000 miles from the Yellow Sea to the Black, overnight lodging, supply cart, draft animals, and a reserve of three million horses in Mongolia alone. The service lasted seven centuries in Mongolia, where the last relay stations were decommissioned in 1949. By comparison, the American Pony Express lasted only eighteen months and completed only 616 runs.
13. T. Severin, *The Oriental Adventure: Explorers of the East* (Boston: Little, Brown, 1978), p. 24.
14. W. McNeill, *Plagues and Peoples* (New York: Anchor Books, 1998). Plague first spread to Middle Eastern and European populations from A.D. 165 to 180. In the third century, it ravaged Carthage, Egypt, and Libya and defeated Justinian's efforts to establish imperial unity in the Mediterranean. Outbreaks from A.D. 542 until 750 prefaced the advance of Islam out of Arabia in 643. Much of Mongolia and the Asian steppe is still a reservoir for plague, the source of the worst outbreak in modern times which spread along the caravan routes of northern China in 1911 and killed upward of sixty thousand people. It was during the so-called Manchurian Plague in 1911 that marmots (a rabbit-sized relative of woodchucks, gophers, prairie dogs, and hyraxes) were identified as carriers of the disease, along with steppe dogs, mice, and rats, whose fleas and ticks transmit the disease to humans. Mongolians knew this since the time of Genghis Khan, and still call the plague "marmot sickness." William of Rubruck reported in 1255 that when a Mongol was very sick, a white flag on his tent warned others to stay away, a quarantine precaution still practiced by modern herders. When marmots were drowsy and not alert to the hunter's approach, the Mongols knew it was time to clear out and head for new pastures. Although most of the world's plague outbreaks now occur in Africa, there was an outbreak in Kazakhstan in 1990.
15. For a fuller discussion of Muslim philosophy toward illness and Islam's adaptation to the Black Death, see my earlier book, *Black Death: AIDS in Africa* (New York: Palgrave Macmillan, 2003).
16. Timur had been raised north of Samarkand in a clan of nomadic Turkic Mongols who were members of the Chagatai military elite. After becoming lord of the Kish in 1360, he was wounded in an attack on a fortified town and the arrow in his hip left his right leg rigid and shorter than the left. Although he was uneducated and illiterate, he spoke three languages, was an excellent chess player, loved listening to history, and had a passion for sumptuously decorated tents.

17. O. Wild, "The Silk Road," 1992, www.ess.uci.edu/~oliver/silk.html.
18. H. Mayell, "Genghis Khan a Prolific Lover, DNA Data Implies," *National Geographic News*, February 14, 2003.
19. C. Thubron, *The Silk Road: Beyond the Celestial Kingdom* (New York: Simon and Schuster, 1989), p. 8.
20. Information Office, State Council of the People's Republic of China, "National Minorities Policy and Its Practice in China," September 1999.
21. D. Gladney, *Dislocating China: Muslims, Minorities and Other Subaltern Subjects* (Chicago: University of Chicago Press, 2004).
22. M. Edwards, "Han Dynasty," *National Geographic Magazine* (February 2004): 2–29. Other useful references on Chinese history include C. Mason, *A Short History of Asia* (New York: Palgrave Macmillan, 2000); "History of China," www.chaos.umd.edu/history/.
23. A. Andrea and J. Overfield, eds., *The Human Record: Sources in Global History*, 3rd ed. (Boston: Houghton Mifflin Company, 1998), pp. 26–28.
24. N. Kristof, "Why We Speak English," in *Thunder from the East: Portrait of a Rising Asia* (New York: Alfred A. Knopf, 2000); G. Menzies, *1421: The Year China Discovered America* (New York: William Morrow, 2002).
25. A. Kroeber, "The Hot Zone," *WIRED* (October 2002): 205.
26. "Rebellions," www.tse.dyndns.org/~sktse/rebels.htm. Peasant rebellions were also common in Europe where, according to Engels, "the stick and the whip ruled the agricultural districts" ever since the Thirty Years War. From the late 1700s, relatively continuous violence also marred Europe's industrial age.
27. J. Chan, "Rural Revolts in China Reveal Widespread Disaffection over Tax Burdens," *World Socialist Web Site*, May 25, 2001, www.wsws.org.
28. UNAIDS, *HIV/AIDS: China's Titanic Peril* (Geneva: June, 2002).
29. Human Rights Watch, "Locked Doors: The Human Rights of People Living with HIV/AIDS in China," *Human Rights Watch* 15, no. 7 (Washington, DC: Asia Division, September 2003), p. 3.
30. T. McGirk and S. Jakes, "Stalking a Killer," *Time Asia*, September 30, 2002.
31. A. Kroeber, "The Hot Zone."
32. Human Rights Watch, 2003.
33. A. Park, "China's Secret Plague," *Time Asia*, December 15, 2003.
34. U.S. Embassy, "Keeping China's Blood Supply Free of HIV," April 1997; see also Centers for Disease Control, *Report of an HIV/AIDS Assessment in China*, 2001, www.usembassy-china.org.

CHAPTER FOUR

1. Quoted in Ooi Keat Gin's "The White Rajah's Rule," *The Star Online*, November 19, 2001, http://thestar.com.my/lifestyle/story. Brooke's life is the subject of a 2003 biography by Nigel Barley, *The White Rajah* (Boston: Little, Brown); for more information on Wallace and Brooke see the introduction to C. Smith, 2004, *Alfred Russel Wallace: Writings on Evolution, 1843–1912* (Thoemmes Continuum, January 2004) and P. Spencer, "I wanna be like you," *CNNTraveller*, Issue 1, 2004, www.cnntraveller.com.
2. These figures are from N. Kristof and S. WuDunn, *Thunder from the East: Portrait of a Rising Asia* (New York: Alfred A. Knopf, 2000), chapter 2, "Why We Speak English."

3. WHO/New Delhi, "Strategy for Safe Blood Transfusion," www.w3.whosea.org.
4. M. Specter, "India's Plague," *New Yorker*, December 17, 2001, p. 77.
5. All recent figures on the epidemic and HIV/AIDS knowledge come from the Population Foundation of India and the Population Reference Bureau chartbook, *HIV/AIDS in India* (New Delhi, 2003) available from the Population Reference Bureau web site.
6. "India's AIDS Epidemic," PBS online newsletter, August 6, 2003; P. Raghunath, "Andhra District Worst Hit by HIV/AIDS," *Gulf News* online edition, November 30, 2003.
7. A. Mozes, "Tainted Blood Supply Spread HIV/AIDS in Poor Nations," Reuters Health, 2002, www.rense.com.
8. R. Devraj, "India: Get Your Upper Class Blood Here," *Asia Times*, June 26, 2002.
9. S. Dube, *Sex, Lies and AIDS* (New Delhi: HarperCollins India, 2000).
10. D. Mukerjee, "Should There Be Job Reservations in Pvt Sector?," *Business Standard*, June 16, 2004.
11. T. O'Neill, "Untouchables," *National Geographic* (June 2003), www.nationalgeographic.com.
12. 'EVP', "A Financial Passage to India," *Khaleej Times* online, May 17, 2004, www.khaleejtimes.com.
13. J. Keay, *India: A History* (New York: HarperCollinsPublishers, 2000), p. 383.
14. K. Meyer, *The Dust of Empire* (New York: Century Foundation, 2003), p. 90.
15. S. Wolpert, *Gandhi's Passion* (New York: Oxford University Press, 2001).
16. Ibid., p. 91.
17. J. McCarry, "The Promise of Pakistan," *National Geographic* (October 1997): 56.
18. K. Meyer, *The Dust of Empire*, p. 89.
19. K. Hall, *A History of South East Asia*, 4th ed. (London: Macmillan, 1981).
20. J. Barwise and N. White, *A Traveller's History of South East Asia* (New York: Interlink Books, 2002).
21. A. Konstam, *Historical Atlas of Exploration, 1492–1600* (New York: Checkmark Books, 2002), p. 60.
22. J. Barwise and N. White, *A Traveller's History of Southeast Asia*.
23. K. Meyer, *The Dust of Empire: The Race for Mastery in the Asian Heartlands* (New York: Century Foundation, 2003), p. 9.
24. Quoted in Barwise and White, 2002, p. 168.
25. T. Dahlby, "Indonesia: Living Dangerously," *National Geographic* (March 2001): 80.
26. A. Lake, *Six Nightmares: Real Threats in a Dangerous World and How American Can Meet Them* (2001).
27. "Indonesia's Insulation from HIV/AIDS Wears Thin," Deutsche Press-Agentur, June 19, 2003.
28. C. Garnett, "NLM History Lecture Examines 'Death in the Cannibal Islands,'" NIH Record, www.nih.gov; A. Salmond, *The Trial of the Cannibal Dog: The Remarkable Story of Captain Cook's Encounters in the South Seas* (New Haven, CT: Yale University Press, 2003); N. Thomas, *Cook: The Extraordinary Voyages of Captain James Cook* (New York: Walker & Company, 2003).
29. Amnesty International, *Myanmar: The Rohingya Minority: Fundamental Rights Denied*, 2004, www.amnestyusa.org/new/document, pp. 5–6.
30. C. Beyrer, "HIV/AIDS: Accelerating and Disseminating Across Asia," *The Washington Quarterly* (Winter 2001): 211 ff.

31. J. Barwise and N. White, *A Traveller's History of Southeast Asia* (New York: Interlink Books, 2002).

32. United Nations/Vietnam, 2002, *Millennium Development Goals: Bringing the MDGs Closer to the People* (Hanoi: United Nations Country Team), p. 31.

33. Department for MCH/FP, *Assessment Survey Report on Pregnants' Knowledge, Opinion and Attitude on HIV/AIDS and HIV/AIDS Prevention of Local Health Services* (Hanoi: Ministry of Health, 2002), p. 54.

34. AIDWatch, "Project Profile: Sepon Mine in Laos and EFIC," www.aidwatch.org.

35. R. Skeldon, "Population Mobility and HIV Vulnerability in South East Asia: An Assessment and Analysis" (Bangkok, Thailand: UNDP South East Asia HIV and Development Project, 2000), pp. 10–11.

36. Human Rights Watch, "Not Enough Graves: The War on Drugs, HIV/AIDS, and Violations of Human Rights in Thailand," *Human Rights Watch* (June 2004) 16, no. 8 (C).

37. A. Holt, "Thailand's Troubled Border: Islamic Insurgency or Criminal Playground?" *Asia Media*, May 20, 2004, www.asianmedia.ucla.edu.

CHAPTER FIVE

1. A. Berry, *Infinite Tropics: An Alfred Russel Wallace Anthology* (New York: Verso, 2002), p. 14. Other references on the Darwin-Wallace controversy include B. Beddall, ed., *Wallace and Bates in the Tropics: An Introduction to the Theory of Natural Selection* (London: Macmillan, 1969); A. Brackman, *A Delicate Arrangement: The Strange Case of Charles Darwin and Alfred Russel Wallace* (New York: Times Books, 1980); L. Brooks, *Just Before the Origin: Alfred Russel Wallace's Theory of Evolution* (New York: Columbia University Press, 1984); J. Camerini, ed., *The Alfred Russel Wallace Reader: A Selection of Writings from the Field* (Baltimore: Johns Hopkins University Press, 2002); W. George, *Biologist Philosopher: A Study of the Life and Writings of Alfred Russel Wallace* (New York: Abelard-Schuman, 1964); P. Raby, *Alfred Russel Wallace: A Life* (Princeton, NJ: Princeton University Press, 2001); C. Aydon, *Charles Darwin: The Naturalist Who Started a Scientific Revolution* (New York: Carroll & Graf Publishers, 2002); J. Browne, *Charles Darwin: Voyaging, vol. 1*, and Browne, *Charles Darwin: A Sense of Place, vol. 2* (New York: Alfred A. Knopf, 1995 and 2002); C. Darwin, *The Voyage of the Beagle* (New York: Collier, 1937); C. Darwin, *The Origin of the Species By Means of Natural Selection or The Preservation of Favored Races in the Struggle for Life* (New York: Modern Library, 1993); and C. Darwin, *The Descent of Man and Selection in Relation to Sex* (New York: Collier Books, 1962); and W. Karp, *Charles Darwin and the Origin of the Species* (New York: Harper & Row, 1968).

2. A. McCoy, *The Politics of Heroin: CIA Complicity in the Global Drug Trade*, Revised Edition (New York: HarperCollins Publishers, 2003).

3. R. Davenport-Hines, *The Pursuit of Oblivion: A Global History of Narcotics* (New York: W. W. Norton, 2002), p. 60. This book is the source of most of the material on the history of opium in this chapter.

4. Ibid., p. 263.

5. Ibid., p. 424.

6. Near the end of the French-Indochinese war in 1954, the Vietnamese seized a ton of raw opium from a French military warehouse on the Vietnam coast that

supplied addicts in New York through Europe, a network known as the French Connection.

7. E. Girardet, "Afghanistan: Between War and Peace," *National Geographic* (November 2003): 40.

8. E. Griswold, "Where the Taliban Roam: Dodging the Jihad in Pakistan's Tribal Lands," *Harper's Magazine* (September 2003): 59.

9. S. Bose, *Kashmir: Roots of Conflict, Paths to Peace* (Cambridge, MA: Harvard University Press), p. 16.

10. L. Simons, "Kashmir: Trapped in Conflict," *National Geographic* (September 1999): 16.

11. A. Rashid, *Jihad: The Rise of Militant Islam in Central Asia* (New Haven, CT: Yale University Press, 2002), p. xi.

12. M. Edwards, "A Broken Empire: After the Soviet Union's Collapse," *National Geographic* (March 1993): 29.

13. Rashid, 2002, p. 25.

14. Human Rights Watch, *Fanning the Flames: How Human Rights Abuses are Fueling the AIDS Epidemic in Kazakhstan*, June 2003.

15. F. Hill and C. Gaddy, *The Siberian Curse: How Communist Planners Left Russia Out in the Cold* (Washington, DC: The Brookings Institution, 2003), pp. 1–2.

16. T. Severin, "Conquistadors of Siberia," in *The Oriental Adventure: Explorers of the East* (Boston: Little, Brown, 1976), p. 40.

17. A. Reid, *The Shaman's Coat: A Native History of Siberia* (New York: Walker & Company, 2002), p. 2.

18. A. Parshev, *Poschemu rossiya ne Amerika: kniga dlya tekh, kto ostayetsya zeds [Why Russia Is Not America: A Book for Those Who Remain Here]* (Moscow: Krymskiy Most–9D, 2000), p. 106.

19. F. Montaigne, "Russia Rising," *National Geographic* (December 2001): 18.

20. R. Denber, "'Glad to be Deceived': The International Community and Chechnya," *Human Rights Watch World Report 2004*, www.hrw.org/wr2k4/.

21. N. Eberstadt, "Russia: Too Sick to Matter?"*Policy Review* (June 1999).

22. J. Csete, *Lessons Not Learned: Human Rights Abuses and HIV/AIDS in the Russian Federation*, Human Rights Watch vol. 16, no. 5 (April 2004).

23. N. Walsh, "Russia Dumps its Children on the Streets," *The Observer*, April 18, 2004.

24. P. Landesman, "Arms and the Man," *New York Times Magazine*, August 17, 2003, pp. 28–57.

25. UN Office on Drugs and Crime, *Global Illicit Drug Trends, 2002* (New York: United Nations, 2003), p. 7.

CHAPTER SIX

1. While the conversation in this passage is an invention, the thoughts attributed to Mr. Darwin and Mr. Wallace are not. Darwin's comparison of man's best friends is taken from N. Barlow, ed., *The Autobiography of Charles Darwin, 1809–1882* (New York: W.W. Norton). The two quotes from Wallace have the following sources: From "Hereditary and Pre-Natal Influences: An Interview with Dr. Alfred Russel Wallace, *Humanitarian* vol. 4 (1984): 87, and a letter by Wallace to *The London Times*, February 11, 1909, p. 10d.

2. S. Begley, "The Roots of Hatred," *AARP Magazine*, May & June 2004, p. 48.

3. M. Nussbaum, *Women and Human Development: The Capabilities Approach* (Cambridge: Cambridge University Press, 2000), p. 4.
4. E. Guest, *Children of AIDS: Africa's Orphan Crisis* (London: Pluto Press, 2001), p. 1.
5. H. Epstein, "The Hidden Cause of AIDS," *The New York Review* (May 9, 2002), pp. 43–49.
6. B. Flowers, *The Prostitution of Women and Girls* (McFarland, 1998).
7. L. Brown, *Sex Slaves: The Trafficking of Women in Asia* (London: Virago Press, 2001), p. 33.
8. B. Crossette, "U.N. Finds AIDS Knowledge Still Lags in Stricken Nations," *The New York Times* (June 23, 2002), p. 10.
9. C. Breyer, "Accelerating and Disseminating Across Asia," *Washington Quarterly* (Winter 2001): 212.
10. Human Rights Watch, "Just Die Quietly: Domestic Violence and Women's Vulnerability to HIV in Uganda," *Human Rights Watch*, August 2003.
11. Human Rights Watch, "Women and HIV/AIDS," June 7, 2004, www.hrw.org/women/aids.html.
12. UNAIDS, *Women and HIV/AIDS: Confronting the Crisis* (Geneva and New York: UNAIDS, UNFPA, and UNIFEM, 2004).
13. The information in this section comes from UNAIDS, *Gender and AIDS: UNAIDS Technical Update* (Geneva: UNAIDS, 1998); and N. Feinstein and B. Prentice, *Gender and AIDS Almanac* (Geneva: UNAIDS, 2001). For more information on the biological basis of sexuality and sexually transmitted diseases, see my earlier book, *Black Death: AIDS in Africa* (New York: Palgrave Macmillan, 2003).
14. Asian Society, *AIDS in Asia: Leadership Initiatives in India*, teleconference held October 14, 2003, www.kaisernetwork.org.
15. L. Rofel, "The Outsider Within: Margery Wolf and Feminist Anthropology," *American Anthropologist* 105, no.3: 596–604.
16. L. Rebhun, "Sexuality, Color, and Stigma among Northeast Brazilian Women," *Medical Anthropology Quarterly* 18, no. 2 (2004). 183–199.
17. V. Lukere, *Gender, Women and Mothers: HIV/AIDS and the Pacific*, Gender Relations Center, Australian National University Working Paper No. 7.
18. "South Africa: HIV/AIDS Threatens to Undermine Democracy," UN Integrated Regional Information Networks, April 9, 2004, www.allafrica.com.
19. "Women's History Month 2004: Treaties, Voting Rights and Activism," www.seeingblack.com.
20. "Global Women's Issues Scorecard on the Bush Administration," August 26, 2003, www.genderhealth.org.
21. Human Rights Watch, "The Philippines Unprotected: Sex, Condoms and the Human Right to Health," *Human Rights Watch* 16, no. 6 (May 2004).
22. This figure is quoted from Tim Severin, *In Search of Genghis Khan* (New York: Atheneum/Macmillan, 1991), p. 23.
23. S. Soucek, *A History of Inner Asia* (Cambridge: Cambridge University Press, 2000), p. 298.
24. C. Janes and O. Chuluundorj, "Free Markets and Dead Mothers: The Social Ecology of Maternal Mortality in Post-Socialist Mongolia," *Medical Anthropology Quarterly* 18, no. 2 (2004): 230–257.
25. M. Komroff, ed., *The Travels of Marco Polo* (New York: Heritage Press, 1934), p. 251.

26. P. Iyer, *Sun After Dark*, (New York: Random House, 2004), p. 124.
27. S. Gopalan, "Women's Entitlement to Property," *India Times*, Internet, 2004, http://timesfoundation.indiatimes.com, p. 1.
28. S. Agarwal, *Genocide of Women in Hinduism*, www.dallistan.org/books/gowh/gowh-i.html, p. 2.
29. K. Armstrong, *Buddha* (New York: Penguin Books, 2001), p. 95.
30. L. Poon, "History of China," 2004, www.chaos.umd.edu/history/. Poon stresses his reliance on the electronic version of the U.S. *Army Area Handbook*, which can be accessed at the Library of Congress website, http://lcweb2.loc.gov/frd/cs/cntoc.html.
31. J. Barwise and N. White, *A Traveller's History of Southeast Asia* (New York: Interlink Books, 2002), p. 40.
32. C. Hirschman and B. Teerawichitchainan, "Culture and Socioeconomic Influences on Divorce During Modernization: Southeast Asia, 1940s to 1960s," *Population and Development Review* 29, no. 2(june 2003): 215–253.
33. Human Rights Watch, "Women and HIV/AIDS," www.hrw.org/women/aids.html.
34. D. Whelan, *Gender and AIDS: Taking Stock of Research and Programmes* (Geneva: UNAIDS, 1999), p. 30.
35. N. Eberstadt, "Population, Public Health, and Globalization: Four Unexpected Surprises," American Enterprise Institute presentation, December 1, 2003, www.aei.org.
36. N. Eberstadt, "Missing Girls Bode Ill for China in Future Decades," American Enterprise Institute, February 16, 2004, www.aei.com.

CHAPTER SEVEN

1. E. Pankhurst, "Why We Are Militant," Speech at Cooper Union, October 13, 1913, www.cooper.edu/humanities/core/hss3/e_panhurst.html.
2. Material on Goldstein comes from B. Crain, "Australian Feminism and the British Militant Suffragettes," Monash University, www.aph.gov.au/senate/pubs/occ_lect/transcripts/311003.pdf.
3. USAID/UNAIDS, *Children on the Brink 2002* (Washington, DC, 2002), www.synergyaids.com. Much of the material in this section comes from *Children on the Brink 2000* (Washington, DC, 2000), www.synergyaids.com, which I coauthored with John Williamson.
4. "AIDS: China's State Secret," *Guardian Unlimited*, January 7, 2003, www.guardian.co.uk.
5. A. Park, "China's Secret Plague," *Time Asia*, December 15, 2003.
6. In *Black Death: AIDS in Africa*, I describe the development of these responses in a story drawn from my experiences in sixteen African countries that runs through the book.
7. WHO, *Adults on Antiretroviral Treatment by World Region* (World Health Organization, November 2003), www.avert.org/aidsdrugsafrica2.htm.
8. For street children, see the Kaiser Daily HIV/AIDS Report, May 28, 2002; N. Ansell and L. Young, "Young AIDS Migrants in Southern Africa," 2003, DFID Contract R 7896; C. Lockhart, "*Kunyenga*, "Real Sex," and Survival," *Medical Anthropological Quarterly* 16, no. 3 (2002).
9. 'UNICEF Demands Action on AIDS Orphan Crisis," Reuters NewMedia, November 26, 2002.

10. ILO, *Helping Hands or Shackled Lives?* (Geneva: International Labor Organization, 2004).

11. Human Rights Watch, "Small Change: Bonded Child Labor in India's Silk Industry," *Human Rights Watch* 15, no. 2 (January 2003), p. 9.

12. Human Rights Watch, "Locked Doors: The Human Rights of People Living with HIV/AIDS in China," *Human Rights Watch* 15, no. 7 (September 2003).

13. E. Stuer, "Phone Fiction," *WIRED* (June 2004): 56.

14. UNICEF, "Many Young Asians Ignorant about AIDS Risks," Bangkok, June 1, 2004, www.chinapost.com.

15. C. Mason, *A Brief History of Asia* (New York: Palgrave Macmillan, 2000), p. 83.

16. Human Rights Watch, "Easy Targets: Violence Against Children Worldwide," *Human Rights Watch*.

CHAPTER EIGHT

1. UNAIDS, "A Globally Effective HIV Vaccine Requires Greater Participation of Women and Adolescents in Clinical Trials," press release, August 31, 2004, Geneva.

2. B. Sterling, "New World Disorder," *WIRED* (July 2003).

3. P. Jennings, "Need for renewed regional focus," *The Australian*, May 20, 2004.

4. T. Weinberg, "'Bold Steps' Are Needed in the AIDS Fight, Doctor Says," *Palm Beach Sun-Sentinel*, March 28, 2004.

5. PlusNews, "Sanlam Warns of AIDS Economic Time Bomb," *PlusNews Daily News Briefs*, June 23, 2004, UN Office for Coordination of Humanitarian Affairs.

6. L. Moonze, "AIDS Has Put Zambia into an Uncharted Territory," *Lusaka Post*, April 4, 2004.

7. B. Rau and J. Collins, "The Impact of HIV/AIDS," *Population and Development Strategies*, no. 9 (New York: UN Population Fund, August 2003), p. xv.

8. L. Kaggwa, "AIDS Amplifies Cancer Cases in Uganda," *New Vision*, April 12, 2004.

9. Reference to be added later.

10. For drug access and vaccines see World Trade Organization, 2003, "TRIPS: Counsel Discussion on Access to Medicines, Developing Country Group's Paper," June 20, 2001; K. Baldwin, "Latin American AIDS Activists Turn on Brazil," Reuters, May 25, 2002; SRI Media, "HIV/AIDS: TRIPPS and President Bush's 'Emergency Plan for AIDS Relief'"; O. Jablonski, "Accelerating Access: Serving Pharmaceutical Companies and Corrupting Health Systems," Act Up-Paris, May 14, 2002; S. Gottlieb, "Drug Companies Maintain 'Astounding' Profits," BMJ New York, May 4, 2002; SRI Media, "AIDS Drug Will Cost each Patient $20,000 a Year," February 24, 2003; R. Carroll, "Africa's AIDS Drugs Trapped in the Laboratory,"*The Guardian*, May 21, 2003; M. Specter, "The Vaccine," *The New Yorker*, February 3, 2003; SRI Media, "AIDS Vaccine Dramatic Findings," February 24, 2003.

11. P. Farmer, *Pathologies of Power* (2003).

INDEX

Afghanistan
  base for radical Islamic movement,
    162–163, 167
  CIA involvement, 156–158
  communist period and Soviet Union,
    156–157
  impact of war, 157
  opium production, 157–158
antiretroviral therapy
  availability in developing countries,
    225
  China, 224
  manufacture in developing countries,
    225
  opportunistic infections, 228
  pharmaceutical industry, 262–263
  resistance, 227
  types and regimens, 226–227
Asia
  colonialism, 102–104
  delayed development and AIDS,
    104–106
  early history, 58–61
  geography, 61–62
  nomads, impact, 60–61, 72–77
    see also specific groups
  spice trade, 142
    see also individual countries

Bangladesh
  causes of AIDS epidemic, 118
  independence, 116–117
  social characteristics, 117–118
Brooke, Rupert, 100–102
Brunei, 128
bubonic plague, 71
Burma, *see Myanmar*

Cambodia, 130–131

Canada, syphilis outbreak, 8
Central Asia
  AIDS epidemics, 167
  Great Game, 163
  impact of Afghanistan war, 162–163,
    166
  Islamic revival, 165–166
  Islamic extremists, 167
  Russian conquest, 163
  Soviet exploitation, 163–165
China
  AIDS epidemics, 90–95
  blood scandal, 92–94
  Communist China, 87–88
  Han dynasty, 81, 83
  liberalization, 90
  Manchus, 85–86
  mandarinate, 81–82
  Ming dynasty, 84–85
  minorities, 78–79, 80–81
  Muslims, 79–80
  orphans, 221–222
  opium wars, 86
  peasant rebellions, 88–90
  relationship with non-Hans, 77–78
children
  vulnerability to infection, 239–241
  HIV-infected children, 236–237
  infection rates, 239
  prevention of mother-to-child
    transmission, 237–238
  stigma, 236
  vulnerability to HIV infection,
    238–239
    see also orphans
condoms
  effectiveness, 31, 188
  female condoms, 188
  history of male condom, 31–32

100 percent condom use, 132
political attacks on effectiveness,
    32–33,
popularity in U.S. and Europe,
    144–146
    see also Philippines

Darwin, Charles
    and Wallace, 99–100, 141–142
    position on women, 181–182
Drugs
    British East India Company, 143
    CIA involvement, 152–154, 156–158,
        175
    English colonial exploitation,
        142–143, 146–147
    French colonial exploitation, 148–149
    growth of global drug trade, 174–175
    heroin emergence, 151
    history, 142–146
    international control efforts, 150–152,
        154, 175–177
    Myanmar government involvement,
        153–154
    Philippines, 149–150
    Thai government involvement, 148
    Yunnan and the Panthays, 148–149

Eastern Europe
    AIDS epidemics, 8–11
    breakup of Soviet Union, 173–174

Gladstone, Herbert, 5, 255–257
Gladstone, William, 182–183

HIV/AIDS, Asia
    conflict of tradition and modernity, 58
    control and prevention, 15
    history, 59
    impact of colonialism, 15, 134–135
    projections, 9, 36–40
    reasons for rapid spread, 40–42
    responsibility of leaders, 59–60
    role of religions, 60
HIV/AIDS, global epidemic
    compared to other STD epidemics, 34
    compared to terrorism, 8
    compared to war, 26
    early years of pandemic, 26–27

global infection rates and projections,
    7–8, 27
human rights organizations,
    266–267
life expectancy reduction, 14
migration and tourism, 44–47
military, 47–49
mutation to respiratory infection, 12
pharmaceutical companies, 262–263
poverty, 12–13, 49–51
social impact, 30–31, 259–260
U.S. role, 263–266
vaccine, 260–261
women, 16, 21–23, 42–44
young people, 16, 44
    see also HIV/AIDS, Asia
HIV virus
    discovery and description, 28–29
    transmission routes, 31, 33, 35–36

India
    AIDS epidemics, 106–107
    AIDS prevention, 108–109
    Bengal partition, 113–114
    blood scandal, 107–108
    caste system, 110–111
    child labor, 234–235
    Clive, Robert, 112, 143
    colonial exploitation, 112–115
    minorities, 110
    Mogul dynasty, 111–112
    Partition of India, 115–116
    social trends and AIDS, 109–110
Indochina, 128–129
Indonesia
    causes of AIDS, 124
    Dutch rule, 121–122
    ethnic conflicts, 123–124
    independence, 122
    social characteristics, 122–124

Jammu-Kashmir, 160–162

Laos
    ethnic minorities, 131
    independence, 130–131
    migration, 131–132
    modernization, 131
    sex trade, 184

Malaysia, 127–128
male circumcision, 35–36
Mongols
   alliance with Christian Europe, 67
   Batu, 66–67
   decline of empire, 71
   Genghis Khan, 62–63, 65–66, 77
   Hulegu, 67–68
   Kublai, 68–70
   Mongke, 67
   Ogudai, 66–67
   Timur or Tamerlane, 71–7
   see also Asia, nomads
Mongolia
   end of Mongol empire, 200
   Soviet control, 201–202
   Buddhism, 200–202
   social trends, 202
Muslims
   AIDS epidemic, 207–208
   Dar al-Islam, 63
   empire, 64–65
   Mohammed and women, 206
   slavery, 206–207
Myanmar
   causes of AIDS, 127
   colonial conquest, 125
   human rights abuses, 125 126
   military regime, 125–126

orphans
   attachment disorder, 244–246
   child-headed households, 229
   child labor, 234–236
   Chu Yuan-chung, 249
   community care, 228–231
   European orphanages, 223–224
   Genghis Khan, 249–250
   government response, 232–233
   grandparents, 243
   Little Orphan Annie, 248
   Muhammad, 250
   need for international assistance, 233
   number, 222, 250
   Orphan Trains, 246–248
   problems, 222–223, 230–231
   social responses, 223–224
   trafficking, 233–234
   violence against children, 251

Pakistan
   independence, 116, 159
   impact of Afghanistan war, 158–159
   nuclear weapons trade, 160
   Partition, 115–116
   separation of Bangladesh, 116–117
Pankhurst, Emmeline
   Cat and Mouse Act, 5
   early years, 23–25
   Goldstein, Vida, 220
   marriage to Richard, 25–26, 57
   militancy, 56–57, 218–220
   Poor Law Guardian, 57
   separation from Labour Party, 57–58
   unsexed viragoes, 5
   war babies, 221
   white slavery, 220
Philippines
   AIDS epidemic, 197–199
   condoms, 198–199
   human rights violations, 198
   independence, 197
   Spanish conquest, 197

religions
   animist, 199–200
   Buddhism, 210–213
   Hinduism, 208–210
   HIV/AIDS and religions, 203–216
   Islam, 206–208
   Sangha Mehta, 212–213
   Tibetan Buddhism, 203–204
Russia
   AIDS epidemic, 173
   Chechnyan crisis, 172–173
   early history, 167–170
   impact of liberalization, 172
   size and economic potential, 170–172
   Yermak, 168–170

Sex Sector
   ILO study, 194
   impact on society, 196–197
   international trafficking, 195–196
   rural remittances by sex workers,
     195
   sex as an industry, 193–194
   sex and gross domestic product,
     194

sexually transmitted diseases
    and AIDS, 33
    increase in prevalence, 34
    types of, 33–34
Singapore, 128
Sri Lanka, 125
South East Asia
    colonial conquest, 119–121
    early empires, 118–119
    see also individual countries
stories of HIV/AIDS
    Binh, 137–139
    Kamilika, 253, 255
    Molly, 21, 53–54
    Phet, 1–4,217–218
    Rageena, 97–99, 179–181
    Safia, 253–254
    Sumi, 18
    Surendra (orphan), 241–243
    Vladimir, 179
    Zacharia, 255
Sub-Saharan Africa
    HIV infection rates, 8
    HIV impact on society, 8

Thailand
    AIDS epidemic, 133
    early history, 133
    illegal drugs, 134
    100 percent condom use, 132
Tibet
    early history, 202–204
    Panchen Lama, 205
    Red Guards, 205

Ukraine, 174
United Kingdom, HIV infections, 7
United States
    foreign policy and HIV/AIDS,
        263–266
    infections among college students, 7
    HIV fifth leading cause of death, 7

Philippines HIV/AIDS epidemic,
    197–199
pornographic movie industry, 7
    *see also Drugs, CIA involvement and
        international control*

Vietnam
    resistance to French, 120
    social evils approach to AIDS
        prevention, 129

Wallace, Alfred Russel
    and Rupert Brooke, 100–102
    Banda Islands, 139–140
    drugs and women, 182–183
    position on women, 182
    species collecting, 140–141
Women's Social and Political Union,
    5–6
women
    biological vulnerability, 188
    Convention on the Elimination of All
        Forms of Discrimination Against
        Women, 185
    economics, 188–189, 261263–266
    Global Coalition on Women and
        HIV/AIDS, 184
    global statistics, 184–186
    HIV/AIDS statistics, 187–188
    Hinduism, 208–210
    knowledge of HIV/AIDS, 186
    microbicides,188
    Nepal, 185, 210
    right to refuse sex, 186–187
    political vulnerability, 192–193
    sex ratios in Asia, 216
    sex slaves, 186
    social and cultural vulnerability,
        189–191
    violence, 187
    vulnerability, 258
    see also Sex Sector